Dietary Pattern and Health Volume 1

Special Issue Editor
Zumin Shi

MDPI • Basel • Beijing • Wuhan • Barcelona • Belgrade

MDPI

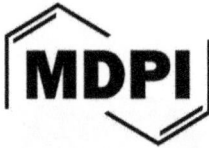

Special Issue Editor
Zumin Shi
University of Adelaide
Australia

Editorial Office
MDPI AG
St. Alban-Anlage 66
Basel, Switzerland

This edition is a reprint of the Special Issue published online in the open access journal *Nutrients* (ISSN 2072-6643) from 2015–2016 (available at: http://www.mdpi.com/journal/nutrients/special_issues/dietary-pattern-health).

For citation purposes, cite each article independently as indicated on the article page online and as indicated below:

Author 1; Author 2. Article title. *Journal Name* **Year**, *Article number*, page range.

First Edition 2017

Volume 1
ISBN 978-3-03842-587-8 (Pbk)
ISBN 978-3-03842-588-5 (PDF)

Volume 2
ISBN 978-3-03842-595-3 (Pbk)
ISBN 978-3-03842-596-0 (PDF)

Volume I – Volume II
ISBN 978-3-03842-597-7 (Pbk)
ISBN 978-3-03842-610-3 (PDF)

Table of Contents

About the Special Issue Editor

Zumin Shi is an associate professor at the University of Adelaide. He got his medical degree in Beijing Medical University in 1988. From 1988 to 2001, he worked at Jiangsu Provincial Center for Disease Control and Prevention, China. Having 13 years' experience in nutrition and foodborne disease prevention, he started his master in international community health in University of Oslo in 2001. He was conferred a PhD in the area of epidemiology from University of Oslo in Feb 2007. After his PhD he had his postdoc in University of Newcastle, and University of Oslo. In 2009, he joined SA Health and University of Adelaide. Dr. Shi's main research interest is the relationship between food intake, lifestyles and chronic diseases. He also has interests in food safety and foodborne disease prevention. He has published over 150 journal articles and authored a number of books.

Preface to "Dietary Pattern and Health"

This special issue is divided into two volumes based on how dietary patterns were constructed for use in dietary studies: Volume 1 contains studies considering the relationship between posteriori dietary patterns and health outcome (18 papers) while Volume 2 includes studies considering: a priori dietary patterns and health outcome (20 papers).

In Volume 1, a posteriori dietary patterns based on factor analysis/principal component analysis (PCA, 15 papers), cluster analysis (2 papers), reduced rank regression (RRR, 2 papers) and various health outcomes are covered. Seven papers from China, Spain, the Netherlands and South Africa focus on dietary patterns and obesity. Six papers have assessed the association between dietary patterns and metabolic diseases in Ghana, Australia, China, Qatar, and USA. Studies on the associations between dietary patterns and cognitive function, atopic dermatitis and general health are also included. Most of the studies use a comprehensive food frequency questionnaire (FFQ) to assess food intake. A small number of studies use a short version of FFQ.

Three papers use data from national representative studies including the National Health and Nutrition Examination Survey (NHANES) in the USA, China Kadoorie Biobank survey, and Australian Health Survey 2011.

There are three pioneering papers in terms of methodology in the volume. Using principal component analysis, Pisa et al. construct nutrient patterns and find a positive association between animal-based nutrient pattern and obesity among rural South African adolescents. Thani et al. construct lifestyle patterns by incorporating dietary habits and lifestyle factors among Qatari women of childbearing age. Similarly, Perez-Rodrigo et al. combine factor analysis and cluster analysis to assess the association between lifestyle patterns and obesity among Spanish children and adolescents. This novel data-driven approach highlighted the synergistic effect of the clustering of dietary habits and other lifestyles. It can be used as an alternative to the priori healthy lifestyle scores.

In Volume 2, there are four sections. In the review and perspective section, four papers focus on Mediterranean diet. Davis et al. systematically review the definition of Mediterranean diet used in population based research. Hoffman et al discuss the influence of food processing techniques on nutritional values (e.g. phytochemicals) in the Mediterranean diet. This is an important area but often neglected in the research or promotion of Mediterranean diet. It may help to understand the association between diet and health in populations with different cooking practices. D'Alessandro et al review population studies on the association between Mediterranean diet and cardiovascular diseases. The review by Fito discusses the role of nutritional genomics in the association between Mediterranean diet and cardiovascular disease.

In section 2, seven original research papers describe the association between priori dietary pattern scores (e.g. Mediterranean diet score, Nordic Food Index, diet quality score) and health outcomes (bone mineral density, polycystic ovary syndrome, diabetes, cardiovascular disease, nasopharyngeal carcinoma, and general health).

Three papers are included in the clinical trial section focusing on 1) the effect of weight loss on leptin and adiponectin; 2) sex difference in the effect of Mediterranean diet on LDL, and 3) feasibility of recruiting families in intervention program based on dietary patterns.

The last section of Volume 2 focuses on the food and nutrients intake as well as the associations with health outcomes. Some of the papers may help to understand the association between dietary patterns and health outcomes. For example, a study by Cao et al. assesses the association between macronutrient intake and obstructive sleep aponea among Australian men and found high fat intake is associated with daytime sleepiness. Using data from the 2008/2009 New Zealand Adult Nutrition Survey, Brow et al. find that nut consumption was associated with more favorable body composition and cardiometabolic profiles.

The collection of papers suggest that dietary pattern analysis is an area of growing interest. Findings from the papers show the importance of overall dietary patterns. The dietary pattern analysis approach takes into account the synergetic effects of food and nutrients. Factor analysis/PCA is the most commonly used method in the posteriori dietary pattern research. Currently, all the studies using RRR method were conducted using SAS software. As the free RRR packages became available in R (e.g. rrr package, rrpack), more studies in this area will be expected.

Zumin Shi
Special Issue Editor

nutrients

MDPI

Article

Major Dietary Patterns in Relation to General and Central Obesity among Chinese Adults

Canqing Yu [1], Zumin Shi [2], Jun Lv [1], Huaidong Du [3], Lu Qi [4,5], Yu Guo [6], Zheng Bian [6], Liang Chang [7], Xuefeng Tang [8], Qilian Jiang [9], Huaiyi Mu [10], Dongxia Pan [11], Junshi Chen [12], Zhengming Chen [3] and Liming Li [1,5,*]

[1] Department of Epidemiology and Biostatistics, School of Public Health, Peking University Health Science Center, 38 Xueyuan Road, Beijing 100191, China; E-Mails: yucanqing@pku.edu.cn (C.Y.); lvjun@bjmu.edu.cn (J.L.)

[2] Discipline of Medicine, University of Adelaide, SAHMRI, North Terrace, Adelaide, South Australia 5000, Australia; E-Mail: zumin.shi@adelaide.edu.au

[3] Clinical Trial Service Unit and Epidemiological Studies Unit (CTSU), Nuffield Department of Population Health, University of Oxford, Richard Doll Building, Old Road Campus, Oxford OX3-7LF, UK; E-Mails: huaidong.du@ctsu.ox.ac.uk (H.D.); zhengming.chen@ctsu.ox.ac.uk (Z.C.)

[4] Department of Nutrition, Harvard School of Public Health, 665 Huntington Ave, Boston, MA 02115, USA; E-Mail: nhlqi@channing.harvard.edu

[5] Channing Division of Network Medicine, Department of Medicine, Brigham and Women's Hospital and Harvard Medical School, 75 Francis Street, Boston, MA 02115, USA

[6] Chinese Academy of Medical Sciences, Fuwai Hospital Xishan Branch Court, Western Feng Cun, Mentougou, Beijing 102308, China; E-Mails: guoyu@kscdc.net (Y.G.); bianzheng@kscdc.net (Z.B.)

[7] Henan Center for Disease Control and Prevention, 105 Nongye East Road, Zhengzhou 450016, China; E-Mail: hnchangliang@sina.com

[8] Sichuan Center for Disease Control and Prevention, 6 Zhongxue Road, Chengdu 610041, China; E-Mail: sccdctxf@163.com

[9] Department of Non-communicable Diseases, Liuzhou Center for Disease Control and Prevention, 1-1 Tanzhong West Road, Liuzhou 545007, China; E-Mail: lzjiangqn@163.com

[10] Department of Non-communicable Diseases, Nangang Center for Disease Control and Prevention, 225 Wenchang Street, Haerbin 150040, China; E-Mail: ztmhy@126.com

[11] Department of Non-communicable Diseases, Tongxiang Center for Disease Control and Prevention, 64 Maodun East, Wutong Town, Tongxiang 314500, China; E-Mail: dongxia0724_pan@163.com

[12] China National Center for Food Safety Risk Assessment, 37 Guangqu Road, Beijing 100738, China; E-Mail: chenjunshi@cfsa.net.cn

* Author to whom correspondence should be addressed; E-Mail: lmlee@vip.163.com; Tel.: +86-10-82801528 (ext. 321); Fax: +86-10-82801528 (ext. 322).

Received: 25 May 2015 / Accepted: 8 July 2015 / Published: 15 July 2015

Abstract: Limited evidence exists for the association between diet pattern and obesity phenotypes among Chinese adults. In the present study, we analyzed the cross-sectional data from 474,192 adults aged 30–79 years from the China Kadoorie Biobank baseline survey. Food consumption was collected by an interviewer-administered questionnaire. Three dietary patterns were extracted by factor analysis combined with cluster analysis. After being adjusted for potential confounders, individuals following a traditional southern dietary pattern had the lowest body mass index (BMI) and waist circumference (WC); the Western/new affluence dietary pattern had the highest BMI; and the traditional northern dietary pattern had the highest WC. Compared to the traditional southern dietary pattern in multivariable adjusted logistic models, individuals following a Western/new affluence dietary pattern had a significantly increased risk of general obesity (prevalence ratio (PR): 1.06, 95% confidence interval (CI): 1.03–1.08) and central obesity (PR: 1.07, 95% CI: 1.06–1.08). The corresponding risks for the traditional northern dietary pattern were 1.05 (1.02–1.09) and 1.17 (1.25–1.18), respectively. In addition, the associations were modified by lifestyle behaviors, and the combined effects with alcohol drinking, tobacco smoking, and physical activity were analyzed. Further prospective studies are needed to elucidate the diet-obesity relationships.

Keywords: dietary pattern; general obesity; central obesity; body mass index; waist circumference; cross-sectional study

---

1. Introduction

General obesity, defined by body mass index (BMI), is associated with multiple comorbidities, including cardiovascular disease, diabetes and cancer, and a higher risk of all-cause mortality [1]. Central obesity, defined by waist circumference (WC), is an independent predictor of morbidity and mortality [2]. The cause of obesity is multifactorial and reflects the balance between dietary intake and energy expenditure, such as physical activity [3].

Dietary patterns characterize how foods and nutrients are consumed in combinations, reflect the effects of overall diet, and are more realistic and predictive in analysis of the relationship of diet with health and disease than individual foods or nutrients [4]. Several studies have reported the association of the major dietary patterns with general and central obesity [5–9], and the dietary patterns vary hugely across different countries, culture, or ethnic groups. In general, dietary patterns with greater intakes of high-fiber cereal, fruit, vegetables, and reduced-fat dairy products were inversely associated with obesity, while the dietary patterns with greater intakes of meat, potatoes, and sweets, were positively associated with obesity measures. However, few data are available from developing countries, especially from China, where people have different food culture from other countries and is experiencing an accelerating nutrition transition due to rapid economic, social and cultural changes [10,11], and where the prevalence of general and central obesity has increased greatly during the past decades [12].

Previous studies conducted among the Chinese population reported that dietary patterns and food factors are associated with the presence of glucose tolerace abnormalities [13], metabolic syndrome [14,15], and cardiovascular disease risk factors such as hypertension, hyperglycemia, triglyceride [15]. As to obesity, this association was observed among Chinese men aged 18–59 years for central obesity [15] and among Chinese young women aged 18–44 years for general obesity and central obesity [16]. In the present study, we aimed to examine the associations of dietary patterns with general and central obesity in a large sample of Chinese adults aged 30–79 years from the China Kadoorie Biobank (CKB). We also investigated the joint effects of dietary patterns and lifestyle factors including alcohol drinking, smoking and physical activity.

2. Methods

2.1. Study Population

The CKB is an ongoing prospective study that was designed to investigate the relationship between socioeconomic status, lifestyle behavior, and environmental factors and their association with chronic diseases such as ischemic heart disease, stroke and cancer. Detailed study objectives and designs are described elsewhere [17,18]. In brief, 512,891 men and women were recruited at a baseline survey in 2004–2008 from the general population residing in five urban areas (Qingdao, Harbin, Haikou, Suzhou and Liuzhou) and five rural areas (Sichuan, Gansu, Henan, Zhejiang and Hunan). Selection of the survey areas was based on local patterns of disease and exposure to certain risk factors, population stability, quality of death and disease registries, and local commitment and capacity. These 10 geographically defined areas were further divided into two groups, southern and northern areas, along the Qinling Mountains-Huaihe River line. Much difference exists in the natural geography, geology and culture between two groups (Supplemental Figure S1).

In each study area, about 100–150 administrative units (rural villages or urban residential communities) were selected for the study based on local records. Invitation letters and study information leaflets were delivered door-to-door by local community leaders or health workers after extensive publicity campaign. The target population of the study was restricted to permanent residents aged 30 years or more because of their higher disease outcomes and lower population mobility than younger adults. Eligible residents were invited to participate in the baseline survey at local assessment centers which were set up in each administrative unit specifically for the study. A team of about 15 full-time staff with medical qualifications and fieldwork experience in each study area was established for the survey. In the present analysis, we excluded participants with a prior history of coronary heart disease (n = 15,472), diabetes (n = 16,162), cancer (n = 2577), or stroke (n = 8884); and those with missing value on BMI (n = 2). A total number of 194,276 men and 279,916 women remained.

The project was approved by the ethical committee and research council of the Chinese Centre for Disease Control and Prevention (Beijing, China, 005/2004) and the Oxford Tropical Research Ethics Committee at the University of Oxford (UK, 025-04), and informed written consent was obtained from each participant.

2.2. Data Collection

At the baseline survey, a standardized questionnaire was face-to-face administered by trained interviewers using a laptop-based data-entry system. Detailed information on socio-demographic status, medical history, and lifestyle behaviors such as smoking habits, alcohol consumption, diet and physical activity, was obtained from each participant. The questions on the usual type and duration of activities related to work, commuting, household chores and leisure-time exercise during the past 12 months, were used to quantify the amount of daily physical activity (in metabolic equivalent hours per day (MET-hours/day)) [19].

Dietary data covered 12 major food groups in China: rice, wheat, other staples, meat, poultry, fish, eggs, fresh fruit, fresh vegetables, preserved vegetables, soybean and dairy products; each with five frequency levels of habitual consumption (never/rarely, monthly, 1–3 days/week, 4–6 days/week or daily) during the past 12 months. Each food intake was recoded as days/week: 0, 0.5, 2, 5, and 7 respectively. In addition, the frequency and quantity of beverages consumption were also recorded, including four types of tea (green/jasmine tea, oolong tea, black tea or other tea) and five types of alcohol (beer, rice wine, wine, spirit with ⩾40% alcohol or spirit with <40% alcohol). Thus, the average consumption (in g/week) was calculated [20].

A repeat questionnaire survey was performed within a year after baseline among 926 participants (mean delay of 5.4 months), good reproducibility of the food questionnaire was shown for most of food groups except for fresh vegetables. This is likely due to seasonal availability of fresh vegetables (Supplemental Table S1).

2.3. Dietary Patterns

Dietary patterns from the 12 aforementioned food and nine beverage groups were constructed using factor analysis combined with cluster analysis [21,22]. We first applied factor analysis using a principal component method to identify the major common food factors; then, an orthogonal (varimax) rotation was performed to achieve the structure with independent factor and greater interpretability. The number of factors retained by eigenvalue (>1), scree plot, factor interpretability and the variance explained (5%) by each factor. In the end, we chose the two-factor solution. The pattern loadings (see Supplementary Table S2) showed that the first factor, termed "staple food", showed a negative high loading on rice, and high loadings for wheat and other staple foods. The second factor has high loadings on various "western" and "newly affluent" foods, such as meat, poultry, fish, eggs, soybean,

3

fresh fruit and dairy products (cut-off point: ⩾0.4). Totally, these two factors explained 24.38% of the whole variance of food intake frequency scores.

Subsequently, the factor scores for each factor, calculated by summing the consumption of each food group that was weighted by a factor loading, were used in a cluster analysis. Because we had a large number of participants (n = 474,192), a two-step approach was applied. First, we performed hierarchical cluster analysis by randomly selecting 1% of the total cases to help identify the appropriate numbers of clusters and to determine reasonable initial cluster centers for a subsequent K-means cluster analysis. In the end, the K-means cluster analysis identified three distinct clusters. To minimize any effect of the ordering of samples, five random variables were created and used to sort the data file in ascending and descending order. Cluster assignment was robust across the ten runs; 99.19% to 99.68% of the participants were assigned to the same cluster in all runs. Furthermore, we ran analysis of variance to test the validity of the classification, which indicated that the segmentation of the three clusters was quite satisfactory (Supplemental Table S3).

2.4. Assessment of Anthropometric Measures

Anthropometric measures were also assessed by a baseline survey by trained technicians according to standard protocols. Participants did not wear shoes during the measurements of height and weight. Standing height was measured to the nearest 0.1 cm using a manufactured instrument. Weight was measured to the nearest 0.1 kg using a TANITA TBF-300GS body composition analyzer (Tanita Corp., Tokyo, Japan). BMI was calculated as weight in kilograms divided by the square of the standing height in meters. WC was measured midway between the iliac crest and the lower rib margin at the end of normal expiration. In the present study, we defined general obesity as BMI ⩾ 28 kg/m², and central obesity as WC ⩾ 80 cm in women and WC ⩾ 85 cm in men [23].

2.5. Statistical Analysis

The characteristics were compared between the dietary patterns using the logistic models for categorical variables or a general linear model for the continuous variables to adjust for age and sex. Values are presented as mean ± standard error (SE) or proportion respectively. The crude and multivariable-adjusted means and their 95% confidence intervals (CI) of BMI and WC between different dietary patterns were estimated using a generalized linear model. Considering that odds ratio can overestimate the effect in cross-sectional studies with high-prevalence binary outcomes [24], prevalence ratios (PR) and their 95% CI for were estimated using log-binomial regression [25], adjusting for age (continuous), sex (men, or women), study area (north area or urban area, both yes or no), marital status (married, or unmarried), education level (no formal school, primary school, middle school, high school, or college/university), household income (<10,000, 10,000–19,999, ⩾20,000 Yuan RMB/year), alcohol consumption (never drinker, occasional drinker, ex-drinker, or current regular drinker), tobacco smoking (never smoker, occasional smoker, ex-smoker, or current regular smoker), and physical activity level in MET-hours/day (continuous). In order to eliminate the reverse effect of unmeasured conditions, we performed two sensitivity analyses. First, we excluded a total number of 4175 participants who died within two years after baseline enrollment, and compared the associations with the whole sample. Second, we excluded a total number of 6029 participants who tried to reduce weight by dieting or using weight-loss drugs in the past 12 months, and reevaluate the association of dietary patterns with general and central obesity.

We also performed joint analyses to compare effects of the combination of dietary patterns and conventional lifestyle behaviors, such as alcohol drinking, tobacco smoking, and physical activity, in relation to general and central obesity. We tested the interaction between dietary patterns and lifestyle factors by creating categorical interactions terms and performed a likelihood ratio test to compare the difference of models with and without the interactions terms. All statistical analyses were performed with SAS version 9.3 (SAS Institute Inc., Cary, NC, USA). Significance was defined as $p < 0.05$.

4

Table 1. Dietary patterns identified by K-means cluster procedure [1].

	Dietary Patterns						Overall Mean (SD)
	Traditional Southern Dietary Pattern		Traditional Northern Dietary Pattern		Western/New Affluence Dietary Pattern		
Food group, day/week							
Rice	7.0	+ +	1.4	– – –	5.6	=	5.3 (2.6)
Wheat	1.7	– –	7.0	+ + +	5.0	+	3.7 (2.9)
Other staple foods	0.4	–	4.0	+ + +	1.2	–	1.4 (2.3)
Meat	3.9	=	1.4	– –	5.5	+ +	3.7 (2.5)
Poultry	0.8	=	0.1	– –	1.4	+ +	0.8 (1.0)
Fish	1.5	=	0.1	– –	2.3	+ +	1.4 (1.6)
Eggs	1.8	–	2.4	=	4.2	+ +	2.5 (2.2)
Fresh vegetables	6.9	=	6.6		7.0	+	6.8 (0.8)
Soybean	1.6	=	0.9	–	2.6	+ +	1.7 (1.6)
Preserved vegetables	2.3	=	1.5	–	2.5	+	2.2 (2.4)
Fresh fruit	1.9	– –	1.3	– –	5.3	+ + +	2.6 (2.5)
Dairy products	0.2	– –	0.4	–	3.2	+ + +	0.9 (2.1)
Beverage group, g/week							
Beer	1.2	=	0.9	=	14.4	+	4.1 (33.6)
Rice wine	5.9	=	<0.1	=	1.1	=	3.5 (35.3)
Wine	<0.1	=	<0.1	=	0.4	=	0.1 (3.6)
Heavy spirit (≥40%)	31.1	=	10.8	–	22.3	=	24.3 (113.0)
Light spirit (<40%)	13.9	=	6.1	=	4.4	=	9.9 (68.4)
Green tea	5.8	=	3.5	–	11.3	+	6.5 (15.9)
Oolong tea	0.5	=	<0.1	=	0.6	=	0.4 (4.5)
Black tea	1.8	+	<0.1	=	0.2	–	1.0 (7.6)
Other tea	<0.1	=	<0.1	=	<0.1	=	0.0 (0.7)

[1] SD, standard deviation; The sign – indicates variation below the mean frequency of intake, while + indicates variation above the mean frequency of intake. For example, we used + (or –) for 0.1–0.49 SD units (SDUs); + + (or – –) for 0.5–0.99 SDUs; and + + + (or – – –) for 1.0–1.99 SDUs; The sign = means equal to mean frequency of intake; For example, for "rice", the "traditional southern dietary pattern" had a mean intake of 7.0 days/week, which is 0.65 (*i.e.*, (7.0–5.3)/2.6) SDUs above the mean intake, so the corresponding sign (+ +) is used to indicate 0.5–0.99 SDUs above the mean.

3. Results

Three unique dietary patterns were identified in the present Chinese population (Table 1). The first cluster, the traditional southern dietary pattern, represented a typical traditional diet in South China, characterized by high intakes of rice but low intakes of wheat as staples. The second cluster was a traditional northern dietary pattern that, on the other hand, was characterized by high intakes of wheat and other staples, but low intakes of rice, meat, poultry, fish and fresh fruit. The third cluster, labeled as the Western/new affluence dietary pattern, was characterized by high consumption of fresh fruit and protein products such as meat, poultry, fish, eggs and dairy products.

Among the study population, 53.9% of the participants followed the traditional southern dietary pattern, 23.4% followed the traditional northern dietary pattern, and 22.7% followed the Western/new affluence dietary pattern. Participants who followed the Western/new affluence dietary pattern had better education and higher household income, were more likely to be a current drinker but less likely to be a current smoker, and were slightly less physically active (Table 2). Not surprisingly, those clustered into the traditional northern dietary pattern mainly lived in northern rural areas, while those with the traditional southern dietary patterns mainly lived in the southern rural areas.

Table 2. Selected characteristics of Chinese adults aged 30–79 according to dietary patterns [1].

	Traditional Southern Dietary Pattern	Traditional Northern Dietary Pattern	Western/New Affluence Dietary Pattern
n (%)	255,758 (53.9)	110,962 (23.4)	107,472 (22.7)
Female, %	59.3	59.2	58.4
Age, years	51.7 ± 0.02	49.8 ± 0.03	50.4 ± 0.03
Urban area, %	40.1	6.8	85.2
Southern area, %	94.2	0.7	43.6
Married, %	93.0	92.9	93.6
High school and above, %	38.3	38.0	83.6
Annual household income, %			
<10,000 Yuan RMB	24.2	56.5	8.3
10,000–19,999 Yuan RMB	27.7	33.2	27.6
⩾20,000 Yuan RMB	48.1	10.3	64.1
Current drinker, %	8.1	3.2	10.3
Current smoker, %	13.3	11.4	8.8
Physical activity, Met-hour/day	22.7 ± 0.03	23.0 ± 0.04	18.9 ± 0.04

[1] Values are age and sex adjusted percent or mean ± standard error (SE); All values in rows except sex are statistically different, *p* < 0.05; Met: metabolic equivalent task; Yuan RMB: unit of Chinese money.

Age and sex adjusted means of anthropometric measures for three dietary patterns are presented in Figure 1. In general, the individuals who followed the traditional southern dietary pattern had the lowest BMI and WC, and those following a Western/new affluence dietary pattern had the highest BMI and WC (*p* values < 0.05). The differences remained statistically significant after adjustment for potential confounders, except in those following a traditional northern dietary pattern, who had the highest multivariable adjusted WC (Supplemental Table S4). The associations of dietary patterns with general and central obesity were similar (Table 3). Compared with the individuals following the traditional southern dietary pattern, those following the Western/new affluence dietary pattern were more likely to be generally obese (PR = 1.70; 95% CI = 1.67–1.74) and centrally obese (PR = 1.38; 95% CI = 1.37–1.40), and those following traditional northern dietary patterns were more likely to be generally obese (PR = 1.39; 95% CI = 1.36–1.42) and centrally obese (PR = 1.21; 95% CI = 1.20–1.22). The associations for both general and central obesity were attenuated after controlling for potential confounders but were still significant. Furthermore, such associations did not materially change when we further excluded deaths within two years after the baseline enrollment or the participants who tried to reduce weight during the last 12 months (data not shown).

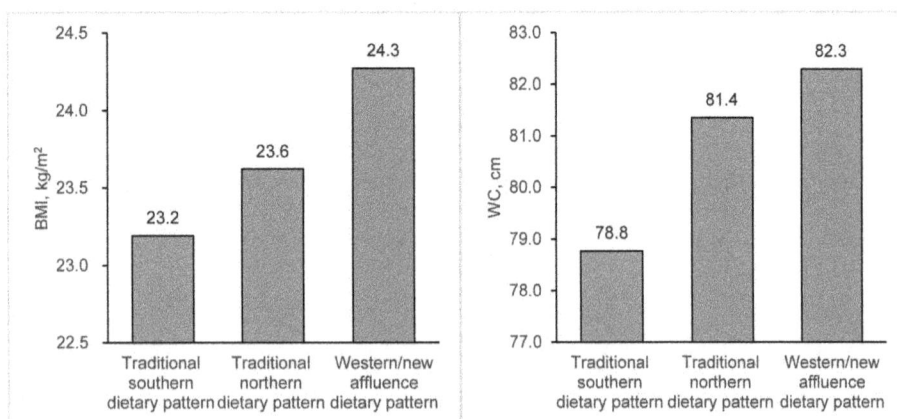

Figure 1. Age and sex adjusted means of body mass index (BMI) and waist circumference (WC) by dietary patterns in Chinese adults aged 30–79 years.

We also assessed the joint effects of dietary patterns with conventional lifestyle behaviors (Table 4), the multivariable-adjusted associations of dietary patterns with general and central obesity were modified by alcohol drinking, tobacco smoking, and physical activity (all p values for interaction <0.05). A 28% and 24% excessive risk of general and central obesity respectively were observed among the current drinkers who had a Western/new affluence dietary pattern compared with a non-current drinker who had a traditional southern dietary pattern ($p < 0.05$). Furthermore, a 7% of elevated risk of central obesity was observed among current smokers who had a Western/new affluence dietary pattern (95% CI: 1.05–1.09); in spite of that, current smokers were generally associated with a significantly lower risk of general and central obesity compared with those without these lifestyle behaviors in each dietary pattern. Physical activity was negatively associated with general and central obesity in each dietary pattern (all p values for trend <0.05). Participants with a traditional northern dietary pattern combined with the most active ($\geqslant$25.31 MET-hours/day), had the lowest risk of general obesity (PR = 0.59, 95% CI = 0.56–0.62), and those with the traditional southern dietary pattern in this group had the lowest risk of central obesity (PR = 0.82, 95% CI = 0.81–0.83).

Table 3. Multivariate adjusted prevalence ratios for general and central obesity by dietary patterns in Chinese adults aged 30–79 years [1,2].

	Traditional Southern Dietary Pattern	Traditional Northern Dietary Pattern	Western/New Affluence Dietary Pattern
General obesity			
No. of cases (%)	20,512 (8.02)	12,404 (11.18)	14,678 (13.66)
Crude	1.00	1.39 (1.36–1.42)	1.70 (1.67–1.74)
Model 1	1.00	1.41 (1.38–1.44)	1.71 (1.68–1.75)
Model 2	1.00	1.05 (1.01–1.09)	1.08 (1.05–1.10)
Model 3	1.00	1.05 (1.02–1.09)	1.06 (1.03–1.08)
Central obesity			
No. of cases (%)	90,783 (35.50)	47,694 (42.98)	52,813 (49.14)
Crude	1.00	1.21 (1.20–1.22)	1.38 (1.37–1.40)
Model 1	1.00	1.24 (1.23–1.25)	1.40 (1.39–1.41)
Model 2	1.00	1.17 (1.16–1.19)	1.08 (1.07–1.10)
Model 3	1.00	1.17 (1.15–1.18)	1.07 (1.06–1.08)

[1] Values are prevalence ratios and 95% CIs unless specified. General obesity: BMI $\geqslant$ 28 kg/m^2, Central obesity: WC $\geqslant$ 85 cm for men, $\geqslant$80 cm for women; [2] Crude: unadjusted model. Model 1: adjusted for age and sex. Model 2: model 1 + study area, marital status, education level, household income. Model 3: model 2 + alcohol consumption, smoking status, and physical activity.

Table 4. Joint effect of dietary patterns and lifestyle factors in relation to general obesity and central adiposity among Chinese adults aged 30–79 years [1,2].

	Traditional Southern Dietary Pattern	Traditional Northern Dietary Pattern	Western/New Affluence Dietary Pattern	P for Interaction
General obesity				
Current drinker				
No	1.00	1.04 (1.00–1.08)	1.03 (1.00–1.06)	<0.001
Yes	1.06 (1.02–1.10)	1.19 (1.12–1.28)	1.28 (1.23–1.34)	
Current smoker				
No	1.00	1.10 (1.06–1.14)	1.00 (0.97–1.03)	<0.001
Yes	0.69 (0.67–0.72)	0.56 (0.53–0.60)	0.92 (0.88–0.96)	
Physical activity				
T1	1.00	1.28 (1.23–1.33)	1.20 (1.16–1.24)	
T2	0.93 (0.90–0.96)	0.98 (0.93–1.03)	0.95 (0.91–0.98)	<0.001
T3	0.85 (0.82–0.87)	0.59 (0.56–0.62)	0.78 (0.74–0.81)	
Central adiposity				
Current drinker				
No	1.00	1.11 (1.10–1.13)	1.02 (1.01–1.03)	<0.001
Yes	1.03 (1.01–1.04)	1.19 (1.16–1.22)	1.24 (1.22–1.26)	
Current smoker				
No	1.00	1.19 (1.18–1.21)	1.00 (0.99–1.01)	<0.001
Yes	0.81 (0.80–0.82)	0.84 (0.82–0.86)	1.07 (1.05–1.09)	
Physical activity				
T1	1.00	1.16 (1.14–1.17)	1.10 (1.09–1.11)	
T2	0.92 (0.90–0.93)	1.11 (1.09–1.13)	0.95 (0.94–0.97)	<0.001
T3	0.82 (0.81–0.83)	0.98 (0.96–1.00)	0.87 (0.85–0.88)	

[1] General obesity: Body mass index (BMI) $\geq$ 28 kg/m^2; Central obesity: Waist circumference (WC) $\geq$ 85 cm for men, $\geq$80 cm for women; Physical activity was categorized into tertiles, T1: <12.29 metabolic equivalent task (MET-) hours/day, T2: 12.29–25.30 MET-hours/day, T3: $\geq$25.31 MET-hours/day; [2] Values are presented as prevalence ratios (95% CI) adjusted for age, sex, study area, marital status, education level, household income, alcohol consumption, smoking status, and physical activity.

4. Discussion

In the present study of a large sample of Chinese adults, we found that the traditional southern dietary pattern, characterized by high intakes of rice but low intakes of wheat as staple foods, was associated with the lowest risk of general and central obesity. Compared with the traditional southern dietary pattern, the traditional northern dietary pattern was characterized by high intakes of wheat as a staple food, but low intakes of rice, meat, poultry, fish, and fresh fruit, was associated with an elevated risk of general and central obesity. The Western/new affluence dietary pattern, characterized by high consumption of fresh fruit and protein products such as red meat, poultry, fish, eggs and dairy products, was also associated with an increased risk of general and central obesity. These associations were independent of the socio-demographic and conventional lifestyle behaviors.

The dietary patterns in this present study were constructed using cluster analysis combined with factor analysis, which derived more reproducible and interpretable results. The three dietary patterns fully captured the geographical, socioeconomic and dietary characteristics in the Chinese population, and were consistent with previously reported results from a large-scale, nationally representative sample of Chinese adults with a validated semi-quantitative food frequency questionnaire [13–15]. Similar dietary patterns were also reported from three consecutive 24-hours recalls of dietary intake among young Chinese women aged 18–44 years [16].

The risk differences between the traditional southern dietary pattern and traditional northern dietary pattern in terms of general and central obesity were reported in previous cross-sectional studies [14–16,26]. In a five-year prospective study conducted in Jiangsu, Shi *et al.* [27] reported that adoption of a traditional southern dietary pattern was associated with less weight gain. These two traditional Chinese dietary patterns, which mainly differ in taking rice or wheat as a staple, had remarkably different distributions in northern and southern China. Previous prevalence studies on obesity also revealed this geographic difference [28,29]. One study that used the percentage of rice in the staple food as an index of a staple food pattern, reported that the index was inversely related to weight gain [30]. The underlying mechanism is unclear; it may have some connection with lipid alteration caused by carbohydrate intake [31,32] and insufficiency of micronutrients [33] in the traditional northern dietary pattern.

The Western/new affluence dietary pattern was suggested to be associated with an elevated risk of general and central obesity. This is consistent with a body of literature conducted in different countries and ethnicities [14,15,34–39]. Meat consumption, one of the key features of the Western/new affluence dietary pattern, was reported to be strongly associated with weight gain in several prospective studies [3,40,41]. The mechanism underlying the positive association is unclear: several hypotheses have been made regarding energy density in appetite control and an underlying detrimental lifestyle beyond the dietary patterns [40]. However, in the present study, which took into account conventional behavioral factors as potential confounders in this relationship, the associations were only slightly attenuated.

Previous studies reported that lifestyle behaviors, such as alcohol drinking [42–44] and tobacco smoking [45,46], were associated with BMI or measures of obesity. These associations were observed in the present study. In addition, we found that the associations of dietary patterns in relation to general and central obesity were modified by these lifestyle factors. Current drinkers and current smokers who have a Western/new affluence dietary pattern have the highest risk of general and central obesity. Physical activity as a form of energy expenditure, is often regarded as a standard clinical recommendation for generally or centrally obese individuals [47]. Previous studies reported regular physical activity had a protective effect against long-term gain in weight [3,48,49], BMI [50], or central obesity [15]. This protective effect was stronger among individuals who followed a traditional northern dietary pattern for general obesity, and those who followed a Western/new affluence dietary pattern for central obesity according the joint analysis. The energetics of diet composition may explain this difference. The carbohydrate from wheat and other staple food contributes major dietary energy intake in the traditional northern dietary pattern, while protein-rich diet components, such as meat, poultry, fish, egg, and dairy products, provide most of dietary energy in the Western/new affluence dietary pattern. Evidence has shown that high protein diets produced greater improvements than high carbohydrate diets in both short and long term weight maintenance. The former was shown to be associated with an increased ratio of fat/muscle loss and positive changes of blood lipids profile, such as lowing triacylglycerols (TAG) and ratio of TAG/high density lipoprotein cholesterol (HDL-C) [51,52]. Similar to these findings, we found that individuals who followed a Western/new affluence dietary pattern with higher physical activity, were associated a lower risk of central obesity as comparing to those followed a traditional northern dietary pattern with the same physical activity level. Proposed mechanisms include increased hunger, lower satiety, or great calorie intake after consuming carbohydrates *vs.* a protein-rich diet [53]. This information could be helpful when it was translated into diet recommendations in weight control programs.

The present study is thus far the largest study of the dietary patterns on general and central obesity with objective anthropometric measurement in the Chinese population. However, some points should be considered in interpreting our findings. First, the nature of cross-sectional design limits causal inference. However, the observed associations remained after a further exclusion of participants who tried to reduce weight by dieting and using weight-loss drugs during the last 12 months and those who had chronic conditions at baseline survey. Secondly, the limitation of our questionnaires should be considered. We only assessed 12 crude food groups that are common in the Chinese diet; other food groups that may be related to general and central obesity were not collected, such as sweets, other than non-alcoholic beverages. Although the major dietary patterns in Chinese adults were well captured in our study, only the frequencies but not the quantity of the major food groups were collected. Thus, it was difficult to calculate and adjust for total energy intake. However, according to a previous study in Iranian women, additional adjustment of energy intake could not affect the magnitude and significance of BMI and WC, or use general and central obesity as an outcome [39]. In addition, shifting the quantitative focus on food calories to qualitative focus on consuming foods of different types, could address different food-induced physiological pathways and different metabolic effects [54]. Thirdly, although we excluded the participants who had chronic conditions at the baseline and adjusted for a wide range of socio-demographic and behavioral variables in present analysis, the possibility of residual confounding, such as ethnicity, could not be excluded. We didn't collect detailed dietary information on food processing, which limited our ability to comprehensively adjust for other specific dietary factors. Furthermore, we constructed the major three dietary patterns, which captured the most typical diet habits in Chinese population. However, some minor dietary patterns might also be associated with general and central obesity.

5. Conclusions

In conclusion, we found that the traditional southern dietary pattern was related to a lower risk of general and central obesity independent of socio-demographic and lifestyle behavior factors, while the Western/new affluence dietary pattern was associated with increased risk of these conditions. Although the differences in physical measures and the risk of general and central obesity were very moderate, a slight difference in the population level may have important public health significance. Hence, the results from the present study could be integrated into community-based health promotion and intervention programs of chronic diseases. Furthermore, future studies are required to elucidate the mechanisms beyond the well-known risk factors of obesity.

Acknowledgments: This work is supported by grants (81202266, 81390541, 81390544) from the National Natural Science Foundation of China; by a grant (2011BAI09B01, 2012-14) from the National Key Technologies Research and Development Program in the 12th Five-Year Plan, Chinese Ministry of Science and Technology; by a grant (088158/Z/09/Z) from the Wellcome Trust in the UK; by a grant from the Kadoorie Charitable Foundation in Hong Kong. Qi is supported by NIH grants from the National Heart, Lung, and Blood Institute (HL071981, HL034594, HL126024), the National Institute of Diabetes and Digestive and Kidney Diseases (DK091718, DK100383, DK078616), the Boston Obesity Nutrition Research Center (DK46200), and United States-Israel Binational Science Foundation Grant 2011036. Qi was a recipient of the American Heart Association Scientist Development Award (0730094N). The funders had no role in the study design, data collection, data analysis and interpretation, writing of the report, or the decision to submit the article for publication.

Author Contributions: The authors' contributions were as follows: Liming Li and Zhengming Chen had full access to all the data in the study and take responsibility for the integrity of the data and the accuracy of the data analysis. Study concept and design: Liming Li, Zhengming Chen and Junshi Chen; Acquisition of data and quality control: Yu Guo, Zheng Bian, Liang Chang, Xuefeng Tang, Qilian Jiang, Huaiyi Mu and Dongxia Pan; Analysis and interpretation of data: CanqingYu, Zumin Shi and Lu Qi; Drafting of the manuscript: Canqing Yu; Critical revision of the manuscript for important intellectual content: Zumin Shi, Qi Lu, Huaidong Du and Zhengming Chen; Statistical analysis: Canqing Yu and Jun Lv; Obtained funding: Liming Li and Zhengming Chen.

China Kadoorie Biobank Collaborative Group

International Steering Committee: Junshi Chen, Zhengming Chen, Rory Collins, Liming Li (PI), Richard Peto. **International Co-ordinating Centre, Oxford:** Derrick Bennett, Yumei Chang, Yiping Chen, Zhengming Chen, Robert Clarke, Huaidong Du, Xuejuan Fan, Haiyan Gao, Simon Gilbert, Andri Iona, Rene Kerosi, Ling Kong, Om Kurmi, Garry Lancaster, John McDonnell, Winnie Mei, Iona Millwood, Qunhua Nie, Jayakrishnan Radhakrishnan, Paul Ryder, Sam Sansome, Dan Schmidt, Paul Sherliker, Margaret Smith, Rajani Sohoni, Robin Walters, Jenny Wang, Lin Wang, Alex Williams, Ling Yang, Xiaoming Yang. **National Coordinating Centre, Beijing:** Zheng Bian, Ge Chen, Lei Guo, Yu Guo, Bingyang Han, Can Hou, Peng Liu, Jun Lv, Pei Pei, Shuzhen Qu, Yunlong Tan, Canqing Yu, Huiyan Zhou. **10 Regional Coordinating Centres: Qingdao** Qingdao CDC: Zengchang Pang, Shaojie Wang, Yun Zhang, Kui Zhang. Licang CDC: Silu Liu, Wei Hou. **Heilongjiang** Provincial CDC: Zhonghou Zhao, Shumei Liu, Zhigang Pang. Nangang CDC: Weijia Feng, Shuling Wu, Liqiu Yang, Huili Han, Hui He, Bo Yu. **Hainan** Provincial CDC: Xianhai Pan, Shanqing Wang, Hongmei Wang. Meilan CDC: Xinhua Hao, Chunxing Chen, Shuxiong Lin, Xiangyang Zheng. **Jiangsu** Provincial CDC: Xiaoshu Hu, Minghao Zhou, Ming Wu, Ran Tao. Suzhou CDC: Yeyuan Wang, Yihe Hu, Liangcai Ma, Renxian Zhou, Guanqun Xu, Yan Lu. **Guangxi** Provincial CDC: Baiqing Dong, Naying Chen,

Ying Huang. Liuzhou CDC: Mingqiang Li, Jinhuai Meng, Zhigao Gan, Jiujiu Xu, Yun Liu, Jingxin Qing. **Sichuan** Provincial CDC: Xianping Wu, Yali Gao, Ningmei Zhang. Pengzhou CDC: Guojin Luo, Xiangsan Que, Xiaofang Chen. **Gansu** Provincial CDC: Pengfei Ge, Jian He, Xiaolan Ren. Maiji CDC: Hui Zhang, Enke Mao, Guanzhong Li, Zhongxiao Li, Jun He, Yulong Lei, Xiaoping Wang. **Henan** Provincial CDC: Guohua Liu, Baoyu Zhu, Gang Zhou, Shixian Feng. Huixian CDC: Yulian Gao, Tianyou He, Li Jiang, Jianhua Qin, Huarong Sun. **Zhejiang** Provincial CDC: Liqun Liu, Min Yu, Yaping Chen, Ruying Hu. Tongxiang CDC: Zhixiang Hu, Jianjin Hu, Yijian Qian, Zhiying Wu, Chunmei Wang, Lingli Chen. **Hunan** Provincial CDC: Wen Liu, Guangchun Li, Huilin Liu. Liuyang CDC: Xiangquan Long, Xin Xu, Youping Xiong, Zhongwen Tan, Xuqiu Xie, Yunfang Peng, Weifang Jia.

Conflicts of Interest: The authors declare no conflict of interest.

References

1. Flegal, K.M.; Kit, B.K.; Orpana, H.; Graubard, B.I. Association of all-cause mortality with overweight and obesity using standard body mass index categories: A systematic review and meta-analysis. *JAMA* **2013**, *309*, 71–82. [CrossRef] [PubMed]
2. Carmienke, S.; Freitag, M.H.; Pischon, T.; Schlattmann, P.; Fankhaenel, T.; Goebel, H.; Gensichen, J. General and abdominal obesity parameters and their combination in relation to mortality: A systematic review and meta-regression analysis. *Eur. J. Clin. Nutr.* **2013**, *67*, 573–585. [CrossRef] [PubMed]
3. Mozaffarian, D.; Hao, T.; Rimm, E.B.; Willett, W.C.; Hu, F.B. Changes in diet and lifestyle and long-term weight gain in women and men. *N. Engl. J. Med.* **2011**, *364*, 2392–2404. [CrossRef] [PubMed]
4. Hu, F.B. Dietary pattern analysis: A new direction in nutritional epidemiology. *Curr. Opin. Lipidol.* **2002**, *13*, 3–9. [CrossRef] [PubMed]
5. McNaughton, S.A.; Mishra, G.D.; Stephen, A.M.; Wadsworth, M.E. Dietary patterns throughout adult life are associated with body mass index, waist circumference, blood pressure, and red cell folate. *J. Nutr.* **2007**, *137*, 99–105. [PubMed]
6. Newby, P.K.; Muller, D.; Hallfrisch, J.; Qiao, N.; Andres, R.; Tucker, K.L. Dietary patterns and changes in body mass index and waist circumference in adults. *Am. J. Clin. Nutr.* **2003**, *77*, 1417–1425. [PubMed]
7. Newby, P.K.; Muller, D.; Hallfrisch, J.; Andres, R.; Tucker, K.L. Food patterns measured by factor analysis and anthropometric changes in adults. *Am. J. Clin. Nutr.* **2004**, *80*, 504–513. [PubMed]
8. Van Dam, R.M.; Grievink, L.; Ocke, M.C.; Feskens, E.J. Patterns of food consumption and risk factors for cardiovascular disease in the general dutch population. *Am. J. Clin. Nutr.* **2003**, *77*, 1156–1163. [PubMed]
9. Maskarinec, G.; Novotny, R.; Tasaki, K. Dietary patterns are associated with body mass index in multiethnic women. *J. Nutr.* **2000**, *130*, 3068–3072. [PubMed]
10. Zhai, F.Y.; Du, S.F.; Wang, Z.H.; Zhang, J.G.; Du, W.W.; Popkin, B.M. Dynamics of the Chinese diet and the role of urbanicity, 1991–2011. *Obes. Rev.* **2014**, *15*, 16–26. [CrossRef] [PubMed]
11. Wang, Z.H.; Zhai, F.Y.; Wang, H.J.; Zhang, J.G.; Du, W.W.; Su, C.; Zhang, J.; Jiang, H.R.; Zhang, B. Secular trends in meat and seafood consumption patterns among Chinese adults, 1991–2011. *Eur. J. Clin. Nutr.* **2015**, *69*, 227–233. [CrossRef] [PubMed]
12. Xi, B.; Liang, Y.; He, T.; Reilly, K.H.; Hu, Y.; Wang, Q.; Yan, Y.; Mi, J. Secular trends in the prevalence of general and abdominal obesity among Chinese adults, 1993–2009. *Obes. Rev.* **2012**, *13*, 287–296. [CrossRef] [PubMed]
13. He, Y.; Ma, G.; Zhai, F.; Li, Y.; Hu, Y.; Feskens, E.J.; Yang, X. Dietary patterns and glucose tolerance abnormalities in Chinese adults. *Diabetes Care* **2009**, *32*, 1972–1976. [CrossRef] [PubMed]
14. He, Y.; Li, Y.; Lai, J.; Wang, D.; Zhang, J.; Fu, P.; Yang, X.; Qi, L. Dietary patterns as compared with physical activity in relation to metabolic syndrome among Chinese adults. *Nutr. Metab. Cardiovasc. Dis.* **2013**, *23*, 920–928. [CrossRef] [PubMed]
15. Wang, D.; He, Y.; Li, Y.; Luan, D.; Zhai, F.; Yang, X.; Ma, G. Joint association of dietary pattern and physical activity level with cardiovascular disease risk factors among Chinese men: A cross-sectional study. *PLoS ONE* **2013**, *8*, e66210. [CrossRef] [PubMed]

16. Zhang, J.G.; Wang, Z.H.; Wang, H.J.; Du, W.W.; Su, C.; Zhang, J.; Jiang, H.R.; Zhai, F.Y.; Zhang, B. Dietary patterns and their associations with general obesity and abdominal obesity among young Chinese women. *Eur. J. Clin. Nutr.* **2015**. [CrossRef] [PubMed]

17. Chen, Z.; Chen, J.; Collins, R.; Guo, Y.; Peto, R.; Wu, F.; Li, L.; China Kadoorie Biobank Collaborative Group. China Kadoorie Biobank of 0.5 million people: Survey methods, baseline characteristics and long-term follow-up. *Int. J. Epidemiol.* **2011**, *40*, 1652–1666. [CrossRef] [PubMed]

18. Chen, Z.; Lee, L.; Chen, J.; Collins, R.; Wu, F.; Guo, Y.; Linksted, P.; Peto, R. Cohort profile: The Kadoorie Study of chronic disease in China (KSCDC). *Int. J. Epidemiol.* **2005**, *34*, 1243–1249. [CrossRef] [PubMed]

19. Du, H.; Bennett, D.; Li, L.; Whitlock, G.; Guo, Y.; Collins, R.; Chen, J.; Bian, Z.; Hong, L.S.; Feng, S.; *et al.* Physical activity and sedentary leisure time and their associations with BMI, waist circumference, and percentage body fat in 0.5 million adults: The China Kadoorie Biobank Study. *Am. J. Clin. Nutr.* **2013**, *97*, 487–496. [CrossRef] [PubMed]

20. Millwood, I.Y.; Li, L.; Smith, M.; Guo, Y.; Yang, L.; Bian, Z.; Lewington, S.; Whitlock, G.; Sherliker, P.; Collins, R.; *et al.* Alcohol consumption in 0.5 million people from 10 diverse regions of China: Prevalence, patterns and socio-demographic and health-related correlates. *Int. J. Epidemiol.* **2013**, *42*, 816–827. [CrossRef] [PubMed]

21. Zhang, X.; Dagevos, H.; He, Y.; van der Lans, I.; Zhai, F. Consumption and corpulence in China: A consumer segmentation study based on the food perspective. *Food Policy* **2008**, *33*, 37–47. [CrossRef]

22. Li, Y.; He, Y.; Lai, J.; Wang, D.; Zhang, J.; Fu, P.; Yang, X.; Qi, L. Dietary patterns are associated with stroke in Chinese adults. *J. Nutr.* **2011**, *141*, 1834–1839. [CrossRef] [PubMed]

23. Zhou, B.F. Predictive values of body mass index and waist circumference for risk factors of certain related diseases in Chinese adults—Study on optimal cut-off points of body mass index and waist circumference in Chinese adults. *Biomed. Environ. Sci.* **2002**, *15*, 83–96. [PubMed]

24. Barros, A.J.; Hirakata, V.N. Alternatives for logistic regression in cross-sectional studies: An empirical comparison of models that directly estimate the prevalence ratio. *BMC Med. Res. Methodol.* **2003**, *3*, 21. [CrossRef] [PubMed]

25. Skov, T.; Deddens, J.; Petersen, M.R.; Endahl, L. Prevalence proportion ratios: Estimation and hypothesis testing. *Int. J. Epidemiol.* **1998**, *27*, 91–95. [CrossRef] [PubMed]

26. Kim, J.H.; Lee, J.E.; Jung, I.K. Dietary pattern classifications and the association with general obesity and abdominal obesity in Korean women. *J. Acad. Nutr. Diet.* **2012**, *112*, 1550–1559. [CrossRef] [PubMed]

27. Shi, Z.; Yuan, B.; Hu, G.; Dai, Y.; Zuo, H.; Holmboe-Ottesen, G. Dietary pattern and weight change in a 5-year follow-up among Chinese adults: Results from the jiangsu nutrition study. *Br. J. Nutr.* **2011**, *105*, 1047–1054. [CrossRef] [PubMed]

28. Reynolds, K.; Gu, D.; Whelton, P.K.; Wu, X.; Duan, X.; Mo, J.; He, J.; For the InterASIA Collaborative Group. Prevalence and risk factors of overweight and obesity in China. *Obesity* **2007**, *15*, 10–18. [CrossRef] [PubMed]

29. Yu, Z.; Lin, X.; Haas, J.D.; Franco, O.H.; Rennie, K.L.; Li, H.; Xu, H.; Pang, X.; Liu, H.; Zhang, Z.; *et al.* Obesity related metabolic abnormalities: Distribution and geographic differences among middle-aged and older Chinese populations. *Prev. Med.* **2009**, *48*, 272–278. [CrossRef] [PubMed]

30. Shi, Z.; Taylor, A.W.; Hu, G.; Gill, T.; Wittert, G.A. Rice intake, weight change and risk of the metabolic syndrome development among Chinese adults: The jiangsu nutrition study (JIN). *Asia Pac. J. Clin. Nutr.* **2012**, *21*, 35–43. [PubMed]

31. Mittendorfer, B.; Sidossis, L.S. Mechanism for the increase in plasma triacylglycerol concentrations after consumption of short-term, high-carbohydrate diets. *Am. J. Clin. Nutr.* **2001**, *73*, 892–899. [PubMed]

32. Kondo, I.; Funahashi, K.; Nakamura, M.; Ojima, T.; Yoshita, K.; Nakamura, Y. Association between food group intake and serum total cholesterol in the Japanese population: NIPPON DATA 80/90. *J. Epidemiol.* **2010**, *20*, S576–S581. [CrossRef] [PubMed]

33. Garcia, O.P.; Ronquillo, D.; Caamano Mdel, C.; Camacho, M.; Long, K.Z.; Rosado, J.L. Zinc, vitamin A, and vitamin C status are associated with leptin concentrations and obesity in Mexican women: Results from a cross-sectional study. *Nutr. Metab.* **2012**, *9*, 59. [CrossRef] [PubMed]

34. Murtaugh, M.A.; Herrick, J.S.; Sweeney, C.; Baumgartner, K.B.; Guiliano, A.R.; Byers, T.; Slattery, M.L. Diet composition and risk of overweight and obesity in women living in the Southwestern United States. *J. Am. Diet. Assoc.* **2007**, *107*, 1311–1321. [CrossRef] [PubMed]

35. Pala, V.; Sieri, S.; Masala, G.; Palli, D.; Panico, S.; Vineis, P.; Sacerdote, C.; Mattiello, A.; Galasso, R.; Salvini, S.; *et al.* Associations between dietary pattern and lifestyle, anthropometry and other health indicators in the elderly participants of the EPIC-Italy cohort. *Nutr. Metab. Cardiovasc. Dis.* **2006**, *16*, 186–201. [CrossRef] [PubMed]

36. Haidari, F.; Shirbeigi, E.; Cheraghpour, M.; Mohammadshahi, M. Association of dietary patterns with body mass index, waist circumference, and blood pressure in an adult population in Ahvaz, Iran. *Saudi Med. J.* **2014**, *35*, 967–974. [PubMed]

37. Cho, Y.A.; Shin, A.; Kim, J. Dietary patterns are associated with body mass index in a Korean population. *J. Am. Diet. Assoc.* **2011**, *111*, 1182–1186. [CrossRef] [PubMed]

38. Paradis, A.M.; Godin, G.; Perusse, L.; Vohl, M.C. Associations between dietary patterns and obesity phenotypes. *Int. J. Obes.* **2009**, *33*, 1419–1426. [CrossRef] [PubMed]

39. Esmaillzadeh, A.; Azadbakht, L. Major dietary patterns in relation to general obesity and central adiposity among Iranian women. *J. Nutr.* **2008**, *138*, 358–363. [PubMed]

40. Vergnaud, A.C.; Norat, T.; Romaguera, D.; Mouw, T.; May, A.M.; Travier, N.; Luan, J.; Wareham, N.; Slimani, N.; Rinaldi, S.; *et al.* Meat consumption and prospective weight change in participants of the EPIC-PANACEA study. *Am. J. Clin. Nutr.* **2010**, *92*, 398–407. [CrossRef] [PubMed]

41. Wang, Z.; Zhang, B.; Zhai, F.; Wang, H.; Zhang, J.; Du, W.; Su, C.; Zhang, J.; Jiang, H.; Popkin, B.M. Fatty and lean red meat consumption in China: Differential association with Chinese abdominal obesity. *Nutr. Metab. Cardiovasc. Dis.* **2014**, *24*, 869–876. [CrossRef] [PubMed]

42. Wannamethee, S.G.; Shaper, A.G.; Whincup, P.H. Alcohol and adiposity: Effects of quantity and type of drink and time relation with meals. *Int. J. Obes.* **2005**, *29*, 1436–1444. [CrossRef] [PubMed]

43. Schroder, H.; Morales-Molina, J.A.; Bermejo, S.; Barral, D.; Mandoli, E.S.; Grau, M.; Guxens, M.; de Jaime Gil, E.; Alvarez, M.D.; Marrugat, J. Relationship of abdominal obesity with alcohol consumption at population scale. *Eur. J. Nutr.* **2007**, *46*, 369–376. [CrossRef] [PubMed]

44. Lukasiewicz, E.; Mennen, L.I.; Bertrais, S.; Arnault, N.; Preziosi, P.; Galan, P.; Hercberg, S. Alcohol intake in relation to body mass index and waist-to-hip ratio: The importance of type of alcoholic beverage. *Public Health Nutr.* **2005**, *8*, 315–320. [CrossRef] [PubMed]

45. Dare, S.; Mackay, D.F.; Pell, J.P. Relationship between smoking and obesity: A cross-sectional study of 499,504 middle-aged adults in the UK general population. *PLoS ONE* **2015**, *10*, e0123579. [CrossRef] [PubMed]

46. Xu, F.; Yin, X.M.; Wang, Y. The association between amount of cigarettes smoked and overweight, central obesity among Chinese adults in Nanjing, China. *Asia Pac. J. Clin. Nutr.* **2007**, *16*, 240–247. [PubMed]

47. Weinsier, R.L.; Hunter, G.R.; Heini, A.F.; Goran, M.I.; Sell, S.M. The etiology of obesity: Relative contribution of metabolic factors, diet, and physical activity. *Am. J. Med.* **1998**, *105*, 145–150. [CrossRef]

48. Hankinson, A.L.; Daviglus, M.L.; Bouchard, C.; Carnethon, M.; Lewis, C.E.; Schreiner, P.J.; Liu, K.; Sidney, S. Maintaining a high physical activity level over 20 years and weight gain. *JAMA* **2010**, *304*, 2603–2610. [CrossRef] [PubMed]

49. Schulze, M.B.; Fung, T.T.; Manson, J.E.; Willett, W.C.; Hu, F.B. Dietary patterns and changes in body weight in women. *Obesity* **2006**, *14*, 1444–1453. [CrossRef] [PubMed]

50. Bottai, M.; Frongillo, E.A.; Sui, X.; O'Neill, J.R.; McKeown, R.E.; Burns, T.L.; Liese, A.D.; Blair, S.N.; Pate, R.R. Use of quantile regression to investigate the longitudinal association between physical activity and body mass index. *Obesity* **2014**, *22*, E149–E156. [CrossRef] [PubMed]

51. Layman, D.K.; Boileau, R.A.; Erickson, D.J.; Painter, J.E.; Shiue, H.; Sather, C.; Christou, D.D. A reduced ratio of dietary carbohydrate to protein improves body composition and blood lipid profiles during weight loss in adult women. *J. Nutr.* **2003**, *133*, 411–417. [PubMed]

52. Clifton, P.M.; Condo, D.; Keogh, J.B. Long term weight maintenance after advice to consume low carbohydrate, higher protein diets—A systematic review and meta analysis. *Nutr. Metab. Cardiovasc. Dis.* **2014**, *24*, 224–235. [CrossRef] [PubMed]

53. Ludwig, D.S. Dietary glycemic index and obesity. *J. Nutr.* **2000**, *130*, 280s–283s. [PubMed]
54. Lucan, S.C.; DiNicolantonio, J.J. How calorie-focused thinking about obesity and related diseases may mislead and harm public health. An alternative. *Public Health Nutr.* **2015**, *18*, 571–581. [CrossRef] [PubMed]

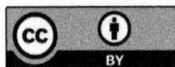

nutrients

MDPI

Article

Association between Dietary Patterns and the Indicators of Obesity among Chinese: A Cross-Sectional Study

Long Shu [1], Pei-Fen Zheng [1,2], Xiao-Yan Zhang [1,*], Cai-Juan Si [1], Xiao-Long Yu [1], Wei Gao [1], Lun Zhang [1] and Dan Liao [1]

[1] Department of Nutrition, Zhejiang Hospital, Xihu district, Hangzhou 310013, Zhejiang, China;
E-Mails: shulong19880920@126.com (L.S.); kuaidou09@163.com (P.-F.Z.); xiaosi_32075001@126.com (C.-J.S.);
xly2008hi@163.com (X.-L.Y.); gaowei05715133@163.com (W.G.); zhanglun306@163.com (L.Z.);
liaodan0203@sina.com (D.L.)

[2] Department of Digestion, Zhejiang Hospital, Xihu district, Hangzhou 310013, Zhejiang, China

* Author to whom correspondence should be addressed; E-Mail: zxy19740804@sina.com;
Tel.: +86-571-8798-5133; Fax: +86-571-8798-0175.

Received: 10 July 2015 / Accepted: 11 September 2015 / Published: 17 September 2015

Abstract: No previous study has investigated dietary pattern in association with obesity risk in a middle-aged Chinese population. The purpose of this study was to evaluate the associations between dietary patterns and the risk of obesity in the city of Hangzhou, the capital of Zhejiang Province, east China. In this cross-sectional study of 2560 subjects aged 45–60 years, dietary intakes were evaluated using a semi-quantitative food frequency questionnaire (FFQ). All anthropometric measurements were obtained using standardized procedures. The partial correlation analysis was performed to assess the associations between dietary patterns and body mass index (BMI), waist circumference (WC), and waist to hip ratio (WHR). Multivariate logistic regression analysis was used to examine the associations between dietary patterns and obesity, with adjustment for potential confounders. Four major dietary patterns were extracted by means of factor analysis: animal food, traditional Chinese, western fast-food, and high-salt patterns. The animal food pattern was positively associated with BMI (r = 0.082, 0.144, respectively, p < 0.05) and WC (r = 0.102, 0.132, respectively, p < 0.01), and the traditional Chinese pattern was inversely associated with BMI (r = −0.047, −0.116, respectively, p < 0.05) and WC (r = −0.067, −0.113, respectively, p < 0.05) in both genders. After controlling for potential confounders, subjects in the highest quartile of animal food pattern scores had a greater odds ratio for abdominal obesity (odds ratio (OR) = 1.67; 95% confidence interval (CI): 1.188–2.340; p < 0.01), in comparison to those from the lowest quartile. Compared with the lowest quartile of the traditional Chinese pattern, the highest quartile had a lower odds ratio for abdominal obesity (OR = 0.63; 95% CI: 0.441–0.901, p < 0.05). Conclusions: Our findings indicated that the animal food pattern was associated with a higher risk of abdominal obesity, while the traditional Chinese pattern was associated with a lower risk of abdominal obesity. Further prospective studies are warranted to confirm these findings.

Keywords: dietary patterns; obesity; China; cross-sectional study; factor analysis

---

1. Introduction

Obesity is a health risk factor for chronic diseases such as cardiovascular diseases, type 2 diabetes, hypertension and several types of cancers [1], and has become a major concern in all populations worldwide [2]. According to the World Health Organization (WHO) statistics, 39% of adults aged 18 years and over were overweight in 2014, and 13% were obese [3]. In China, the prevalence of obesity in Chinese adults has increased dramatically from 7.1% in 2002 to approximately 12.0% in 2010 [4]. It is well known that obesity is considered a complex multifactorial chronic disease that may be associated with some factors, including genetic and environmental factors, and especially dietary factors [5].

Over the past several decades, some previous epidemiological studies specifically focused on diet modification as an important role for the prevention of obesity, and they have reported the associations between the intakes of individual nutrients or foods and food groups and the risk of obesity [6,7]. Nonetheless, due to the complexity of diets and the potential interactions between food components [8], these analyses revealed the limited impact of diets on the occurrence of obesity. Consequently, the analysis of dietary patterns has been increasingly used in nutritional epidemiology. Furthermore, because of its ability to examine the holistic effect of diet, dietary pattern analysis also has been used to determine the associations between diet and some chronic diseases [9,10].

More recently, due to rapid economic, social, and cultural changes in China, the dietary pattern is shifting from the traditional pattern with a high consumption of staple food, coarse grains, vegetables, and fruits, to the western pattern with a high consumption of animal foods and other high energy-dense foods [11]. Following the dietary transition, chronic diseases (e.g., obesity, hypertension) are accelerating in China [12]. Therefore, it is important to examine the dietary pattern and its association with obesity in the Chinese population, especially in the middle-aged and elderly population, who are more prone to be influenced by some non-communicable chronic diseases. In fact, the relationship between dietary patterns and obesity has scarcely been reported in the Chinese population [13,14]. To the best of our knowledge, no previous study has reported the relationship between dietary patterns and obesity in Chinese adults aged 45–60 years. Therefore, the aim of the study was to identify major dietary patterns among a Chinese population aged 45–60 years, and evaluate the associations of these patterns with the indicators of obesity.

2. Subjects and Methods

2.1. Study Population

During the period of July 2014 through June 2015, this cross-sectional study was carried out in Hangzhou, the capital of Zhejiang Province, east China. The study sample was taken from eight areas (Gongshu, Shangcheng, Xiacheng, Jianggan, Xihu, Bingjiang, Xiaoshan, and Yuhang) and five counties (Fuyang, Tonglu, Chunan, Jiande, and Linan) by a stratified cluster random-sampling method. We chose one residential village or community from every county or area randomly, according to resident health records, with participants aged between 45 and 60 years residing in the selected villages or communities. A total of 2734 eligible participants (1440 male, 1294 female) were invited to attend a health examination at the Medical Center for Physical Examination, Zhejiang Hospital, where the participant was face-to-face interviewed by a trained interviewer using written questionnaires. We excluded an additional 36 participants because of incomplete anthropometric information, as well as 138 participants who provided missing or incomplete information on their dietary intake. Finally, 2560 participants were included in our analyses. The protocol of this study was approved by the institutional review and ethics committee of Zhejiang Hospital, Zhejiang Province, China, and written informed consent was obtained from all participants.

2.2. Assessment of Dietary Intake

The 58 food items in the semi-quantitative food frequency questionnaire (FFQ) were divided into 33 food groups based on the roles of food in diet and nutritional characteristics (Table S1). This FFQ was based on the food frequency questionnaire used in the 2010 China National Nutrition and Health Survey (CNNHS). Participants were asked to recall the frequency of each food item over the previous 12 months and the estimated portion size, using local weight units (1 Liang = 50 g) or natural units (cups). The frequency of food intake was measured using nine categories: never, <12 times/year, 1–3 times/month, 1–2 times/week, 3–4 times/week, 5–6 times/week, 1 time/day,

2 times/day, and 3 times/day. The selected frequency category for each food item was converted into a daily intake.

2.3. Identification of Dietary Patterns

The Kaiser-Meyer-Olkin Measure of Sample Adequacy and the Bartlett Test of Sphericity were used to assess data adequacy for factor analysis. We used the factor analysis (principal component) to identify the dietary patterns. The factors were rotated by orthogonal transformation (varimax rotation) to maintain the uncorrelated nature of the factors and greater interpretability; the eigenvalue and scree plot were applied to decide which factors remained [15]. After evaluating the eigenvalues, the scree plot test, and interpretability, eigenvalues $\geqslant 2.0$ were retained. Factor groups with a factor loading $\geqslant |0.4|$ were considered to significantly contribute to the pattern in this study. The labeling of dietary patterns was based on the interpretation of foods with high factor loadings for each dietary pattern [16]. According to these criteria, four major dietary patterns were identified. The animal food pattern was characterized by high intakes of rice, mushroom, red meat, fish and shrimp, seafood, and fats/oils. The traditional Chinese pattern was characterized by high intakes of rice, steamed bun/noodles, coarse grains, tubers, fresh vegetables and fruits, fish and shrimp, miscellaneous beans and tea. The western fast-food pattern was characterized by high intakes of fast foods, snacks, chocolates, coffee, and drinks. The high-salt pattern was characterized by high intakes of pickled vegetables, processed and cooked meat, bacon and salted fish and bean sauce.

2.4. Assessment of Anthropometric Measurements

Height was measured to the nearest 0.1 cm with subjects standing without shoes. Body weight in light clothes was measured to the nearest 0.1 kg using a digital scale. Body mass index (BMI) was calculated as weight in kilograms divided by squared height in meters. waist circumference (WC) was measured halfway between the lower rib edge and the upper iliac crest by means of a metric measure with an accuracy of 1 mm [17] and hip circumstance was measured at the maximum level over light clothing by using an inelastic plastic tape [18]. All measurements were performed by nurses trained to use standardized procedures.

2.5. Assessment of Other Variables

The validity of the questionnaire in assessing physical activity was described elsewhere [19]. The physical activity levels were expressed as metabolic equivalents in hours per week (MET-h/week). Information on smoking status included the categories of never smokers, current smokers, and former smokers. The educational level was categorized in three classes: primary school or below, middle and high school, junior college or above. Total energy intake was estimated through the FFQ, expressed in kilocalorie per day (kcal/day) and categorized according to quartile.

2.6. Definition of Terms

Obesity was defined by BMI $\geqslant 28$ kg/m^2 and abdominal obesity was defined as (male: WC $\geqslant 85$ cm; female: WC $\geqslant 80$ cm) in a Chinese population [20].

2.7. Statistical Analyses

Factor scores were categorized into quartiles (quartile1 represented a low consumption of this food pattern while quartile 4 represented a high consumption of this food pattern). The total participants numbered 2560 in our analyses. Thus, the number of participants in each quartile of each dietary pattern is 640. The characteristics of the study participants were calculated across quartiles of each dietary pattern. Data are presented as the mean ± standard deviation (SD) for continuous variables and as a sum (percentages) for categorical variables. We used analysis of variance (ANOVA) to describe mean differences by continuous variables and the chi-squared test to evaluate the difference between categorical variables. Analysis of covariance was used to compare the difference of BMI, WC, and waist to hip ratio (WHR) in the highest categories compared with the lowest categories of different dietary patterns. The partial correlation analysis was performed to assess the associations between dietary patterns and BMI, WC, and WHR. Multivariate logistic regression analysis was used to examine the associations between dietary patterns and obesity, with adjustment for age, smoking status, economic income, educational level, physical activity level, and total energy intake.

Statistical analyses were performed using the SPSS software package version 16.0 for Windows (SPSS Inc., Chicago, IL, USA). Two-sided p-values < 0.05 were considered statistically significant.

3. Results

Both the Kaiser-Meyer-Olkin index (0.798) and Bartlett's test ($p < 0.001$) showed that the correlation among the variables was sufficiently strong for a factor analysis [21]. Four major dietary patterns were extracted by means of the factor analysis: animal food, traditional Chinese, western fast-food, and high-salt patterns. These factors explained 27.9% of the whole variance. In addition, the factor-loading matrixes for these dietary patterns were shown in Table 1.

Table 1. Factor-loading matrix for major dietary patterns among 2560 Chinese adults aged 45–60 years *.

Food Groups	Dietary Patterns			
	Animal Food	Traditional Chinese	Western Fast-Food	High-Salt
Rice	0.476	0.560	-	-
Steamed bun/noodles	-	0.411	-	-
Coarse grains	-	0.544	-	-
Tubers	-	0.535	-	-
Fresh vegetables and fruits	-	0.540	-	-
Pickled vegetables	-	-	-	0.561
Mushroom	0.462	-	-	-
Red meat	0.650	-	-	-
Processed and cooked meat	-	-	-	0.517
Fish and shrimp	0.599	0.530	-	-
Seafood	0.568	-	-	-
Bacon and salted fish	-	-	-	0.601
Miscellaneous bean	-	0.535	-	-
Bean sauce	-	-	-	0.436
Fats/oils	0.402	-	-	-
Fast foods	-	-	0.467	-
Snacks	-	-	0.456	-
Chocolates	-	-	0.485	-
Coffee	-	-	0.450	-
Drinks	-	-	0.561	-
Tea	-	0.438	-	-
Variance of intake explained (%)	7.5	7.2	7.2	6.0

* Absolute values < 0.4 were excluded for simplicity.

The characteristics of study participants across quartile categories of the dietary pattern scores were shown in Table 2. Participants in the top quartile of the animal food pattern were more likely to be smokers, significantly younger, and had a higher prevalence of general and abdominal obesity, and higher education level, income, and physical activity. Conversely, compared with those in the lowest quartile, individuals in the highest quartile of the traditional Chinese pattern were more likely to be female, less likely to be smokers, significantly older, and had a lower prevalence of general and abdominal obesity and hypertension and higher economic income. In addition, participants in the highest quartile of the western fast-food pattern were more likely to be female, significantly younger, and had higher economic income than those in the lowest quartile. In contrast, participants in the highest quartile of the high-salt pattern were more likely to be smokers, male, and had a lower education level and economic income than those in the lowest quartile.

Table 2. Characteristics of the study participants by quartile (Q) categories of dietary pattern scores in the Hangzhou.

	Animal Food			Traditional Chinese			Western Fast-Food			High-Salt		
	Q1 (n = 640)	Q4 (n = 640)	*p	Q1 (n = 640)	Q4 (n = 640)	*p	Q1 (n = 640)	Q4 (n = 640)	*p	Q1 (n = 640)	Q4 (n = 640)	*p
Age (year)	51.8 ± 0.3	50.3 ± 0.2	<0.001	50.0 ± 0.2	51.9 ± 0.3	<0.001	51.5 ± 0.2	49.7 ± 0.2	<0.001	50.7 ± 0.2	51.0 ± 0.2	0.789
Gender (%)			<0.001			<0.001			<0.001			<0.001
Male	328(51.2)	454(70.9)		543(84.8)	208(32.5)		433(67.6)	336(52.5)		323(50.5)	413(64.5)	
Female	312(48.8)	186(29.1)		97(15.2)	432(67.5)		207(32.4)	304(47.5)		317(49.5)	227(35.5)	
Obesity (%)	65(10.1)	108(16.8)	<0.001	113(17.6)	53(8.3)	<0.001	99(15.5)	68(10.7)	0.01	79(12.3)	95(14.9)	0.374
Abdominal obesity (%)	215(33.6)	258(40.3)	0.002	254(39.7)	211(33.0)	0.004	248(38.8)	229(35.8)	0.149	225(35.2)	232(36.3)	0.600
Hypertension (%)	196(30.7)	223(34.9)	0.213	261(40.8)	176(27.5)	<0.001	210(32.8)	162(25.3)	0.035	171(26.7)	215(33.6)	0.030
Smoking status (%)			<0.001			<0.001			0.708			0.011
Current	121(18.9)	253(39.5)		319(49.9)	68(10.7)		176(27.5)	184(28.8)		148(23.2)	195(30.4)	
Former	7(1.1)	11(1.7)		5(0.8)	5(0.8)		4(0.6)	6(0.9)		6(0.9)	7(1.1)	
Never	512(80.0)	376(58.8)		316(49.3)	567(88.5)		460(71.9)	450(70.3)		486(75.9)	438(68.5)	
Education level (%)			<0.001			0.551			0.588			<0.001
<High school	230(36.0)	91(14.2)		162(25.3)	143(22.4)		152(23.7)	133(20.8)		116(18.1)	177(27.7)	
High school	222(34.7)	172(26.9)		200(31.2)	196(30.7)		191(29.9)	191(29.9)		189(29.6)	203(31.7)	
>High school	188(29.3)	377(58.9)		278(43.5)	301(46.9)		297(46.4)	316(49.3)		335(52.3)	260(40.6)	
Average monthly income per person (%)			<0.001			<0.001			<0.001			<0.001
≤2000 (RMB)	261(40.8)	111(17.3)		218(34.1)	160(25.0)		207(32.4)	141(22.1)		123(19.2)	225(35.2)	
2000-3000 (RMB)	268(41.9)	244(38.1)		257(40.1)	245(38.3)		269(42.1)	219(34.2)		244(38.2)	253(39.5)	
>3000 (RMB)	111(17.3)	285(44.6)		165(25.8)	235(36.7)		164(25.5)	280(43.7)		273(42.6)	162(25.3)	
Physical activity (%)			<0.001			0.116			0.550			0.346
Light	452(70.7)	568(88.8)		506(79.1)	535(83.6)		517(80.8)	532(83.1)		543(84.8)	516(80.7)	
Moderate	143(22.3)	66(10.3)		106(16.6)	95(14.9)		103(16.1)	96(15.0)		76(11.9)	102(15.9)	
Vigorous	45(7.0)	6(0.9)		28(4.3)	10(1.5)		20(3.1)	12(1.9)		21(3.3)	22(3.4)	
Total energy intake (Kcal/day)	1707.1 ± 254.8	1757.6 ± 289.1	0.457	1830.6 ± 323.5	1631.6 ± 224.2	<0.001	1738.4 ± 269.7	1724.5 ± 311.8	0.513	1620.7 ± 224.8	1840.2 ± 320.0	<0.001

Categorical variables are presented as sum and percentages, and continuous variables are presented as Mean ± standard deviation (SD). * p values for continuous variables (analysis of variance) and for categorical variables (chi-square test). Quartiles of dietary pattern score are presented by Q1, Q2, Q3, Q4, n = 640. p < 0.05 was considered statistically significant. Monthly income per person (RMB) was presented as mean.

19

The difference of BMI, WC, and WHR by quartile (Q) categories of dietary pattern scores using analysis of covariance model was shown in Table 3. After controlling for gender, age, smoking status, economic income, educational level, physical activity level, and total energy intake, those participants in the highest quartile of the animal food pattern had significantly higher BMI and WC ($p < 0.05$). Conversely, participants in the highest quartile of the traditional Chinese pattern had lower BMI, WHR, and WC than those in the lowest quartile ($p < 0.05$).

After adjusting for age, smoking status, economic income, educational level, physical activity and total energy intake, partial correlation analysis indicated that: in men, the animal food pattern had a positive correlation with BMI and WC ($r = 0.082, 0.102$, respectively, $p < 0.05$); the traditional Chinese pattern was inversely associated with BMI, WC, and WHR ($r = -0.047, -0.067, -0.062$, respectively, $p < 0.05$). In women, the animal food pattern had a positive correlation with BMI ($r = 0.144$, $p < 0.01$) and WC ($r = 0.132$, $p < 0.01$); the traditional Chinese pattern was inversely associated with BMI ($r = -0.116$, $p < 0.05$) and WC ($r = -0.113$, $p < 0.05$); the high-salt pattern had a positive correlation with BMI ($r = 0.104$, $p < 0.05$). Although the coefficients of correlation were statistically significant, the association between dietary pattern score and the indicators of obesity was weak (Table 4).

Table 3. Analysis of covariance model to evaluate the difference of BMI, WC, and WHR by quartile (Q) categories of dietary pattern scores.

	BMI (kg/m^2)	*p*	WHR	*p*	WC (cm)	*p*
Animal food pattern						
Q1 ($n = 640$)	24.27 ± 2.81	**0.035**	0.87 ± 0.08	0.533	84.02 ± 8.68	**0.002**
Q4 ($n = 640$)	25.10 ± 3.12		0.89 ± 0.06		87.35 ± 9.04	
Traditional Chinese pattern						
Q1 ($n = 640$)	25.13 ± 2.95	**0.023**	0.89 ± 0.06	**0.030**	87.78 ± 8.90	**<0.001**
Q4 ($n = 640$)	24.01 ± 2.76		0.86 ± 0.08		82.63 ± 8.45	
Western fast-food pattern						
Q1 ($n = 640$)	24.93 ± 3.00	0.217	0.89 ± 0.07	0.078	86.97 ± 8.58	0.193
Q4 ($n = 640$)	24.43 ± 2.93		0.87 ± 0.06		84.85 ± 8.91	
High-salt pattern						
Q1 ($n = 640$)	24.40 ± 3.11	0.259	0.87 ± 0.06	0.986	84.79 ± 9.63	0.777
Q4 ($n = 640$)	24.83 ± 2.96		0.88 ± 0.06		85.98 ± 8.61	

Adjusted for gender, age, physical activity, smoking status, economic income, educational level, and total energy intake. Abbreviation: BMI, body mass index; WHR, waist hip rate; WC, waist circumference. $p < 0.05$ was considered statistically significant; Q4: the highest quartile of dietary patterns, Q1: the lowest quartile of dietary.

Table 4. Partial correlation analysis for the relationship between dietary pattern score and BMI, WC, and WHR.

	BMI (kg/m^2)	*p*	WC (cm)	*p*	WHR	*p*
Animal food pattern						
Males	0.082	**0.018**	0.102	**0.009**	0.055	0.261
Females	0.144	**0.004**	0.132	**0.008**	0.024	0.637
Traditional Chinese pattern						
Males	−0.047	**0.042**	−0.067	**0.031**	−0.062	**0.035**
Females	−0.116	**0.039**	−0.113	**0.045**	−0.007	0.826
Western fast-food pattern						
Males	−0.031	0.318	−0.022	0.344	−0.013	0.711
Females	−0.023	0.649	−0.046	0.360	−0.078	0.120
High-salt pattern						
Males	0.002	0.945	0.008	0.806	0.027	0.517
Females	0.104	**0.039**	0.024	0.632	0.019	0.807

Abbreviation: BMI, body mass index; WC, waist circumference; WHR, waist to hip ratio. Adjusted for age, smoking status, economic; income, educational level, physical activity level, and total energy intake.

The association between dietary patterns and the risk of abdominal obesity by multivariate logistic regression was shown in Table 5. After adjusting for potential confounders, subjects in the highest quartile of the animal food pattern scores had a greater odds ratio for abdominal obesity (OR = 1.67; 95% CI: 1.188–2.340; $p < 0.01$), in comparison to those from the lowest quartile; compared with the lowest quartile of the traditional Chinese pattern, the highest quartile had a lower odds ratio for abdominal obesity (OR = 0.63; 95% CI: 0.441–0.901, $p < 0.05$); Nevertheless, the western fast-food and high-salt patterns showed no association with the risk of abdominal obesity.

Table 5. Multivariate adjusted odds ratios (95% CI) for abdominal obesity across quartile (Q) categories of dietary patterns scores.

	Animal Food Pattern Score			Traditional Chinese pattern Score			Western Fast-Food Pattern Score			High-Salt Pattern Score		
	Q1	Q4	p	Q1	Q4	p	Q1	Q4	p	Q1	Q4	p
						Abdominal obesity						
Model 1	1.00	1.55 (1.144, 2.107)	0.005	1.00	0.68 (0.488, 0.936)	0.018	1.00	0.85 (0.628, 1.153)	0.297	1.00	1.03 (0.764, 1.382)	0.856
Model 2	1.00	1.67 (1.191, 2.345)	0.003	1.00	0.63 (0.438, 0.891)	0.009	1.00	0.88 (0.541, 1.143)	0.358	1.00	0.98 (0.705, 1.352)	0.886
Model 3	1.00	1.67 (1.188, 2.340)	0.003	1.00	0.63 (0.441, 0.901)	0.011	1.00	0.88 (0.625, 1.225)	0.437	1.00	0.94 (0.673, 1.320)	0.731

Model 1: adjusted for sex and age; Model 2: further adjusted for physical activity level; Model 3: additionally adjusted for total energy intake. Q4: the highest quartile of dietary patterns, Q1: the lowest quartile of dietary patterns; CI: confidence interval.

4. Discussion

In this cross-sectional study, we identified four dietary patterns: animal food, traditional Chinese, western fast-food, and high-salt patterns. Our findings suggested that the animal food pattern was positively associated with BMI and WC, and the traditional Chinese pattern was inversely associated with BMI and WC. However, the association of dietary patterns with BMI and WC was very weak. Moreover, further analysis indicated that the animal food pattern was associated with a higher risk of abdominal obesity, while the traditional Chinese pattern was associated with a lower risk of abdominal obesity. To the best of our knowledge, this is the first investigation from a middle-aged Chinese population to report the association of major dietary patterns with the indicators of obesity.

The animal food pattern was characterized by high intakes of rice, mushroom, red meat, fish and shrimp, seafood and fats/oils. In this study, we found a positive relationship between the animal food pattern and abdominal obesity. The results of this study were consistent with previous studies reporting a significant inverse association between food consumption in the western pattern and the risk of obesity [22–24]. The positive association between the animal food pattern and obesity may partly be attributable to this pattern's unhealthy constituents (red meat and fats/oils). Red meat containing amounts of saturated fat and cholesterol, is considered an energy-dense food and the excess consumption may contribute to a surplus intake of energy, which may increase the risk of obesity [25]. In addition, higher intakes of meat were reported to be associated with weight gain in the European Prospective Investigation into Cancer and Nutrition-Potsdam Study [26]. Togo *et al.* also found that high consumption of meat is positively associated with BMI and WC [27]. Furthermore, in the present study, a higher intake of meat may reflect some undetected dietary behavior or lifestyle contributing to weight gain. Overall, these findings underscore the importance of animal food in the alarming prevalence of obesity in a Chinese population.

The traditional Chinese pattern, characterized by a high consumption of rice, steamed bun/noodles, coarse grains, tubers, fresh vegetables and fruits, fish and shrimp, miscellaneous beans and tea, is generally considered a healthy pattern. In the present study, we found an inverse relationship between this pattern and WC, BMI, and obesity. However, it should be noted that the association between this pattern and WC, and BMI is very weak. Our findings are consistent with previously reported findings in Chinese studies [28], suggesting that the "traditional" dietary pattern was negatively associated with weight gain in Chinese adults. The protective effect of the traditional Chinese pattern could be attributed to this pattern's healthy constituents (e.g., whole grains, fresh vegetable and fruits, and beans) (Table S2). Whole grains and fresh vegetables and fruits contain large amounts of dietary fiber. Previous studies have found that the high consumption of dietary fiber is associated with a decreased risk of obesity [29]. In addition, some foods (e.g., whole grains and vegetables) in the traditional Chinese pattern have a low glycemic index (GI), which has been found to decrease the risk of obesity [30]. Kong *et al.* reported that low GI was associated with a decreased risk of obesity in the Chinese population [31]. However, a high glycemic index in the traditional Chinese pattern may be present because of a high rice intake. In this pattern, we found that rice had a high factor loading. Recently a study indicated that rice intake was inversely associated with weight gain [32]. Rice is a low-energy food, which may contribute to the buck of the traditional Chinese pattern. Compared with wheat flour, rice absorbs more water when cooked. Thus, the energy density of the rice is lower than the wheat staple diet. Previously some studies have indicated that high energy-dense diets are associated with an increased risk of obesity [33].

The western fast-food pattern was characterized by high intakes of fast foods, snacks, chocolates, coffee, and drinks. We did not find a significant association of this pattern with obesity in this study. The results are inconsistent with existing studies, which found that a high consumption of fast food was associated with the risk of overweight and obesity in the urban Chinese population [34]. The complex nature of this pattern may explain this finding to some extent. On the one hand, compared with the western dietary pattern (high consumption of refined grains, red meat, butter, high-fat dairy products, sweets and desserts, pizza and soft drinks) [23], the western fast-food pattern is characterized by high intakes of fast foods, snacks, chocolates, coffee, and drinks, and low intakes of red meat, butter, and high-fat dairy products in our study. Several studies have also suggested that the consumption of red meat is associated with an increased risk of obesity [35,36]. On the other hand, the study participants were predominately a group of Chinese population aged 45–60 years, who rarely consumed fast food, snacks, and drinks. In addition, epidemiological evidence and experimental studies have demonstrated that drinking tea is associated with a lower risk of obesity and related diseases [37,38]. Furthermore, no significant association could also be due to the reverse causality. Study participants with a risk of obesity might have been advised to reduce their fat intake, thereby changing dietary habits. This possibility cannot be excluded in a cross-sectional study.

The high-salt pattern was characterized by high intakes of pickled vegetables, processed and cooked meat, bacon, salted fish, and bean sauce in our analyses. Although a positive association of this pattern with BMI was found in women, the association was very weak. Moreover, we found no association of the high-salt pattern in relation to abdominal obesity. No significant association could be attributed to the complex constituents in this pattern. On the one hand, the unhealthy constituents (e.g., processed meat, cooked meat, and bacon) have been reported to be associated with a higher risk of obesity [39]. In addition, previous studies have shown that a high salt intake was associated with an increased risk of hypertension, an important risk factor for obesity [40]. On the other hand, some healthy foods such as vegetables and fish were also loaded in this pattern and could interact with other foods to counteract the adverse effect on obesity. As previously reported [29], high consumption of dietary fiber is associated with a decreased risk of obesity. Meanwhile, the omega-3 polyunsaturated fatty acid (omega-3PUFA) contained in fish has been reported to have a protective role against obesity [41]. Furthermore, physical activity as a form of energy expenditure, has been considered as a standard clinical recommendation for obese individuals [42]. In our analyses, participants in the highest quartile of the high-salt pattern have higher physical activity level than those in the lowest quartile. Some studies demonstrated that a higher levels of physical activity had a protective effect against long-term gain in weight [43,44].

5. Strengths and Limitations

The present study holds its strengths and limitations. Firstly, to our knowledge, this is the first study examining the associations between dietary patterns and the indicators of obesity among a middle-aged Chinese population. Because of unique diet cultures and backgrounds, our findings further identify the special dietary patterns of the middle-aged Chinese population. Secondly, the use of a validated semi-quantitative FFQ by a face-to-face interview ensured that the data we collected are accurate. Thirdly, we have adjusted for potential known confounders for reliability in the present study. Nevertheless, several potential limitations should be considered in this study. Firstly, given the cross-sectional design of this study, we are unable to assess the causal relationship between dietary patterns and obesity. Thus, our findings need to be confirmed in a future prospective study. Secondly, several subjective and arbitrary decisions in the use of factor analysis need to be considered [45]. Finally, the study participants are restricted to the middle-aged Chinese population in the city of Hangzhou, Zhejiang Province, east China. Thus, the conclusions may not be extrapolated to the entire Chinese population.

6. Conclusions

In conclusion, our findings suggested that the animal food pattern was associated with a higher risk of abdominal obesity, while the traditional Chinese pattern was associated with a lower risk of abdominal obesity among a Chinese population aged 45–60 years. Nevertheless, more prospective studies are required to clarify whether the causal associations exist between dietary patterns and the risk of obesity.

Acknowledgments: This study was supported by the Joint construction of projects by provinces and the ministry of education (Grant No. 2014PYA002). We thank all participants from Department of Nutrition, Zhejiang Hospital for their assistance and support. We also acknowledge the Medical Center for Physical Examination, Zhejiang Hospital for their important contributions to collection of data in this study.

Author Contributions: Long Shu, Xiao-Yan Zhang and Pei-Fen Zheng conceived and designed the experiments. Cai-Juan Si, Xiao-Long Yu, Wei Gao, Lun Zhang and Dan Liao conducted research. Xiao-Yan Zhang and Long Shu analyzed data and wrote the paper. All authors read and approved the final manuscript.

Conflicts of Interest: The authors declared no conflict of interest.

References

1. Zalesin, K.C.; Franklin, B.A.; Miller, W.M.; Peterson, E.D.; McCullough, P.A. Impact of obesity on cardiovascular disease. *Endocrinol. Metab. Clin. N. Am.* **2008**, *37*, 663–684. [CrossRef] [PubMed]
2. Park, J.H.; Yoon, S.J.; Lee, H.; Jo, H.S.; Lee, S.I.; Kim, Y.; Kim, Y.I.; Shin, Y. Burden of disease attributable to obesity and overweight in Korea. *Int. J. Obes. (Lond.)* **2006**, *30*, 1661–1669. [CrossRef] [PubMed]
3. World Health Organization. *WHO Global Status Report 2014*; World Health Organization: Geneva, Switzerland, 2015.
4. Li, X.Y.; Jiang, Y.; Hu, N.; Li, Y.C.; Zhang, M.; Huang, Z.J.; Zhao, W.H. Prevalence and characteristic of overweight and obesity among adults in China, 2010. *Eup. PubMed Cent.* **2012**, *46*, 683–686.
5. NHLBI; Obeisty Education Initiative Expert Panel on the Identification, Evaluation, and Treatment of Obesity in Adults (US). *Clinical Guidelines on the Identification, Evaluation, and Treatment of Overweight and Obesity in Adults: The Evidence report*; National Heart, Lung, and Blood Institute: Bethesda, MD, USA, 1998; pp. 98–4083.
6. Harnack, L.; Walters, S.A.; Jacobs, D.R., Jr. Dietary intake and food sources of whole grains among US children and adolescents: data from the 1994–1996 Continuing Survey of Food Intakes by Individuals. *J. Am. Diet. Assoc.* **2003**, *103*, 1015–1019. [CrossRef]
7. Tighe, P.; Duthie, G.; Vaughan, N.; Brittenden, J.; Simpson, W.G.; Duthie, S.; Mutch, W.; Wahle, K.; Horgan, G.; Thies, F. Effect of increased consumption of whole-grain foods on blood pressure and other cardiovascular risk markers in healthy middle-aged persons: A randomized controlled trial. *Am. J. Clin. Nutr.* **2010**, *92*, 733–740. [CrossRef] [PubMed]

8. Lancaster, K.J.; Smiciklas-Wright, H.; Weitzel, L.B.; Mitchell, D.C.; Friedmann, J.M.; Jensen, G.L. Hypertension-related dietary patterns of rural older adults. *Prev. Med.* **2004**, *38*, 812–818. [PubMed]

9. Yusof, A.S.; Isa, Z.M.; Shah, S.A. Dietary patterns and risk of colorectal cancer: A systematic review of cohort studies (2000–2011). *Asian Pac. J. Cancer Prev.* **2012**, *13*, 4713–4717. [CrossRef] [PubMed]

10. Li, Y.; He, Y.; Lai, J.; Wang, D.; Zhang, J.; Fu, P.; Yang, X.; Qi, L. Dietary patterns are associated with stroke in Chinese adults. *J. Nutr.* **2011**, *141*, 1834–1839. [PubMed]

11. Zhai, F.; Wang, H.; Du, S.; He, Y.; Wang, Z.; Ge, K.; Popkin, B.M. Prospective study on nutrition transition in China. *Nutr. Rev.* **2009**, *67*, S56–S61. [CrossRef] [PubMed]

12. Du, S.; Lu, B.; Zhai, F.; Popkin, B.M. A new stage of the nutrition transition in China. *Public Health Nutr.* **2002**, *5*, 169–174. [CrossRef] [PubMed]

13. Shang, X.; Li, Y.; Liu, A.; Zhang, Q.; Hu, X.; Du, S.; Ma, J.; Xu, G.; Li, Y.; Guo, H.; *et al.* Dietary pattern and its association with the prevalence of obesity and related cardiometabolic risk factors among Chinese children. *PLoS ONE* **2012**, *7*, e43183. [CrossRef] [PubMed]

14. Zhang, J.; Wang, H.; Wang, Y.; Xue, H.; Wang, Z.; Du, W.; Su, C.; Zhang, J.; Jiang, H.; Zhai, F. Dietary patterns and their associations with childhood obesity in China. *Br. J. Nutr.* **2015**, *113*, 1–7. [CrossRef] [PubMed]

15. Zhang, C.; Schulze, M.B.; Solomon, C.G.; Hu, F.B. A prospective study of dietary patterns, meat intake and the risk of gestational diabetes mellitus. *Diabetologia* **2006**, *49*, 2604–2613. [CrossRef] [PubMed]

16. Newby, P.K.; Tucker, K.L. Empirically derived eating patterns using factor or cluster analysis: A review. *Nutr. Rev.* **2004**, *62*, 177–203. [CrossRef] [PubMed]

17. Esmaillzadeh, A.; Kimiagar, M.; Mehrabi, Y.; Azadbakht, L.; Hu, F.B.; Willett, W.C. Dietary patterns, insulin resistance, and prevalence of the metabolic syndrome in women. *Am. J. Clin. Nutr.* **2007**, *85*, 910–918. [PubMed]

18. Berg, C.M.; Lappas, G.; Strandhagen, E.; Wolk, A.; Torén, K.; Rosengren, A.; Aires, N.; Thelle, D.S.; Lissner, L. Food patterns and cardiovascular disease risk factors: The Swedish INTERGENE research program. *Am. J. Clin. Nutr.* **2008**, *88*, 289–297. [PubMed]

19. Yang, C.Q.; Shu, L.; Wang, S.; Wang, J.J.; Zhou, Y.; Xuan, Y.J.; Wang, S.F. Dietary Patterns Modulate the Risk of Non-Alcoholic Fatty Liver Disease in Chinese Adults. *Nutrients* **2015**, *7*, 4778–4791. [CrossRef] [PubMed]

20. Wang, H.J.; Wang, Z.H.; Yu, W.T.; Zhang, B.; Zhai, F.Y. Changes of waist circumference distribution and the prevalence of adiposity among Chinese adults from 1993 to 2006. *Eup. Pubmed Cent.* **2008**, *29*, 953–958.

21. Cunha, D.B.; de Almeida, R.M.; Sichieri, R.; Pereira, R.A. Association of dietary patterns with BMI and waist circumference in a low-income neighbourhood in Brazil. *Br. J. Nutr.* **2010**, *104*, 908–913. [CrossRef] [PubMed]

22. Haidari, F.; Shirbeigi, E.; Cheraghpou, M.; Mohammadshahi, M. Association of dietary patterns with body mass index, waist circumference, and blood pressure in an adult population in Ahvaz, Iran. *Saudi Med. J.* **2014**, *35*, 967–974. [PubMed]

23. Esmaillzadeh, A.; Azadbakht, L. Major dietary patterns in relation to general obesity and central adiposity among Iranian women. *J. Nutr.* **2008**, *138*, 358–363. [PubMed]

24. Cho, Y.A.; Shin, A.; Kim, J. Dietary patterns are associated with body mass index in a Korean population. *J. Am. Diet. Assoc.* **2011**, *111*, 1182–1186. [CrossRef] [PubMed]

25. Vergnaud, A.C.; Norat, T.; Romaguera, D.; Mouw, T.; May, A.M.; Travier, N.; Luan, J.; Wareham, N.; Slimani, N.; Rinaldi, S.; *et al.* Meat consumption and prospective weight change in participants of the EPIC-PANACEA study. *Am. J. Clin. Nutr.* **2010**, *92*, 398–407. [CrossRef] [PubMed]

26. Schulz, M.; Kroke, A.; Liese, A.D.; Hoffmann, K.; Bergmann, M.M.; Boeing, H. Food groups as predictors for short-term weight changes in men and women of the EPIC-Potsdam cohort. *J. Nutr.* **2002**, *132*, 1335–1340. [PubMed]

27. Togo, P.; Osler, M.; Sorensen, T.I.; Heitmann, B.L. Food intake patterns and body mass index in observational studies. *Int. J. Obes. Relat. Metab. Disord.* **2001**, *25*, 1741–1751. [CrossRef] [PubMed]

28. Shi, Z.; Yuan, B.; Hu, G.; Dai, Y.; Zuo, H.; Holmboe-Ottesen, G. Dietary pattern and weight change in a 5-year follow-up among Chinese adults: Results from the Jiangsu Nutrition Study. *Br. J. Nutr.* **2011**, *105*, 1047–1054. [CrossRef] [PubMed]

29. Murakami, K.; Sasaki, S.; Okubo, H.; Takahashi, Y.; Hosoi, Y.; Itabashi, M. Dietary fiber intake, dietary glycemic index and load, and body mass index: A cross-sectional study of 3931 Japanese women aged 18–20 years. *Eur. J. Clin. Nutr.* **2007**, *61*, 985–995. [CrossRef] [PubMed]

30. Sugiyama, M.; Tang, A.C.; Wakaki, Y.; Koyama, W. Glycemic index of single and mixed meal foods among common Japanese foods with white rice as a reference food. *Eur. J. Clin. Nutr.* **2003**, *57*, 743–752. [CrossRef] [PubMed]

31. Kong, A.P.; Choi, K.C.; Chan, R.S.; Lok, K.; Ozaki, R.; Li, A.M.; Ho, C.S.; Chan, M.H.; Sea, M.; Henry, C.J.; *et al.* A randomized controlled trial to investigate the impact of a low glycemic index (GI) diet on body mass index in obese adolescents. *BMC Public Health* **2014**, *14*, 180. [CrossRef] [PubMed]

32. Shi, Z.; Taylor, A.W.; Hu, G.; Gill, T.; Wittert, G.A. Rice intake, weight change and risk of the metabolic syndrome development among Chinese adults: The Jiangsu Nutrition Study (JIN). *Asia Pac. J. Clin. Nutr.* **2012**, *21*, 35–43. [PubMed]

33. Prentice, A.M.; Jebb, S.A. Fast foods, energy density and obesity: A possible mechanistic link. *Obes. Rev.* **2003**, *4*, 187–194. [CrossRef] [PubMed]

34. Li, M.; Dibley, M.J.; Sibbritt, D.W.; Yan, H. Dietary habits and overweight/obesity in adolescents in Xi'an City, China. *Asia Pac. J. Clin. Nutr.* **2010**, *19*, 76–82. [PubMed]

35. Satija, A.; Hu, F.B.; Bowen, L.; Bharathi, A.V.; Vaz, M.; Prabhakaran, D.; Reddy, K.S.; Ben-Shlomo, Y.; Smith, G.D.; Kinra, S.; *et al.* Dietary patterns in India and their association with obesity and central obesity. *Public Health Nutr.* **2015**, *20*, 1–11. [CrossRef] [PubMed]

36. Rouhani, M.H.; Salehi-Abargouei, A.; Surkan, P.J.; Azadbakht, L. Is there a relationship between red or processed meat intake and obesity? A systematic review and meta-analysis of observational studies. *Obes. Rev.* **2014**, *15*, 740–748. [CrossRef] [PubMed]

37. Nagao, T.; Komine, Y.; Soga, S.; Hase, T.; Tanaka, Y.; Tokimitsu, I. Ingestion of a tea rich in catechins leads to a reduction in body fat and malondialdehyde-modified LDL in men. *Am. J. Clin. Nutr.* **2005**, *81*, 122–129. [PubMed]

38. Dufresne, C.J.; Farnworth, E.R. A review of latest research findings on the health promotion properties of tea. *J. Nutr. Biochem.* **2001**, *12*, 404–421. [CrossRef]

39. Newby, P.K.; Muller, D.; Hallfrisch, J.; Qiao, N.; Andres, R.; Tucker, K.L. Dietary patterns and changes in body mass index and waist circumference in adults. *Am. J. Clin. Nutr.* **2003**, *77*, 1417–1425. [PubMed]

40. Ogihara, T.; Asano, T.; Fujita, T. Contribution of salt intake to insulin resistance associated with hypertension. *Life Sci.* **2003**, *73*, 509–523. [CrossRef]

41. Lorente-Cebrián, S.; Costa, A.G.; Navas-Carretero, S.; Zabala, M.; Martínez, J.A.; Moreno-Aliaga, M.J. Role of omega-3 fatty acids in obesity, metabolic syndrome, and cardiovascular diseases: A review of the evidence. *J. Physiol. Biochem.* **2013**, *69*, 633–651. [CrossRef] [PubMed]

42. Weinsier, R.L.; Hunter, G.R.; Heini, A.F.; Goran, M.I.; Sell, S.M. The etiology of obesity: Relative contribution of metabolic factors, diet, and physical activity. *Am. J. Med.* **1998**, *105*, 145–150. [CrossRef]

43. Hankinson, A.L.; Daviglus, M.L.; Bouchard, C.; Carnethon, M.; Lewis, C.E.; Schreiner, P.J.; Liu, K.; Sidney, S. Maintaining a high physical activity level over 20 years and weight gain. *JAMA* **2010**, *304*, 2603–2610. [CrossRef] [PubMed]

44. Schulze, M.B.; Fung, T.T.; Manson, J.E.; Wille, W.C.; Hu, F.B. Dietary patterns and changes in body weight in women. *Obesity* **2006**, *14*, 1444–1453. [CrossRef] [PubMed]

45. Martinez, M.E.; Marshall, J.R.; Sechrest, L. Invited commentary: Factor analysis and the search for objectivity. *Am. J. Epidemiol.* **1998**, *148*, 17–21. [CrossRef] [PubMed]

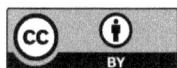

nutrients

MDPI

Article

Dietary Pattern Is Associated with Obesity in Older People in China: Data from China Health and Nutrition Survey (CHNS)

Xiaoyue Xu [1,2,*], John Hall [2], Julie Byles [1] and Zumin Shi [3]

[1] Priority Research Centre for Gender, Health and Ageing, Hunter Medical Research Institute, School of Medicine and Public Health, the University of Newcastle, New Lambton Heights, NSW 2305, Australia; E-Mail: julie.byles@newcastle.edu.au

[2] Centre for Clinical Epidemiology and Biostatistics, Hunter Medical Research Institute, School of Medicine and Public Health, the University of Newcastle, New Lambton Heights, NSW 2305, Australia; E-Mail: john.hall@newcastle.edu.au

[3] School of Medicine, University of Adelaide, Adelaide, SA 5005, Australia; E-Mail: zumin.shi@adelaide.edu.au

* Author to whom correspondence should be addressed; E-Mail: xiaoyue.xu@uon.edu.au; Tel.: +61-2-4042-0767; Fax: +61-2-4042-0043.

Received: 23 June 2015 / Accepted: 17 September 2015 / Published: 23 September 2015

Abstract: Background: No studies have been conducted to explore the associations between dietary patterns and obesity among older Chinese people, by considering gender and urbanization level differences. Methods: We analyzed data from the 2009 China Health and Nutrition Survey (2745 individuals, aged $\geq$ 60 years). Dietary data were obtained using 24 h-recall over three consecutive days. Height, Body Weight, and Waist Circumference were measured. Exploratory factor analysis was used to identify dietary patterns. Multinomial and Poisson regression models were used to examine the association between dietary patterns and Body Mass Index (BMI) status/central obesity. Results: The prevalence of general and central obesity was 9.5% and 53.4%. Traditional dietary pattern (high intake of rice, pork and vegetables) was inversely associated with general/central obesity; modern dietary pattern (high intake of fruit, fast food, and processed meat) was positively associated with general/central obesity. The highest quartile of traditional dietary pattern had a lower risk of general/central obesity compared with the lowest quartile, while an inverse picture was found for the modern dietary pattern. These associations were consistent by gender and urbanization levels. Conclusions: Dietary patterns are associated with general/central obesity in older Chinese. This study reinforces the importance of a healthy diet in promoting healthy ageing in China.

Keywords: dietary pattern; obesity; central obesity; gender; urbanization levels; older Chinese people

1. Introduction

China is ageing rapidly. By the end of 2012, the population aged 60 years or above accounted for 14.3% of the total population. It is predicted that 25% of the population will be aged 60 years and over by 2035. The number of people aged 80 years and over is increasing even more rapidly than the 60–69 and 70–79 year age groups [1]. This change in the age structure in China will have significant impacts, including an increased prevalence of chronic non-communicable diseases (NCDs). NCDs have long duration with slow progression. The four main types of NCDs are cardiovascular diseases, cancers, chronic respiratory diseases, and diabetes [1,2]. Furthermore, recent studies point out that nonalcoholic fatty liver diseases (NFALD) precede the further development of metabolic syndrome and some NCDs, such as type 2 diabetes, especially in the older population [3,4].

China is also facing an obesity epidemic [5,6]. Obesity can be considered a chronic condition, as well as an important biological risk factor for NCDs [7]. During 1992 and 2011, among adults aged from 18 to 75 years, prevalence for overweight has dramatically increased from 14.6% to 45.4%, and has nearly tripled from approximately 5.2% to 15.1% for obesity [8]. In some areas, obesity rates have risen more than three-fold, which results from an increased consumption of more energy-dense, nutrient-poor food with high levels of sugar and saturated fats, combined with reduced physical activity [9].

Dietary patterns can be efficacious indicators of the impact of diet in health outcomes, as they illustrate the combined effects of diet intake. Studies have assessed dietary patterns and obesity among children and adolescents, but the results were not consistent [10,11]. Other studies have indicated dietary patterns are associated with the prevalence of cardiovascular risk factors, hypertension, obesity, body weight, and diabetes among Chinese adults [12,13]. However, research into the association between diet and NCDs among older Chinese is extremely scarce [14,15]. As older people have higher prevalence of NCDs, and have a higher risk of insufficient or unhealthy nutritional status [12,15], it is important to understand the effects of diet among older people. Thus, the aim of this study is to explore the association between dietary patterns and obesity among older Chinese. Moreover, our previous study showed that nutrition changes are linked to an increased burden of obesity and NCDs with considerable geographical variation [14]. Additionally, economic, demographic and related forces operating at different urbanization levels also affect the diet structure [16]. The present study, therefore also assesses the association between Body Mass Index (BMI)/Waist Circumference (WC) according to urbanization levels.

2. Methods

2.1. China Health and Nutrition Survey (CHNS)

CHNS is an ongoing open cohort longitudinal survey of nine waves (1989–2011). The survey uses a multistage random-cluster sampling process to select samples from nine provinces across China [17]. Since the 2000 survey, nine provinces across four regions were included: Northeast (Heilongjiang, Liaoning), East Coast (Shandong, Jiangsu), Central (Hennan, Hubei, Hunan) and West (Gunagxi, Guizhou), which covers all levels of socioeconomic development in China [18]. The selected provinces vary according to geography, economic development and health indicators. Within each province, counties were stratified by different income levels (low, middle, and high), and a weighted sampling scheme was used to randomly select four counties. The provincial capital and one other lower income city were selected when feasible, except that other large cities other than the provincial capitals had to be selected in two provinces. Within each county, one county capital town and three villages within the counties and urban/suburban neighborhoods within the cities were subsequently randomly selected. Finally, twenty households were randomly selected from within each village, town or neighborhood. All individuals in each household were interviewed in the CHNS. Details are described elsewhere [14,17]. In 2009, 15,866 participants aged 18 or over completed the survey. Of these, 2949 participants were aged 60 or above, and 2745 (93%) completed the dietary survey were included in the present study.

Survey protocols, instruments, and the process for obtaining informed consent for CHNS were approved by the institutional review committees of the University of North Carolina at Chapel Hill and the National Institute of Nutrition and Food Safety, China Centre for Disease Control and Prevention. All participants have given their written informed consent [17]. The University of Newcastle, Australia has also approved use of data in this study in 17 December 2013 (Approval Number: H-2013-0360).

2.2. Dietary Assessment and Food Grouping

Dietary assessment is based on a combination of three consecutive 24 h recall at the individual level, and a food inventory taken at the household level over the same three day period. Combination of consecutive three-day 24 h recall and household food inventory can improve the accuracy of recall [19]. Household food consumption was determined by weighing all food consumed by the household over three consecutive randomly selected days. The three consecutive days during which detailed household food consumption data have been collected were randomly allocated from Monday to Sunday and are almost equally balanced across the seven days of the week for each sampling unit. Household food consumption was determined by examining changes in inventory from the beginning to the end of each day, in combination with a weighing and measuring technique. All foods remaining after the last meal before initiation of the survey was weighed and recorded. All purchases as well as home production foods were recorded. Wasted food was estimated when weighing was not possible. At the end of the survey, all remaining food was again weighed and recorded.

To collect individual dietary data, each household member was asked to report all food consumed over the previous 24 h for each of the three days, whether at home or away from home. Interviewers recorded the types and amounts of food consumed at each meal during the previous day. The amount of food in each dish was estimated from the household inventory and the proportion of each dish consumed was reported by each person. Household food inventory was used to collect information of household level food intake and to further estimate the individual salt and oil intake. Extreme dietary data is based on the judgment of the interviewers. For example, if a person reported an intake of 2 kg of rice a day, this was regarded as extreme. Detailed dietary data collection is described elsewhere [14,17]. As the present study does not include calculation of salt and oil intake, we used data of 24 h recall over three consecutive days at the individual level for the analysis. The three-day recall method used in this study has a high correlation with the household food inventory method for each food group (e.g., correlation coefficient was 0.84 for rice, 0.84 for wheat) [19].

The food groups included were based on a food system developed specifically for CHNS and Chinese Food Composition Table [20]. Initially, 33 food groups were included. As some food items were consumed by less than 5% of participants, food intakes were further collapsed into 27 food groups based on similarity of nutritional profiles. The 27 food groups are: rice; wheat flour and wheat noodles; wheat buns and bread; corn and coarse grains; deep-fried wheat; starchy roots and tubers; pork; red meat; organ meat; processed meats; poultry and game; fish and seafood; milk; eggs and egg products; fresh legumes; legume products; dried legumes; fresh vegetables, non-leafy; fresh vegetables, leafy; pickled, salted or canned vegetables; dried vegetables; cakes; fruits; nuts and seeds; beer; liquor and fast food.

Mean consumption of each food group per day was calculated from dietary data, as liang (Chinese ounce, 1 liang = 50 g). Mean consumption of alcoholic beverages, soft drink, and tea was calculated from questionnaire responses. Respondents were asked "do you drink any kind of alcoholic beverage (beer or liquor)?", and were asked further questions on drinking frequency, types and quantity consumed in a week. Also, participants were asked "do you normally drink tea?" and "do you drink soft drinks or sugared fruit drinks?" Further questions on drinking frequency and number of cups consumed per day (a cup is approximately 240 mL) were asked. Energy intake was calculated by CHNS based on Chinese Food Composition Table [21].

2.3. Outcome Variable-Body Composition

Height and body weight were measured based on a standard protocol recommended by the World Health Organization, by trained health workers. Weight in lightweight clothing was measured to the nearest 0.01 kg on a calibrated beam scale, and height was measured to the nearest 0.1 cm without shoes using a portable stadiometer [14,17]. BMI was divided into four categorical levels based on the criteria recommended by the Working Group on Obesity in China which are underweight: BMI < 18.5 kg·m^{-2}; normal: BMI: 18.5–23.9 kg·m^{-2}; overweight: BMI: 24.0–27.9 kg·m^{-2}; general obesity: BMI $\geqslant$ 28.0 kg·m^{-2} [22]. Central obesity was defined as WC $\geqslant$90 cm in men and $\geqslant$80 cm in women according to the International Diabetes Federation criteria [6].

2.4. Other Variables

Education level was allocated into four categories from the six education categories in the questionnaire: illiteracy; low: primary school; medium; junior middle school and high; high middle school or higher. Marital status was categorized as married or other. Work status was divided into two categories (Yes/No). Smokers were identified as people who have at least one cigarette per day (Yes/No), based on the question "how many cigarettes do you smoke per day?" Drinking was allocated to two categories, with the question "last year, did you drink beer or any other alcoholic beverage?" Participants were asked about the time spent for different types of physical activities per week. We calculated Metabolic Equivalent of Task (MET) based on the Compendium of Physical Activities and CHNS [23,24]. Four types of physical activities were included to calculate the MET including domestic activity (e.g., buying food, cooking), occupational activity (e.g., light, moderate, and heavy), transportation activity (e.g., walking from work) and leisure activity (e.g., martial arts). Urbanization is defined by a multidimensional twelve-component urbanization index to capture population density and physical, social, cultural, and economic environments [14,25].

2.5. Statistical Analysis

We only analyzed cross-sectional data collected in 2009. Exploratory factor analysis was used to identify dietary patterns using principal component analysis method in STATA/SE 13.1 (STATA, StataCorp, College Station, TX, USA). The intake (liang or cups) of 27 food groups were included in the factor analysis. Dietary patterns were identified based on the eigenvalue (>1), scree plot, factor interpretability, and the variance explained (>5%). Factors were rotated with varimax to improve the interpretability of factors and minimize the correlation between factors.

Participants were assigned a pattern-specific factor score, which was calculated as the sum of the products of the factor loading coefficients and standardized daily intake of each food associated with that pattern. Factor loadings were included in the calculation of pattern scores.

Factor scores were divided into four quartiles based on their distribution in each stratum. As regions have different levels of socioeconomic development and are therefore a potential factor impacting on the nutrition status [18,26] we included urbanization level in the analysis. Mean and standard deviation (SD) across four quartiles were used to present the average consumptions in each quartile of each food item for each dietary pattern. ANOVAs were used to identify significant differences between the two dietary patterns across four quartiles of food intake. Multinomial regression models were used to examine the associations between BMI status and dietary patterns, stratified by gender. Poisson regression models, instead of logistic regression models [27,28], were used to examine the associations between central obesity (No/Yes) and dietary patterns, stratified by gender. Forest plots [29] were used to show the association between BMI/WC and each dietary pattern, stratified by gender and urbanization levels.

3. Results

Sample characteristics are shown in Table 1. Of 2745 participants with dietary data, 57% ($n = 1563$) were aged 60–69 years and 43% ($n = 1182$) were aged 70 or above. The prevalence of overweight/obesity was 37.5% for men and 42.4% for women. Women (67.5%) had a higher prevalence of central obesity than men (35.7%). 7% of participants ($n = 198$) aged 60 or over have no dietary data. Compared with those with dietary data, people with no dietary data were slightly older (mean: 71.1 *vs.* 69.3), and more lived in a rural area (74.8% *vs.* 63.5%).

Two food patterns were obtained by factor analysis (Figure 1). Traditional dietary pattern (Eigenvalue = 2.25) was loaded heavily on rice, pork, and vegetables, and inversely on wheat flour and wheat buns. Modern dietary pattern (Eigenvalue = 1.75) is characterized by high intake of fruit, dairy, processed food, cakes and fast food, and inversely on rice and wheat flour. The two factors explained the 14.9% of variance in intake.

Table 2 shows food intakes across quartiles of traditional and modern dietary pattern, stratified by gender. For traditional dietary pattern, there were significant increases ($p < 0.001$) in rice, pork, fresh vegetable, fish, poultry and organ meat across quartiles for each gender. Significant decreases were found for corn, wheat flour, and wheat buns ($p < 0.001$). There was no statistically significant difference for energy intake of traditional dietary pattern for men ($p = 0.14$). Energy intakes were different across quartiles for women, but with no clear trend ($p < 0.001$). For the modern dietary pattern, there are significant increases ($p < 0.001$) in fruit, milk fast food, eggs, nuts, cakes, dried vegetables, fish, deep-fried wheat, processed meat, wheat buns, and legume products across quartiles for each gender. Significant decreases were found for rice and wheat flours ($p < 0.001$).

Table 1. Characteristics of study participants.

Factor	Men	Women	*p* Value	N (% of Participants)
	1300 (47.4%)	1445 (52.6%)		2745
Age				
Median (IQR)	67.0 (63.0, 74.0)	69.0 (63.0, 74.0)	0.06	2745 (100%)
Physical activity (MET)				
Median (IQR)	84.1 (62.4; 132.6)	101.8 (79.6; 133.3)	<0.001	2745 (100%)
Marital status *				
Married	1103 (85.6%)	926 (64.7%)	<0.001	2721 (99%)
Other marital status	186 (14.4%)	506 (35.3%)		
Work status *				
No	865 (66.9%)	1145 (79.6%)	<0.001	2731 (99%)
Yes	428 (33.1%)	293 (20.4)		
Education level *				
Illiteracy	176 (13.7%)	642 (44.8%)	<0.001	2721 (99%)
Low	573 (44.5%)	539 (37.6%)		
Medium	282 (21.9%)	140 (9.8%)		
High	256 (19.9%)	113 (7.9%)		
Smoking status *				
No	711 (54.9%)	1351 (93.6%)	<0.001	2739 (99%)
Yes	585 (45.1%)	92 (6.4%)		
Urbanization				
Low	455 (35.1%)	475 (32.9%)	0.39	2739 (99%)
Medium	424 (32.7%)	473 (32.8%)		
High	417 (32.2%)	495 (34.3%)		
BMI *				
Underweight	101 (8.2%)	121 (8.8%)	<0.001	2609 (95%)
Normal	669 (54.3%)	672 (48.8%)		
Overweight	380 (30.8%)	417 (30.3%)		
Obesity	83 (6.7%)	166 (12.1%)		
Central obesity				
No	834 (64.4%)	469 (32.5%)	<0.001	2739 (99%)
Yes	462 (35.7%)	974 (67.5%)		

* Significant differences have been found between physical activity, marital status, work status, education level, smoking status, BMI status and Central obesity ($p < 0.001$).

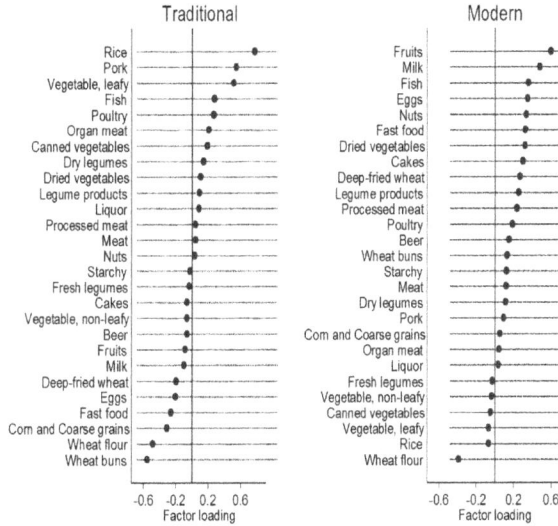

Figure 1. Factor loadings for two food patterns among older Chinese people ($n = 2745$) *. (* Factor loadings of > |0.20| represent the foods which most strongly related to the identified factor).

Table 2. Food intakes across qualities of traditional and modern dietary pattern for men and women.

Food items (Liang per day)	Q1		Q2		Q3		Q4		*p* for Trend
	Mean	SD	Mean	SD	Mean	SD	Mean	SD	
Intake of traditional food pattern									
Men									
Rice	1.36	1.64	3.89	2.07	5.22	2.07	8.01	3.65	<0.001
Pork	0.49	0.67	0.80	0.88	1.35	0.98	2.20	1.68	<0.001
Fresh vegetable, leafy	1.61	1.69	2.01	2.11	2.97	1.86	4.60	2.73	<0.001
Fish	0.18	0.55	0.54	0.97	0.78	1.15	1.12	1.58	<0.001
Poultry	0.11	0.37	0.13	0.46	0.21	0.54	0.48	0.94	<0.001
Organ meat	0.02	0.16	0.03	0.17	0.06	0.22	0.14	0.40	<0.001
Corn and coarse grains	1.03	1.76	0.41	1.07	0.23	0.72	0.11	0.42	<0.001
Wheat flour	3.66	3.27	1.37	1.37	1.21	1.13	0.57	0.91	<0.001
Wheat buns	2.94	2.87	0.99	1.68	0.37	0.81	0.17	0.47	<0.001
Oil (g)	60.4	219.8	45.0	65.3	44.8	45.5	52.5	140.5	0.35
Energy (kJ per day)	8542	8631	7940	3284	8679	2776	10616	6149	0.14

Table 2. *Cont.*

Food items (Liang per day)	Q1		Q2		Q3		Q4		*p* for Trend
	Mean	SD	Mean	SD	Mean	SD	Mean	SD	
Intake of traditional food pattern									
Women									
Rice	3.89	2.07	3.52	1.84	4.79	1.77	7.19	3.31	<0.001
Pork	0.39	0.54	0.74	0.79	1.31	0.90	2.27	1.70	<0.001
Fresh vegetable, leafy	1.50	1.67	2.01	1.76	3.09	1.96	4.62	3.13	<0.001
Fish	0.13	0.41	0.36	0.76	0.69	1.06	1.11	1.74	<0.001
Poultry	0.05	0.20	0.11	0.38	0.23	0.54	0.51	0.92	<0.001
Organ meat	0.02	0.19	0.02	0.13	0.05	0.19	0.15	0.40	<0.001
Corn and coarse grains	0.91	1.70	0.34	0.85	0.15	0.48	0.12	0.52	<0.001
Wheat flour	2.87	2.51	1.25	1.24	0.88	0.97	0.47	0.76	<0.001
Wheat buns	2.25	2.27	0.65	1.19	0.27	0.66	0.19	0.55	<0.001
Oil (g)	52.4	178.7	37.3	39.9	39.2	28.5	53.9	157.0	0.82
Energy (kJ per day)	8140	6967	6797	2454	7442	2066	10616	6149	<0.001
Intake of modern food pattern									
Men									
Fruit	0.04	0.21	0.23	0.68	0.80	1.34	2.45	2.81	<0.001
Milk	0.0	0.0	0.0005	0.009	0.14	0.61	1.07	1.87	<0.001
Fast food	0.01	0.12	0.14	0.54	0.43	0.88	0.92	1.70	<0.001
Eggs	0.24	0.42	0.48	0.58	0.72	0.76	1.01	1.06	<0.001
Nuts	0.003	0.02	0.04	0.17	0.07	0.26	0.29	0.74	<0.001
Cakes	0.008	0.07	0.02	0.14	0.07	0.28	0.32	1.15	<0.001
Dried vegetable	0.009	0.06	0.01	0.07	0.06	0.20	0.16	0.41	<0.001
Fish	0.12	0.38	0.53	0.89	0.92	1.25	1.13	1.63	<0.001
Deep-fried wheat	0.003	0.04	0.03	0.15	0.15	0.39	0.55	1.22	<0.001
Processed meat	0.002	0.02	0.03	0.16	0.08	0.30	0.17	0.58	<0.001
Wheat buns	0.35	1.25	0.74	1.62	1.28	2.29	1.78	2.29	<0.001
Legume products	0.68	1.03	0.91	1.32	1.06	1.32	1.72	1.88	<0.001
Rice	5.91	4.29	5.29	3.12	4.62	3.43	3.63	2.87	<0.001
Wheat flour	2.85	3.29	1.50	1.67	1.35	1.57	0.95	1.34	<0.001
Oil (g)	54.3	136.4	42.0	30.4	55.5	161.0	24.6	170.0	0.85
Energy (kJ per day)	9440	6171	8460	2806	9447	6526	10231	6769	0.001
Intake of modern food pattern									
Women									
Fruit	0.07	0.33	0.33	0.80	0.74	1.31	3.28	3.36	<0.001
Milk	0.005	0.09	0.0012	0.016	0.13	0.55	1.21	1.94	<0.001
Fast food	0.01	0.10	0.12	0.46	0.47	0.85	0.97	1.80	<0.001
Eggs	0.19	0.36	0.49	0.55	0.67	0.63	0.94	0.88	<0.001
Nuts	0.006	0.05	0.03	0.13	0.05	0.18	0.20	0.56	<0.001
Cakes	0.001	0.02	0.02	0.12	0.06	0.23	0.25	0.73	<0.001
Dried vegetable	0.005	0.04	0.01	0.07	0.07	0.23	0.16	0.39	<0.001
Fish	0.12	0.39	0.38	0.71	0.66	1.10	1.06	1.68	<0.001
Deep-fried wheat	0.02	0.15	0.03	0.14	0.21	0.48	0.27	0.54	<0.001
Processed meat	0.005	0.04	0.03	0.15	0.05	0.20	0.13	0.39	<0.001
Wheat buns	0.19	0.75	0.69	1.41	1.41	2.08	1.25	1.63	<0.001
Legume products	0.55	0.80	0.73	1.12	1.16	1.42	1.42	1.81	<0.001
Rice	4.67	3.36	4.41	2.73	3.53	2.89	3.30	2.77	<0.001
Wheat flour	2.33	2.53	1.39	1.57	1.15	1.30	0.73	0.95	<0.001
Oil (g)	45.3	94.1	39.1	48.6	51.7	146.2	44.8	159.0	0.70
Energy (kJ per day)	7597	4375	7355	3096	8148	5849	8719	3504	<0.001

SD: standard deviation; liang: Chinese ounce, 1 liang = 50 g.

The prevalence of overweight and obesity was 29.4% and 8.4% in quartile 4 (Q4) and 34.9% and 11.3% in quartile 1 (Q1) of traditional dietary pattern. For the modern dietary pattern, compared with Q1, people in Q4 have a higher prevalence of being overweight and obese (Overweight: 36.7% in Q4, 23.3% in Q1; Obesity: 13.2% in Q4, 6.5% in Q1). Similar differences were found for central obesity.

The prevalence of central obesity was 45.1% in Q4 and 59.0% in Q1 for traditional dietary pattern; while it was 59.1% in Q4, and 42.2% in Q1 for modern dietary pattern.

Multinomial and Poisson regression models are shown in Table 3. After adjusting for age, marital status, work status, education level, smoking, physical activity, modern diet pattern and energy (Table 3(a), model 2), men in the Q4 of traditional diet had relative risk ratios (RRRs) of 0.64 (95% CI: 0.45; 0.92) for overweight, and 0.66 (95% CI: 0.34; 1.27) for general obesity, compared with people in Q1. Across quartiles of traditional dietary pattern, RRRs for overweight/obesity decreased while RRRs for underweight increased. Similar results were found for women. Additionally, the Prevalence Ratios (PRs) for central obesity also significantly decreased across quartiles of traditional dietary pattern, especially for women (p for trend <0.001).

Modern dietary pattern was positively associated with general obesity for men and women (Table 3(b)). Compared with people with Q1 of modern dietary pattern, people with Q4 had higher RRRs for overweight/obesity; while people in Q4 had lower RRRs for underweight. Similarly, modern dietary pattern was positively, but traditional dietary pattern was inversely, associated with central obesity.

In order to confirm the associations, we also analyzed BMI and WC as continuous outcome variables by linear regression models. The results also show that traditional dietary pattern was inversely associated with BMI and WC, while modern dietary pattern was positively associated with BMI and WC. The association between dietary patterns and BMI was attenuated and became non-significant by adjusting for WC. However, the association between traditional dietary patterns and WC was independent of BMI (Appendix Table A1).

Furthermore, to minimize potential effects for other NCDs on BMI/WC, we performed an additional adjustment for NCDs (known diabetes, myocardial infarction and stroke), and the association between dietary pattern and BMI/WC did not change. Compared with Q1 of traditional dietary pattern, people in Q4 had lower BMI ($\beta = -0.41$, 95% CI: -0.56; -0.27) and lower WC ($\beta = -1.70$, 95% CI: -2.12; -1.29). Compared with Q1 of modern dietary pattern, people in Q4 had higher BMI ($\beta = 0.35$, 95% CI: 0.19; 0.51) and had higher WC ($\beta = 1.43$, 95% CI: 0.96; 1.90). After adjusting for three urbanization levels (model 3, Table 3), the p value changed dramatically, especially for the modern dietary pattern. This may imply that urbanization level is a potential confounding or matching variable. Data were thus stratified by urbanization for further analysis.

Figure 2 shows the adjusted model of the association between BMI/WC (continuous variable) and quartiles of two dietary patterns, stratified by gender and three urbanization levels. The association between traditional dietary and BMI/WC were generally consistent across three urbanization levels for men and women. However, in women a positive association between modern dietary pattern and BMI/WC was only seen among those living in medium urbanization level.

Table 3. Relative Risk Ratios (RRRs)/Prevalence Ratios (PRs) and 95% confidence interval (CI) for traditional and modern dietary pattern, stratified by gender.

BMI	Q1	Q2	Q3	Q4	*p* for Trend
(a) Intake of Traditional Dietary Pattern Quartiles					
RRRs					
Men					
Model 1					
Normal	1	1	1	1	
Underweight	1	1.98 (0.97; 4.02)	1.89 (0.95; 3.76)	1.80 (0.91; 3.53)	0.36
Overweight	1	0.73 (0.51; 1.06)	0.61 (0.42; 0.87)	0.66 (0.47; 0.93)	0.002
Obesity	1	0.94 (0.50; 1.77)	0.61 (0.31; 1.18)	0.68 (0.36; 1.26)	0.26
Model 2 [a]					
Normal	1	1	1	1	
Underweight	1	1.46 (0.69; 3.08)	1.64 (0.81; 3.32)	1.75 (0.87; 3.51)	0.20
Overweight	1	0.69 (0.47; 1.02)	0.58 (0.40; 0.84)	0.64 (0.45; 0.92)	0.001
Obesity	1	0.77 (0.39; 1.51)	0.48 (0.24; 0.98)	0.66 (0.34; 1.27)	0.20
Model 3					
Normal	1	1	1	1	
Underweight	1	1.55 (0.73; 3.31)	1.78 (0.87; 3.67)	1.91 (0.94; 3.86)	0.15
Overweight	1	0.65 (0.43; 0.96)	0.54 (0.36; 0.79)	0.61 (0.42; 0.87)	<0.001
Obesity	1	0.66 (0.33; 1.31)	0.40 (0.19; 0.83)	0.55 (0.28; 1.08)	0.09
(a) Intake of Traditional Dietary Pattern Quartiles					
PRs					
Central obesity					
Model 1					
No	1	1	1	1	
Yes	1	0.82 (0.66; 1.02)	0.69 (0.55; 0.86)	0.80 (0.66; 0.99)	0.01
Model 2 [a]					
No	1	1	1	1	
Yes	1	0.82 (0.66; 1.02)	0.70 (0.55; 0.87)	0.82 (0.67; 1.01)	0.009
Model 3					
No	1	1	1	1	
Yes	1	0.78 (0.63; 0.98)	0.66 (0.52; 0.83)	0.80 (0.64; 0.97)	0.003
Women					
Model 1					
Normal	1	1	1	1	
Underweight	1	1.13 (0.62; 2.04)	1.90 (1.09; 3.32)	1.51 (0.83; 2.76)	0.18
Overweight	1	0.93 (0.67; 1.29)	0.83 (0.59; 1.17)	0.92 (0.64; 1.31)	0.28
Obesity	1	0.81 (0.52; 1.28)	0.72 (0.44; 1.15)	0.79 (0.48; 1.29)	0.05
Model 2 [a]					
Normal	1	1	1	1	
Underweight	1	1.02 (0.55; 1.89)	1.75 (0.97; 3.14)	1.96 (1.03; 3.72)	0.05
Overweight	1	0.97 (0.69; 1.37)	0.86 (0.60; 1.23)	0.80 (0.55; 1.17)	0.06
Obesity	1	0.83 (0.52; 1.33)	0.72 (0.44; 1.19)	0.70 (0.42; 1.18)	0.02
Model 3					
Normal	1	1	1	1	
Underweight	1	1.12 (0.60; 2.10)	1.97 (1.08; 3.59)	2.14 (1.12; 4.11)	0.03
Overweight	1	0.91 (0.64; 1.30)	0.80 (0.55; 1.15)	0.76 (0.52; 1.11)	0.03
Obesity	1	0.77 (0.48; 1.25)	0.67 (0.40; 1.12)	0.68 (0.40; 1.14)	0.01

Table 3. *Cont.*

BMI	Q1	Q2	Q3	Q4	*p* for Trend
			PRs		
Central obesity					
Model 1					
No	1	1	1	1	
Yes	1	0.87 (0.80; 0.96)	0.84 (0.76; 0.93)	0.82 (0.74; 0.92)	<0.001
Model 2 [a]					
No	1	1	1	1	
Yes	1	0.88 (0.80; 0.96)	0.84 (0.76; 0.93)	0.81 (0.72; 0.90)	<0.001
Model 3					
No	1	1	1	1	
Yes	1	0.87 (0.79; 0.96)	0.84 (0.76; 0.93)	0.81 (0.72; 0.90)	<0.001
		(b) Intake of Modern Dietary Pattern Quartiles			
			RRRs		
Men					
Model 1					
Normal	1	1	1	1	
Underweight	1	1.16 (0.69; 1.95)	0.76 (0.42; 1.36)	0.41 (0.21; 0.82)	0.002
Overweight	1	1.44 (0.98; 2.12)	2.03 (1.40; 2.94)	2.17 (1.51; 3.13)	0.001
Obesity	1	2.83 (1.27; 6.33)	2.59 (1.14; 5.89)	4.28 (1.99; 9.21)	<0.001
Model 2 [b]					
Normal	1	1	1	1	
Underweight	1	1.04 (0.60; 1.79)	0.88 (0.48; 1.63)	0.65 (0.31; 1.37)	0.07
Overweight	1	1.51 (1.01; 2.26)	1.86 (1.26; 2.76)	1.78 (1.20; 2.65)	0.05
Obesity	1	3.00 (1.31; 6.88)	2.02 (0.86; 4.75)	2.97 (1.31; 6.74)	0.02
Model 3					
Normal	1	1	1	1	
Underweight	1	1.03 (0.59; 1.78)	0.98 (0.52; 1.87)	0.78 (0.35; 1.73)	0.22
Overweight	1	1.43 (0.95; 2.15)	1.69 (1.12; 2.53)	1.58 (1.03; 2.41)	0.21
Obesity	1	2.59 (1.12; 6.00)	1.53 (0.64; 3.70)	2.07 (0.88; 4.90)	0.17
			PRs		
Central obesity					
Model 1					
No	1	1	1	1	
Yes	1	1.13 (0.86; 1.48)	1.48 (1.15; 1.90)	1.89 (1.50; 2.39)	<0.001
Model 2 [b]					
No	1	1	1	1	
Yes	1	1.15 (0.88; 1.50)	1.35 (1.04; 1.74)	1.60 (1.25; 2.04)	<0.001
Model 3					
No	1	1	1	1	
Yes	1	1.10 (0.84; 1.44)	1.24 (0.95; 1.60)	1.42 (1.10; 1.67)	<0.001
			Women		
Model 1					
Normal	1	1	1	1	
Underweight	1	0.68 (0.42; 1.10)	0.81 (0.49; 1.33)	0.16 (0.06; 0.37)	<0.001
Overweight	1	1.04 (0.73; 1.48)	1.77 (1.25; 2.51)	1.70 (0.19; 2.42)	0.004
Obesity	1	1.02 (0.61; 1.70)	1.62 (0.98; 2.66)	2.00 (1.23; 3.25)	0.004
Model 2 [b]					
Normal	1	1	1	1	
Underweight	1	0.64 (0.39; 1.06)	0.95 (0.56; 1.61)	0.21 (0.08; 0.52)	0.005
Overweight	1	1.01 (0.70; 1.45)	1.62 (1.12; 2.34)	1.43 (0.97; 2.12)	0.16
Obesity	1	0.96 (0.57; 1.62)	1.34 (0.80; 2.26)	1.47 (0.87; 2.51)	0.20

Table 3. *Cont.*

BMI	Q1	Q2	Q3	Q4	*p* for Trend
Model 3					
Normal	1	1	1	1	
Underweight	1	0.67 (0.41; 1.11)	1.06 (0.62; 1.83)	0.24 (0.09; 0.63)	0.03
Overweight	1	0.98 (0.68; 1.41)	1.50 (1.02; 2.18)	1.29 (0.86; 1.95)	0.43
Obesity	1	0.90 (0.53; 1.53)	1.21 (0.71; 2.08)	1.32 (0.76; 2.30)	0.37
			PRs		
Central obesity					
Model 1					
No	1	1	1	1	
Yes	1	1.15 (1.02; 1.29)	1.18 (1.05; 1.32)	1.28 (1.14; 1.43)	0.001
Model 2 [b]					
No	1	1	1	1	
Yes	1	1.14 (1.01; 1.28)	1.12 (1.00; 1.25)	1.19 (1.06; 1.33)	0.09
Model 3					
No	1	1	1	1	
Yes	1	1.13 (1.01; 1.27)	1.11 (0.98; 1.25)	1.18 (1.04; 1.33)	0.14

Model 1 crude model; Model 2 [a] adjusted for age, marital status, work status, education level, smoking, physical activity, modern diet pattern and energy; Model 2 [b] adjusted for age, marital status, work status, education level, smoking, physical activity, traditional diet pattern, and energy; Model 3 adjusted for urbanization levels and model 2.

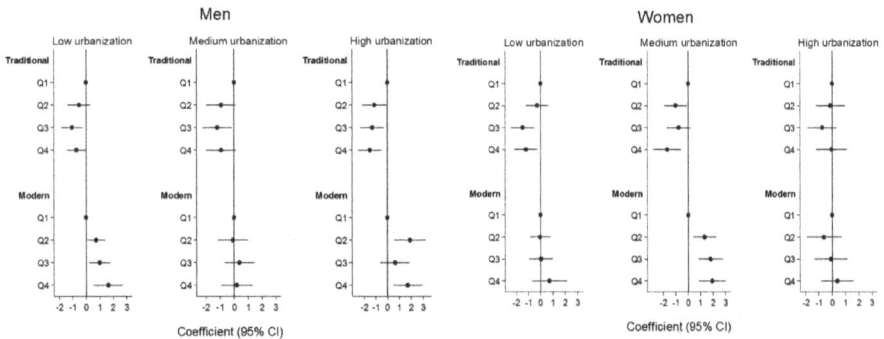

(a)

Figure 2. *Cont.*

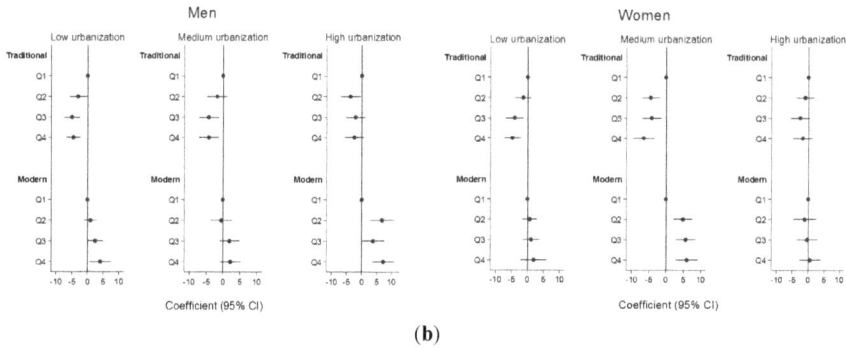

Figure 2. Dietary pattern and BMI/WC by gender, across three urbanization levels *. (* After adjusting for age, marital status, work status, education level, smoking, physical activity and energy). (**a**) Dietary pattern and BMI; (**b**) dietary pattern and WC.

4. Discussion

In this cross-sectional study, we found two distinct dietary patterns for older Chinese people. A traditional dietary pattern was inversely associated with the risk of overweight/obesity and central obesity, whilst positively associated with underweight. By contrast, a modern dietary pattern is significantly related to an increased likelihood of being obese and central obese, and inversely associated with underweight.

Although other dietary patterns have not been consistently identified in previous Chinese studies, the main components (rice, pork, and vegetable) of traditional dietary pattern were similar to those identified in this analysis [12,30]. The key components of traditional dietary pattern include high consumption of rice, pork, vegetables and fish, low consumption of meat, milk and ethanol, similar to the Mediterranean diet (protective against weight gain) [31,32]. We also found that traditional dietary patterns have protective roles for obesity/central obesity. The key components of modern dietary pattern include fruit, milk, processed and fast food. The benefits of intake of fruit are well documented and Chinese Nutrition Society recommends 200–400 g per day [33]. Although fruit is loaded heavily in the modern dietary pattern, the consumption amount is still below the recommended amount, and they are not likely to play a beneficial role in a healthy diet.

Rice is heavily positively loaded in the traditional dietary pattern, and loaded inversely in the modern dietary pattern. A previous systematic review among Asia populations indicated that rice with a high glycemic index was significantly associated with increased risk of developing type 2 diabetes [34]. However, there is still dispute about the association between rice intake and obesity within the Asian population [35,36]. In this study, a traditional dietary pattern that includes high intake of rice can be inversely associated with obesity. Our findings are consistent with studies done in Jiangsu province China, which found that a rice-rich traditional dietary pattern was inversely associated with weight gain [30,37]. As the prevalence of obesity and central obesity in the older Chinese population are high (Table 1), and these are very important biological risk factors for NCDs, our results imply the possibility of a further increase of obesity-related NCDs, such as diabetes, cardiovascular diseases and NAFLD [4,12]. Our study suggests that traditional dietary patterns may have inverse associations for obesity-related NCDs.

A positive association between modern dietary pattern and general/central obesity is consistent with current knowledge. As is shown in Table 2, fast food and processed meat intake increased substantially across quartiles for modern dietary pattern (*p* for trend <0.001). A modern dietary pattern is positively associated with fat and energy intake. The link between fat intake and obesity is well established [38]. However, fat and energy intake does not seem to explain the inverse association between traditional dietary pattern and obesity in the present study.

The discrepancy in the associations between modern dietary pattern and BMI/WC among women living in different urbanization levels may be because the composition of food in modern dietary pattern is different. One of our studies, which examined the association between dietary pattern and hypertension, found the different diet composition for modern dietary pattern at different urbanization levels. For example, the top loading foods are fruit and dairy across three urbanization levels, while the top loading foods are starchy and legumes in the low urbanization level [39]. Another possible reason may be that women living in high urbanization areas may be more concerned about body image and conscious about their health, and also undertake more physical activity than women from other areas.

Underweight is another public health concern among older Chinese people. We found that despite the rapid social and economic development in China, 8.2% of men, and 8.8% of women were still underweight in 2009. Older people are at risk of nutritional deficiency, which increases with age and the decline in a number of physiological functions. Diseases, medication, hospitalization, and other social determinants can also contribute to nutritional inadequacy [40]. It is crucial that dieticians and health professionals encourage older people to consume a healthy and balanced diet [15].

In addition, our results show that the traditional dietary pattern is inversely associated with BMI/WC. We also observed that there may be different food composition in the modern dietary pattern across different urbanization levels. Considering these results, the Chinese dietary guideline should be improved by encouraging healthy diets and the use of available healthy foods at the regional and local levels. Moreover, although the current Chinese guidelines provide general dietary advice to older people, age-specific dietary guidelines for the older Chinese population are needed in the prevention of obesity and NCDs [15,41].

Some limitations need to be addressed in the study. While urbanization level differences are important, the stratified analysis reported here was limited due to study power at the urbanization level. Further studies with larger sample sizes are needed. The association between dietary patterns and obesity may also be confounded by urbanization levels differences in other factors, which were not measured in this study. Although people who have been diagnosed with cancer may have low BMI as well as poor dietary intake, information on cancer was not available in CHNS. Moreover, the cross-sectional design in this study cannot draw conclusions about the etiological link between the two dietary patterns and obesity. However, these limitations do not affect the significance of the study. The present study breaks new ground by exploring dietary patterns and obesity among older populations in China. Strong gender and socioeconomic-specific evidence can inform policy makers and the development of programs for preventing obesity and NCDs in older Chinese people.

5. Conclusions

Prevention of obesity is vital in China, as obesity is a key risk factor for NCDs [7]. This study highlights the importance of a healthy diet for healthy ageing in China. Public awareness, clinical interventions, and nutrition policy are also need to recognize and plan for gender and geographical differences to maximize the success of health promotion approaches. Government should consider regulations and policies that encourage healthy diets and the availability of healthy foods, particularly at the regional and local levels. In addition, healthy dietary guidelines for older people should be developed, as this population group have specific dietary needs and are at higher risk of malnutrition [40].

Acknowledgments: This research received no specific grant from any funding agency in the public, commercial or not-for-profit sectors. This research uses data from China Health and Nutrition Survey (CHNS). We thank the National Institute of Nutrition and Food Safety, China Center for Disease Control and Prevention, Carolina Population Center (5 R24 HD050924), the University of North Carolina at Chapel Hill, the NIH (R01-HD30880, DK056350, R24 HD050924, and R01-HD38700) and the Fogarty International Center, NIH for the CHNS data collection and analysis files from 1989 to 2011 and future surveys, and the China-Japan Friendship Hospital, Ministry of Health for support for CHNS 2009. This research was supported by infrastructure and staff of the

Research Centre for Gender, Health, and Ageing, who are members of the Hunter Medical Research Institute, and by the Australian Research Council Centre of Excellence in Population Ageing Research. The authors thank the University of Newcastle, Australia, for funding Xiaoyue Xu's scholarship in gender, health, and ageing research.

Author Contributions: Xiaoyue Xu, John Hall, Julie Byles and Zumin Shi conceived and designed the study; Xiaoyue Xu performed the data analysis; John Hall, Julie Byles and Zumin Shi contributed materials and analysis tools; Xiaoyue Xu wrote the paper.

Conflicts of Interest: The authors declare no conflict of interest. The founding sponsors had no role in the design of the study; in the collection, analyses, or interpretation of data; in the writing of the manuscript, and in the decision to publish the results.

Appendix

Table A1. Associations between dietary patterns and BMI/WC.

	Q1	Q2	Q3	Q4	*p* for trend
			Coefficients (95% CI)		
			(a) Intake of traditional dietary pattern quartiles		
			BMI *		
			Men		
Model 1 [a]	1	−0.79 (−1.35; −0.24)	−1.14 (−1.68; −0.61)	−0.92 (−1.43; −0.41)	<0.001
Model 1 [a] + WC		−0.01 (−0.38; 0.36)	−0.06 (−0.42; 0.30)	0.11 (−0.23; 0.45)	0.31
			Women		
Model 1 [a]	1	−0.66 (−1.22; −0.10)	−1.09 (−1.67; −0.51)	−1.06 (−1.66; −0.46)	<0.001
Model 1 [a] + WC		0.002 (−0.38; 0.39)	−0.09 (−0.49; 0.31)	0.11 (−0.31; 0.52)	0.96
			WC *		
			Men		
Model 1 [a]	1	−3.13 (−4.81; −1.45)	−4.11 (−5.74; −2.48)	−3.81 (−5.35; −2.26)	<0.001
Model 1 [a] + BMI		−1.30 (−2.41; −0.18)	−1.74 (−2.82; −0.65)	−1.94 (−2.96; −0.91)	<0.001
			Women		
Model 1 [a]	1	−2.69 (−4.24; −1.14)	−3.76 (−5.36; −2.15)	−4.39 (−6.05; −2.72)	<0.001
Model 1 [a] + BMI		−1.17 (−2.23; −0.11)	−1.49 (−2.59; −0.38)	−2.19 (−3.33; −1.04)	<0.001
			(b) Intake of modern dietary pattern quartiles		
			BMI *		
			Men		
Model 1 [b]	1	0.81 (0.28; 1.34)	0.81 (0.26; 1.36)	1.26 (0.68; 1.85)	<0.001
Model 1 [b] + WC		0.38 (0.03; 0.73)	0.07 (−0.30; 0.43)	0.15 (−0.24; 0.54)	0.77
			Women		
Model 1 [b]	1	0.29 (−0.27; 0.85)	0.64 (0.05; 1.23)	1.04 (0.39; 1.69)	0.02
Model 1 [b] + WC		−0.04 (−0.42; 0.34)	0.11 (−0.30; 0.52)	0.27 (−0.18; 0.71)	0.68
			WC *		
			Men		
Model 1 [b]	1	1.74 (0.15; 3.34)	2.72 (1.05; 4.40)	4.27 (2.51; 6.04)	<0.001
Model 1 [b] + BMI		−0.09 (−1.15; 0.97)	1.09 (−0.01; 2.20)	1.61 (0.44; 2.78)	<0.001
			Women		
Model 1 [b]	1	1.65 (0.10; 3.21)	2.33 (0.70; 3.97)	3.22 (1.42; 5.03)	0.002
Model 1 [b] + BMI		0.81 (−0.26; 1.87)	0.85 (−0.27; 1.97)	0.95 (−0.29; 2.19)	0.07

Model 1 [a] after adjusted for age, marital status, work status, education level, smoking, physical activity, modern diet pattern, energy and urbanization levels; model 1 [b] after adjusted for age, marital status, work status, education level, smoking, physical activity, traditional diet pattern, energy and urbanization levels; * BMI: Body Mass Index, * WC: Waist Circumference.

References

1. World Health Organization. Country Health Information Profiles—China. Available online: http://www.wpro.who.int/countries/chn/5CHNpro2011_finaldraft.pdf?ua=1 (accessed on 1 August 2014).
2. World Health Organization. Diet, Nutrition and the Prevention of Chronic Disease: Report of a Joint WHO/FAO Expert Geneva. Available online: http://whqlibdoc.who.int/trs/who_trs_916.pdf (accessed on 21 June 2014).
3. Lonardo, A.; Ballestri, S.; Marchesini, G.; Angulo, P.; Loria, P. Nonalcoholic fatty liver disease: A precursor of the metabolic syndrome. *Dig. Liver Dis.* **2015**, *47*, 181–190. [CrossRef] [PubMed]
4. Bertolotti, M.; Lonardo, A.; Mussi, C.; Baldelli, E.; Pellegrini, E.; Ballestri, S.; Romagnoli, D.; Loria, P. Nonalcoholic fatty liver disease and aging: Epidemiology to management. *World J. Gastroenterol.* **2014**, *20*, 14185–14204. [CrossRef] [PubMed]
5. Yang, G.; Kong, L.; Zhao, W.; Wan, X.; Zhai, Y.; Chen, L.; Koplan, J.P. Emergence of chronic non-communicable diseases in China. *Lancet* **2008**, *372*, 1697–1705. [CrossRef]
6. Shi, Z.; Hu, X.; Yuan, B.; Hu, G.; Pan, X.; Dai, Y.; Byles, J.E.; Holmboe-Ottesen, G. Vegetable-rich food pattern is related to obesity in China. *Int. J. Obes.* **2008**, *32*, 975–984. [CrossRef] [PubMed]
7. Li, Y.; Wang, L.; Jiang, Y.; Zhang, M.; Wang, L. Risk factors for noncommunicable chronic diseases in women in China: Surveillance efforts. *Bull. World Health Organ.* **2013**, *91*, 650–660. [CrossRef] [PubMed]
8. Dai, J.; Sriboonchitta, S.; Zi, C.; Yang, Y. A study on whether economic development and urbanization of areas are associated with prevalence of obesity in Chinese adults: Findings from 2009 China Health and Nutrition Surveys. *Model. Depend. Econ.* **2014**, *251*, 289–305.
9. WHO. Obesity and Overweight. Available online: http://www.who.int/dietphysicalactivity/media/en/gsfs_obesity.pdf (accessed on 6 January 2015).
10. Chan, R.; Chan, D.; Lau, W.; Lo, D.; Li, L.; Woo, J. A cross-sectional study to examine the association between dietary patterns and risk of overweight and obesity in Hong Kong Chinese adolescents aged 10–12 years. *J. Am. Coll. Nutr.* **2014**, *33*, 450–458. [CrossRef] [PubMed]
11. Shang, X.; Li, Y.; Liu, A.; Zhang, Q.; Hu, X.; Du, S.; Ma, J.; Xu, G.; Li, Y.; Guo, H.; *et al.* Dietary pattern and its association with the prevalence of obesity and related cardiometabolic risk factors among Chinese children. *PLoS ONE* **2012**, *7*, e43183. [CrossRef] [PubMed]
12. Sun, J.; Buys, N.J.; Hills, A.P. Dietary pattern and its association with the prevalence of obesity, hypertension and other cardiovascular risk factors among Chinese older adults. *Int. J. Environ. Res. Public Health* **2014**, *11*, 3956–3971. [CrossRef] [PubMed]
13. Batis, C.; Mendez, M.A.; Gordon-Larsen, P.; Sotres-Alvarez, D.; Adair, L.; Popkin, B. Using both principal component analysis and reduced rank regression to study dietary patterns and diabetes in Chinese adults. *Public Health Nutr.* **2015**. [CrossRef]
14. Xu, X.; Byles, J.E.; Shi, Z.; Hall, J.J. Evaluation of older Chinese people's macronutrient intake status: Results from the China Health and Nutrition Survey. *Br. J. Nutr.* **2015**, *113*, 159–171. [CrossRef] [PubMed]
15. Xu, X.; Hall, J.; Byles, J.; Shi, Z. Do older Chinese people's diets meet the Chinese Food Pagoda guidelines? Results from the China Health and Nutrition Survey 2009. *Public Health Nutr.* **2015**, *20*, 1–11. [CrossRef] [PubMed]
16. Popkin, B.M. Urbanization, lifestyle changes and the nutrition transition. *World Dev.* **1999**, *27*, 1905–1916. [CrossRef]
17. Carolina Population Center. China Health and Nutrition Survey. Available online: http://www.cpc.unc.edu/projects/china (accessed on 1 December 2013).
18. Liu, F. New trends in China's regional economic development. In *Regional Economic Development in China*; Swee-Hock, S., Wong, J., Eds.; Singapore Institute of Southeast Asian Studies: Kent Ridge, Singapore, 2009; pp. 9–14.
19. Li, Y.; He, Y.; Zhai, F.; Yang, X.; Hu, X.; Zhao, W.; Ma, G.S. Comparison of assessment of food intakes by using 3 dietary survey methods. *Clin. J. Prev. Med.* **2006**, *40*, 273–280.
20. Batis, C.; Sotres-Alvarez, D.; Gordon-Larsen, P.; Mendez, M.A.; Adair, L.; Popkin, B. Longitudinal analysis of dietary patterns in Chinese adults from 1991 to 2009. *Br. J. Nutr.* **2014**, *111*, 1441–1451. [CrossRef] [PubMed]
21. China Institute of Nutrition and Food Safety, China CDC. *China Food Composition Table*; Peking University Medical Press: Beijing, China, 2002.

22. Zhou, B. Predictive values of body mass index and waist circumference for risk factors of certain related diseases in Chinese adults: Study on optimal cut-off points of body mass index and waist circumference in Chinese adults. *Biomed. Environ. Sci.* **2002**, *15*, 83–96. [PubMed]

23. Ainsworth, B.E.; Haskell, W.L.; Herrmann, S.D.; Meckes, N.; Bassett, J.; Tudor-Locke, C.; Greer, J.L.; Vezina, J.; Whitt-Glover, M.C.; Leon, A.S. 2011 Compendium of Physical Activities: A second update of codes and MET values. *Med. Sci. Sports Exerc.* **2011**, *43*, 1575–1581. [CrossRef] [PubMed]

24. Zuo, H.; Shi, Z.; Yuan, B.; Dai, Y.; Hu, G.; Wu, G.; Hussain, A. Interaction between physical activity and sleep duration in relation to insulin resistance among non-diabetic Chinese adults. *BMC Public Health* **2012**, *12*, 247. [CrossRef] [PubMed]

25. Yan, S.; Li, J.; Li, S.; Zhang, B.; Du, S.; Gordon-Larsen, P.; Adair, L.; Popkin, B. The expanding burden of cardiometabolic risk in China: The China Health and Nutrition Survey. *Obes. Rev.* **2012**, *13*, 810–821. [CrossRef] [PubMed]

26. Mukhopadhyay, K.; Thomassin, P.J. Economic impact of adopting a healthy diet in Canada. *J. Public Health* **2012**, *20*, 639–652. [CrossRef]

27. Thompson, M.L.; Myers, J.; Kriebel, D. Prevalence odds ratio or prevalence ratio in the analysis of cross sectional data: What is to be done? *Occup. Environ. Med.* **1998**, *55*, 272–277. [CrossRef] [PubMed]

28. Barros, A.J.; Hirakata, V.N. Alternatives for logistic regression in cross-sectional studies: An empirical comparison of models that directly estimate the prevalence ratio. *BMC Med. Res. Methodol.* **2003**, *3*, 21. [CrossRef] [PubMed]

29. Stata Statistical Software: Release 13; StataCorp LP: College Station, TX, USA, 2013.

30. Shi, Z.; Yuan, B.; Hu, G.; Dai, Y.; Zuo, H.; Holmboe-Ottesen, G. Dietary pattern and weight change in a 5-year follow-up among Chinese adults: Results from the Jiangsu Nutrition Study. *Br. J. Nutr.* **2011**, *105*, 1047–1054. [CrossRef] [PubMed]

31. Sanchez-Villegas, A.; Bes-Rastrollo, M.; Martinez-Gonzalez, M.; Serra-Majem, L. Adherence to a Mediterranean dietary pattern and weight gain in a follow-up study: The SUN cohort. *Int. J. Obes.* **2005**, *30*, 350–358. [CrossRef] [PubMed]

32. Woo, J.; Cheung, B.; Ho, S.; Sham, A.; Lam, T. Influence of dietary pattern on the development of overweight in a Chinese population. *Eur. J. Clin. Nutr.* **2007**, *62*, 480–487. [CrossRef] [PubMed]

33. Chinese Nutrition Society. Pagoda Illustration. Available online: http://www.cnsoc.org/en/nutrition.asp?s=9&nid=806 (accessed on 6 April 2014).

34. Hu, E.; Pan, A.; Malik, V.; Sun, Q. White rice consumption and risk of type 2 diabetes: Meta-analysis and systematic review. *BMJ* **2012**, *344*, e1457. [CrossRef] [PubMed]

35. Kim, J.; Jo, I.; Joung, H. A rice-based traditional dietary pattern is associated with obesity in Korean adults. *J. Acad. Nutr. Diet.* **2012**, *112*, 246–253. [CrossRef] [PubMed]

36. Kolahdouzan, M.; Khosravi-Boroujeni, H.; Nikkar, B.; Zakizadeh, E.; Abedi, B.; Ghazavi, N.; Ayoobi, N.; Vatankhah, M. The association between dietary intake of white rice and central obesity in obese adults. *ARYA Atheroscler.* **2013**, *9*, 140–144. [PubMed]

37. Shi, Z.; Taylor, A.W.; Hu, G.; Gill, T.; Wittert, G.A. Rice intake, weight change and risk of the metabolic syndrome development among Chinese adults: The Jiangsu Nutrition Study (JIN). *Asia Pac. J. Clin. Nitr.* **2012**, *21*, 35–43.

38. Hooper, L.; Abdelhamid, A.; Moore, H.J.; Douthwaite, W.; Skeaff, C.M.; Summerbell, C.D. Effect of reducing total fat intake on body weight: Systematic review and meta-analysis of randomised controlled trials and cohort studies. *BMJ* **2012**, *345*, e7666. [CrossRef] [PubMed]

39. Xu, X.; Hall, J.; Byles, J.; Shi, Z. The University of Newcastle, New Lambton Heights, NSW, Australia. Unpublished work, 2015.

40. Brownie, S. Why are elderly individuals at risk of nutritional deficiency? *Int. J. Nurs. Pract.* **2005**, *12*, 110–118. [CrossRef] [PubMed]

41. Xu, X.; Hall, J.; Byles, J.; Shi, Z. Assessing dietary quality of older Chinese people using the Chinese Diet Balance Index (DBI). *PLoS ONE* **2015**, *10*, e0121618. [CrossRef] [PubMed]

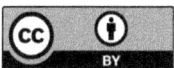

nutrients

MDPI

Article

Clustering of Dietary Patterns, Lifestyles, and Overweight among Spanish Children and Adolescents in the ANIBES Study

Carmen Pérez-Rodrigo [1], Ángel Gil [2], Marcela González-Gross [3], Rosa M. Ortega [4], Lluis Serra-Majem [5], Gregorio Varela-Moreiras [6,7] and Javier Aranceta-Bartrina [8,*]

[1] FIDEC Foundation, University of the Basque Country, Gurtubay s/n, Bilbao 48010, Spain; carmenperezrodrigo@gmail.com
[2] Department of Biochemistry and Molecular Biology II, Institute of Nutrition and Food Sciences, Centre of Biomedical Research, University of Granada, Campus de la Salud, Avda. del Conocimiento, Armilla, Granada 18100, Spain; agil@ugr.es
[3] ImFINE Research Group, Department of Health and Human Performance, Technical University of Madrid, C/Martín Fierro 7, Madrid 28040, Spain; marcela.gonzalez.gross@upm.es
[4] Department of Nutrition, Faculty of Pharmacy, Complutense University of Madrid, Plaza Ramón y Cajal s/n, Madrid 28040, Spain; rortega@ucm.es
[5] Research Institute of Biomedical and Health Sciences, Universidad de Las Palmas de Gran Canaria, Facultad de Ciencias de la Salud, C/Doctor Pasteur s/n, Trasera del Hospital, Las Palmas de Gran Canaria 35016, Spain; lluis.serra@ulpgc.es
[6] Department of Pharmaceutical and Health Sciences, Faculty of Pharmacy, CEU San Pablo University, Urb. Montepríncipe, Crta. Boadilla Km. 5.3, Boadilla del Monte, Madrid 28668, Spain; gvarela@ceu.es or gvarela@fen.org.es
[7] Spanish Nutrition Foundation (FEN), C/General Álvarez de Castro 20. 1a pta, Madrid 28010, Spain
[8] Department of Preventive Medicine and Public Health, University of Navarra, C/Irunlarrea 1, Pamplona 31008, Spain
* Correspondence: jaranceta@unav.es or javieraranceta@bizkaia.eu; Tel.: +34-64-977-7325

Received: 5 November 2015; Accepted: 11 December 2015; Published: 28 December 2015

Abstract: Weight gain has been associated with behaviors related to diet, sedentary lifestyle, and physical activity. We investigated dietary patterns and possible meaningful clustering of physical activity, sedentary behavior, and sleep time in Spanish children and adolescents and whether the identified clusters could be associated with overweight. Analysis was based on a subsample ($n = 415$) of the cross-sectional ANIBES study in Spain. We performed exploratory factor analysis and subsequent cluster analysis of dietary patterns, physical activity, sedentary behaviors, and sleep time. Logistic regression analysis was used to explore the association between the cluster solutions and overweight. Factor analysis identified four dietary patterns, one reflecting a profile closer to the traditional Mediterranean diet. Dietary patterns, physical activity behaviors, sedentary behaviors and sleep time on weekdays in Spanish children and adolescents clustered into two different groups. A *low physical activity-poorer diet* lifestyle pattern, which included a higher proportion of girls, and a *high physical activity, low sedentary behavior, longer sleep duration, healthier diet* lifestyle pattern. Although increased risk of being overweight was not significant, the Prevalence Ratios (PRs) for the *low physical activity-poorer diet* lifestyle pattern were >1 in children and in adolescents. The healthier lifestyle pattern included lower proportions of children and adolescents from low socioeconomic status backgrounds.

Keywords: cluster analysis; dietary patterns; physical activity; sedentary behavior; overweight; children; adolescents

1. Introduction

The prevalence of overweight and obesity has been steadily increasing worldwide over the past decades [1]. Obesity in children is of particular concern because of its rapid rate of increase and the potential negative impact on health and well-being during childhood and beyond.

Childhood obesity rates in Spain are amongst the highest in OECD (Organization for Economic Co-operation and Development) countries [2]. Despite high-quality data that support an overall leveling off of this epidemic among children and adolescents in Australia, Europe, Japan, and the United States, there is evidence for heterogeneity in obesity trends across socioeconomic groups, suggesting less evident leveling off in groups with lower socioeconomic status (SES) [2].

Overweight and obesity result from an imbalance between energy intake and energy expenditure, which leads to weight gain. Identifying important behaviors related to energy balance and their determinants within a specific target group is a key step to design effective obesity prevention interventions [3]. Weight gain has been associated with various specific behaviors related to diet, sedentary lifestyle, and physical activity [4,5]. More recently, sleeping habits have been reported to be possibly relevant for energy balance [6].

Whereas most research has focused on specific nutrient and food intake, overall dietary patterns (DPs) have drawn attention in the past decade because DPs consider all food and nutrient intakes and may account for the cumulative and interactive effects of foods and nutrients [3,7]. Dietary patterns have been used as exposures for many health outcomes [3,8], including obesity [9–14]. A number of studies have investigated DPs in children and adolescents. Several similar DPs have been described across these studies, such as a pattern that includes higher consumption of fruit, vegetables, and fish. A DP combining higher intakes of snacks and other energy-dense foods has also been described in several studies [15,16]. DPs among Spanish children and adolescents were analyzed in the enKid study (Feeding Habits and Nutritional Status in Spanish Children and Youth) in 1998–2000 [17].

No single element can be identified as a universal causal factor in the current obesity epidemic; many distinct behaviors and determinants at different levels influence a more positive energy balance [3]. Many of these behaviors are interrelated and may result in combined effects on health. Clustering, or the co-existence of groups of people who share similar characteristics, is a concept that has been successfully applied to understanding the relationships between different lifestyle behaviors [9,10]. The rationale underlying this approach acknowledges that there are multivariate and interactive influences on lifestyles [18,19].

Exploratory data-driven methods, such as cluster analysis or latent class analysis to investigate lifestyle patterns, have become increasingly common. In recent years a number of studies have used these methods to gain insight and better understand the relationships between diet, physical activity, and sedentary behavior among children and adolescents, as well as the possible cumulative effect of an unhealthy clustering of these behaviors on the development of overweight and obesity [20–23]. However, controversy exists surrounding the co-occurrence as well as their association with children and adolescent overweight [10,18].

To date, limited information is available on health-related behavior patterns among Spanish children and adolescents. Interventions that are appropriately targeted and that effectively consider multiple behavioral changes may be more cost effective and gain adherence from the most in need individuals or groups [24].

The aims of the study were (a) to identify dietary patterns among Spanish children and adolescents; (b) to investigate whether energy balance-related behaviors cluster into meaningful patterns in Spanish children and adolescents; (c) to describe sociodemographic correlates of the identified lifestyle patterns; and (d) to study the association of these correlates with overweight.

2. Methods

Data were obtained from the ANIBES study. ANIBES is an observational cross-sectional survey conducted in a random multistage sample of the Spanish population aged 9–75 years, living in municipalities of at least 2000 inhabitants. The aim of the survey was to evaluate energy intake and energy expenditure in a nationally representative sample of the population in Spain.

Sampling procedures and methods have been described elsewhere in detail [25,26]. Briefly, the sample for the ANIBES Study was designed based on 2012 census data published by the INE (*Instituto Nacional de Estadística*/Spanish Bureau of Statistics) for gender, age, habitat size and region. A multistage stratified sampling procedure was used, with random selection of households within municipalities and age and gender quotas for individuals within households. Interlocked quotas were established for age within region and habitat size within region. The sample selection procedure was based on random routes. In order to ensure the representativeness of the sample, 128 sampling points were used.

The final study sample consisted of 2009 individuals (1013 males, 50.4%; 996 females, 49.6%). In addition, a boost sample was recruited for the youngest age groups (9–12 years; 13–17 years, and 18–24 years) so as to include at least 200 individuals per age group. For this analysis, the final sample plus boost consisted of 213 children aged 9–12 years and 211 adolescents aged 13–17 years. Data were collected between mid-September 2013 and mid-November 2013.

The final protocol was approved by the Ethical Committee for Clinical Research of the Region of Madrid, Spain. Informed parental and student consent was required for each component of the study.

2.1. Measurements

2.1.1. Lifestyle Factors

Diet

Dietary intake was assessed by means of a face-to-face 24-h recall of the one-day intake, as well as with a three-day record kept by means of a tablet device (Samsung Galaxy Tab 2 7.0) on 2 consecutive weekdays and 1 weekend day, which included all foods and beverages consumed at home and away from home. Children were assisted by their parents or guardians to complete the food records and face-to-face interview.

Food record inputs were received in real time, then checked and coded by trained coders who were supervised by dieticians. Food, beverages, and energy and nutrient intakes were calculated using software (VD-FEN 2.1) that was newly developed for the ANIBES study by the Spanish Nutrition Foundation and is based mainly on expanded and updated Spanish food composition tables [27]. A food picture atlas was used to assist in assigning weights to portion sizes of foods consumed. Food and beverage consumption data were grouped into 16 food groups, 45 subgroups, and 754 food items, for in-depth analysis, based on the structure of the food composition database according to similarities in nutrient profile (supplementary materials Table S1). The input variables for dietary pattern analysis were the average weight consumed (g/day) by each individual (three-day food record plus one-day 24-h recall) from 38 food groups. Food groups were used to further collapse dietary intake data in order to avoid missing data from non-consumers of episodically consumed foods. Z-scores for each food group were calculated.

Physical Activity

Physical activity data were collected by face-to-face interview using the validated International Physical Activity Questionnaire (IPAQ) for children and adolescents, modified and validated according to the HELENA (Healthy Lifestyle in Europe by Nutrition in Adolescence) study for children and adolescents [28]. Additionally, objective measurements of physical activity were obtained in a subsample of 167 adults and 39 children, using an ActiGraph accelerometer (models GT3x and GT3x+; ActiGraph, Pensacola, FL, USA) during 3 full consecutive days. The validation of the modified version in HELENA study [28] found significant, but modest correlations (±0.20) comparing the modified IPAQ results with accelerometer data, and a higher validity in the older adolescents in comparison with the younger ones. Preliminary analyses of ANIBES accelerometer data are in line with this, showing modest significant correlations with vigorous physical activity ($r = 0.26$).

Total minutes per week were computed for moderate to vigorous physical activity based on the IPAQ guidelines for data processing and analyses [29]. Data were cleaned and truncated based on IPAQ guidelines and previous research [30]. Additionally, the total minutes per week of commuting-related physical activity (walking, biking) were computed. IPAQ data was used for this analysis. Z-scores of minutes per day for each type of activity were calculated.

Sedentary Behaviors

Sedentary behaviors were assessed using the questionnaire validated in the HELENA study [28]. This questionnaire included daily minutes of the following sedentary activities: television viewing, playing computer games, playing video console games, non-school-related Internet use, school-related Internet use, and studying or homework (not including classroom time). The average time spent per day engaged in these sedentary activities was calculated. Screen time (*i.e.*, time spent in front of a screen, such as that of a computer, tablet, smartphone, or console game) was assessed separately for weekdays and weekend days. Mean television, computer, and total screen time per day were calculated. For the analyses, total minutes per day (min/d) of screen time were considered. Weighted mean duration of each behavior per day (($5 \times$ weekday min/d + $2 \times$ weekend min/d)/7) was derived and summed to provide the measure of screen time used in this analysis.

Sleep Duration

Sleep habits included the number of hours each child or adolescent slept per night, on average, and were reported separately for weekdays and weekend days. In this analysis, only weekdays (h/d of sleep duration) were considered because sleep on weekdays is more likely to be regular and thus more representative of usual sleep duration [31,32].

2.1.2. Body Measurements

Anthropometric measurements were taken individually by trained interviewers, following international standard procedures previously tested in two pilot studies [33], as follows. Height was assessed in triplicate using a stadiometer (model 206; Seca, Hamburg, Germany) and recorded to the nearest 0.1 cm. Weight was assessed while wearing light clothing or underwear, using a Seca 804 weighing scale, and recorded to the nearest 0.1 kg. Waist circumference was assessed in triplicate using a Seca 201 tape measure and recorded to the nearest 0.1 cm. Body mass index (BMI) was calculated as body weight in kilograms divided by the square of body height in meters. Overweight status (overweight, obese) was calculated using age- and sex-specific cutoff values according to the criteria of Cole *et al.* [34], which have been adopted by the International Obesity Task Force.

2.1.3. Covariates

Parental Education

The education levels were established in accordance with the Spanish educational system. After preliminary analysis of the distribution of the variable, categories were collapsed and recoded into a 3-point scale, as follows: (1) low (less than 7 years of education; primary school or less); (2) medium (7–12 years of education; lower to higher secondary education); and (3) high (13 years or more of education; higher vocational, college and university studies).

Socioeconomic Status (SES)

Socioeconomic status was classified based on parental education (six categories) and occupation (12 categories) according to National Association of Opinion and Market Research (ANEIMO) criteria, which adapt to the Spanish context the World Association for Market, Social and Opinion Research (ESOMAR) criteria. This information is then classified into low, mid-low, mid-mid, mid-high, and high socioeconomic class. After preliminary analysis of the distribution of the variable for this analysis, the categories were collapsed and recoded into a 3-point scale, as follows: (1) low; (2) mid-low; and (3) high (mid-mid, mid-high and high) SES levels.

2.2. Data Cleaning

Detailed data cleaning procedures have been previously described [25,26]. Participants were considered fully eligible if verified that their three-day food records had been adequately recorded using the tablet. Provided that participants had fulfilled previous data cleaning stages, they remained in the database if they had successfully completed both face-to-face interviews during fieldwork and had measured weight, height, and waist circumference data. Of the initial sample of 486 children and adolescents recruited, 62 individuals were excluded; 424 individuals (213 children aged 9–12 years and 211 adolescents aged 13–17 years) satisfied the inclusion criteria. Outliers (± 3 SD) for energy intake were excluded in this analysis.

2.3. Data Analysis

All statistical tests were performed using IBM SPSS Statistics for Windows, Version 22.0 (IBM Corp., Armonk, NY, USA). Descriptive statistics were computed for each variable.

2.3.1. Dietary Patterns

Exploratory factor analysis was performed to identify underlying dietary patterns, using the average weight consumed (g/d) by each individual from 38 food groups as input variables. Bartlett's test of sphericity and the Kaiser-Meyer-Olkin (KMO) measure of sampling adequacy were used to verify the appropriateness of factor analysis. To assess the degree of intercorrelations between variables, we adopted a value >0.60 for the KMO. Factors were also orthogonally rotated (the varimax option) to enhance the difference between loadings, which allowed easier interpretability. Factors were retained based on the following criteria: factor eigenvalue >1.4, identification of a break point in the scree plot, the proportion of variance explained, and factor interpretability [35]. The strength and direction of the associations between patterns and food groups were described through a rotated factor loading matrix. Food groups with factor loadings >0.30 and communality >0.20 were retained in the patterns identified. The factor score for each pattern was constructed by summing observed intakes of the component food items weighted by the factor loading. A high factor score for a given pattern indicated high intake of the foods constituting that food factor, and a low score indicated low intake of those foods.

2.3.2. Lifestyle Patterns

To identify clusters with similar dietary patterns, physical activities, sedentary activities, and sleeping habits, a combination of hierarchical and non-hierarchical clustering analysis was used [36]. The variables used had different arithmetic scales; thus, Z-scores were calculated to standardize the data set before clustering, to avoid a greater contribution to the distance of variables having larger ranges than variables with smaller ranges. Univariate and multivariate outliers (>3 SD) were removed. First, hierarchical cluster analysis was performed using Ward's method, based on squared Euclidian distances. Several possible cluster solutions were identified and compared to inform the next step, considering the coefficients and fusion level. A non-hierarchical k-means clustering procedure was used, specifying the number of clusters identified in the first step, using a random initial seed and 10 iterations in order to further refine the preliminary solution by optimizing classification. The final cluster solution was selected based on interpretability and the percent of the study population in each cluster. Reliability and stability of the final cluster solution was tested by randomly taking a subsample (50%) of the total sample and repeating the analyses on this subsample. To check agreement, a kappa statistic was calculated between the cluster solutions of the subsample and that of the total sample.

Pearson's chi-square tests were used to investigate the differences in cluster distribution by gender, parental education level, family SES level, and BMI status. Independent *t*-tests were used to compare physical activities, sedentary behaviors and sleep time across clusters stratified by gender and age group. General linear models were used to estimate multivariate means for food consumption and dietary pattern scores across clusters adjusted for age and energy intake. Logistic regression analysis was used to explore the odds ratios for obesity and overweight among lifestyle patterns. The models were adjusted for energy intake, sex, age, family educational level and socio-economic status (SES). Statistical tests were two-tailed with a 5% level of significance.

3. Results

3.1. Sample Characteristics

After exclusion of outliers and participants with incomplete data, 415 children and adolescents were included in the analysis. Characteristics of the sample are described in the Supplementary Materials Table S2. There was no significant difference in sociodemographic characteristics between children and adolescents. Prevalence of overweight and obesity was significantly higher in children.

3.2. Dietary Patterns

Dietary patterns were computed for the entire sample. Bartlett's test of sphericity and KMO = 0.601 supported the appropriateness of factor analysis. Four major factors were extracted through factor analysis using 38 food groups, which explained 41% of the variance in the model. DP1 (Mediterranean like DP) had high positive loadings on vegetables, olive oil, fish, fruits, yogurt, and fermented milk products, and water and negative loading on sugar-sweetened soft drinks. This pattern is close to the traditional Mediterranean diet. DP2 (Sandwich DP) was characterized by high positive loadings on bread, cold and processed meat products, and cheese. This pattern is closer to a "sandwich-eater" pattern. DP3 (Pasta DP) had high positive loadings on pasta, sauces, and dressings, and baked goods and high negative loadings on legumes. DP4 (Milk-sugary foods DP) showed high positive loadings on milk, sugar, and sugary foods, and food substitutes (Figure 1).

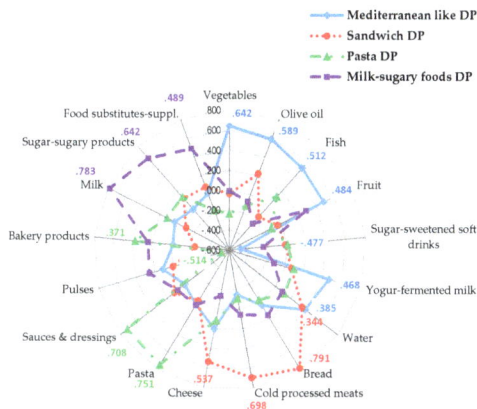

Figure 1. Factor loadings after varimax rotation on identified dietary patterns of food groups retained. Eigenvalues: Mediterranean like Dietary Pattern (DP) = 2.13; Sandwich DP = 1.74; Pasta DP = 1.57; Milk-sugary foods DP = 1.54. % variance explained: Mediterranean like DP: 11.37%; Sandwich DP: 10.0%; Pasta DP: 9.85%; Milk-sugary foods DP: 9.80%. Total variance explained 41.03%. Absolute values less than 0.30 are not shown.

Mediterranean like DP factor scores adjusted for age and energy intake were significantly higher in girls (0.13 ± 0.07 (95% CI: −0.02–0.29)) than boys (−0.07 ± 0.06 (95% CI: −0.19–0.04)).

3.3. Lifestyle Patterns

Based on the four identified DPs, minutes per day of vigorous and moderate physical activity, walking, biking, sedentary screen time, and sleep duration on weekdays, the two-cluster solution was found to be adequate and meaningful regarding the different patterns. Kappa statistic (κ = 0.74) suggested good agreement.

Differential characteristics of each cluster are identified by high (above 0) or low Z-scores (below 0) comparing cluster centers in Z-scores (Figure S1). Children and adolescents aggregated into cluster 1 had low scores on moderate (Z-score = −0.42) and vigorous physical activity (Z-score = −0.30), walking (Z-score = −0.30), biking (Z-score = −0.14), sleep time (Z-score = −0.07), Mediterranean like DP (Z-score = −0.11), and scored positively on sedentary screen time (Z-score = 0.02). Clustering of these behaviors (*low physical activity-poorer diet-Unhealthier lifestyle pattern*) is likely to favor a positive energy balance. Children in cluster 2 scored negatively on sedentary screen time (Z-score = −0.08) and had positive scores for sleep time (Z-score = 0.24), Mediterranean like DP (Z-score = 0.38), moderate physical activity (Z-score = 1.48) and vigorous physical (Z-score = 1.00). Clustering of these behaviors (*high physical activity, low sedentary behavior, longer sleep duration, healthier diet-Healthier lifestyle pattern*) is likely suggestive of healthier energy balance.

Characteristics of the children classified in different clusters are described in Table 1. The Unhealthier lifestyle pattern (*low physical activity-poorer diet*) included 76.9% of the sample and a significant higher proportion of girls than the Healthier lifestyle pattern. There were no significant differences regarding age group, family education, SES level or BMI status, although a higher percentage of children and adolescents included in the Unhealthier lifestyle pattern (*low physical activity-poorer diet*) were from low family SES level and were obese.

Table 1. Gender, age group, family educational and SES levels, and BMI status, by lifestyle pattern [a].

Characteristics	*Unhealthier Lifestyle* **Pattern**	*Healthier Lifestyle* **Pattern**	χ^2
N (%)	319 (76.9%)	96 (23.1%)	
Gender	*N* (%)	*N* (%)	
Boys	186 (58.3%)	72 (75.0%)	8.74 *
Girls	133 (41.7%)	24 (25.0%)	
Age group			2.74
Children (9–12 years)	152 (47.6%)	55 (57.3%)	
Adolescents (13–17 years)	167 (52.4%)	41 (42.7%)	
Parental educational level			1.46
Primary or less	107 (33.5%)	28 (29.2%)	
Secondary	157 (49.2%)	54 (56.3%)	
Higher	55 (17.2%)	14 (14.6%)	
Family SES			2.82
Low	71 (22.3%)	14 (14.6%)	
Mid low	79 (24.8%)	28 (29.2%)	
Mid Mid high-high	169 (53.0%)	54 (56.3%)	
BMI status			1.31
Normal weight	202 (63.3%)	64 (66.7%)	
Overweight	89 (27.9%)	27 (28.1%)	
Obese	28 (8.8%)	5 (5.2%)	

[a] Unhealthier lifestyle pattern: *Low physical activity-poorer diet*. Healthier lifestyle pattern: *High physical activity, low sedentary behavior, longer sleep duration, healthier diet*. Pearson's chi-square tests were used to investigate the differences in lifestyle pattern distribution by gender, parental education level, family SES level, and BMI status; * $p < 0.01$.

Table 2 describes physical activity behaviors, sedentary screen time, sleep time on weekdays, and dietary pattern Z-scores in the final clusters in children and adolescents. Vigorous physical activity, moderate physical activity, walking time as well as Z-scores of Mediterranean like DP, were significantly higher in children and adolescents included in the healthier lifestyle pattern, but not sedentary screen time. Adolescent girls in the healthier lifestyle pattern were significantly older than those in the unhealthier lifestyle pattern.

Consumption of selected food groups and beverages by lifestyle pattern in boys and girls is described on Table 3. Consumption of vegetables, fruit, fish, yogurt, water and juices was significantly higher in boys and girls included in the healthier lifestyle pattern, as well as consumption of cheese among girls. Conversely, consumption of sugar sweetened soft drinks was higher in boys and girls in unhealthier lifestyle pattern.

Prevalence of overweight was compared between lifestyle patterns, adjusting for sociodemographic characteristics and energy intake separately in children and adolescents (Table 4). The prevalence odds ratio (PR) for overweight was not significantly different in children or adolescents allocated into different lifestyle patterns, although PR for adolescents allocated in the unhealthier lifestyle pattern was 2.00 (IC 95% 0.87–4.86) compared to those in the healthier lifestyle pattern. Although not significantly different, both in children and in adolescents the prevalence odds ratio was higher for low–mid low family SES compared to high–mid high SES level and in children, for those from lower family educational level.

Table 2. Physical activity behaviors, sedentary screen time, sleep time on weekdays, and dietary patterns Z-score in the final lifestyle patterns [a] in children and adolescents by gender.

Variables	Boys				Girls			
	Children		Adolescents		Children		Adolescents	
	Unhealthier Lifestyle Pattern	Healthier Lifestyle Pattern	Unhealthier Lifestyle Pattern	Healthier Lifestyle Pattern	Unhealthier Lifestyle Pattern	Healthier Lifestyle Pattern	Unhealthier Lifestyle Pattern	Healthier Lifestyle Pattern
	Mean (SD)	Mean (SD)	Mean (SD)	Mean (SD)	Mean (SD)	Mean (SD)	Mean (SD)	Mean (SD)
Age (year)	10.3 (1.1)	10.3 (1.1)	15.2 (1.5)	14.9 (1.5)	10.5 (1.2)	10.4 (1.2)	14.9 (1.5)	15.9 (1.0) [†]
Sleep time week days (h/d)	8.9 (0.9)	9.1 (1.1)	8.0 (0.8)	8.4 (1.1)	9.0 (0.9)	9.1 (1.0)	7.9 (1.0)	8.3 (1.2)
Sedentary screen time (min/d)	233 (141)	214 (107)	313 (147)	294 (204)	211 (107)	245 (148)	291 (185)	259 (145)
Vigorous PA (min/d)	29 (25)	93 (50) *	30 (31)	72 (57) *	18 (30)	57 (58) *	9 (14)	90 (69) *
Moderate PA (min/d)	27 (24)	114 (51) *	18 (21)	103 (50) *	23 (25)	121 (48) *	13 (14)	98 (38) *
Walking (min/d)	37 (29)	105 (60) *	37 (33)	103 (57) *	42 (30)	90 (54) *	43 (36)	80 (53) *
Biking (min/d)	5 (11)	8 (14)	2 (5)	18 (38) *	1 (4)	9 (18)	1 (4)	1 (2)
Total PA (min/d)	111 (51)	385 (175) *	99 (53)	328 (127) *	98 (51)	385 (175) *	77 (47)	292 (89) *
Mediterranean like DP (Z-score)	−0.08 (0.86)	0.45 (0.95) #	−0.28 (0.88)	0.23 (1.35) #	0.13 (1.0)	0.35 (0.95) #	−0.16 (0.96)	0.62 (0.47) #
Sandwich DP (Z-score)	0.01 (0.94)	−0.11 (0.95)	0.24 (1.05)	0.12 (1.38)	−0.18 (0.95)	−0.26 (0.95)	−0.30 (0.80)	0.01 (0.96)
Pasta DP (Z-score)	0.08 (0.92)	0.03 (1.19)	0.09 (1.16)	0.05 (1.05)	−0.09 (0.87)	0.09 (1.19)	−0.20 (0.81)	−0.19 (0.64)
Milk-sugary foods DP (Z-score)	0.17 (0.81)	0.08 (0.80)	0.19 (1.35)	−0.17 (1.09)	−0.01 (0.76)	0.08 (0.80)	−0.24 (0.89)	−0.59 (0.55)

[a] Unhealthier lifestyle pattern: *Low physical activity-poorer diet*. Healthier lifestyle pattern: *High physical activity, low sedentary behavior, longer sleep duration, healthier diet*. Independent t-tests were used to compare physical activities, sedentary behaviors and sleep time across lifestyle patterns stratified by gender and age group. General linear models were used to estimate multivariate means for dietary pattern scores across lifestyle patterns adjusted for age and energy intake; * $p < 0.05$ for independent t-tests; [†] $p < 0.0001$; # $p < 0.01$ General Linear Models adjusted for age and energy intake.

Table 3. Mean and median consumption of selected food groups and beverages by lifestyle pattern [a] in boys and girls [b].

Food Groups	Boys				Girls			
	Unhealthier Lifestyle Pattern		Healthier Lifestyle Pattern		Unhealthier Lifestyle Pattern		Healthier Lifestyle Pattern	
	Mean (SEM)	Median	Mean (SEM)	Median	Mean (SEM)	Median	Mean (SEM)	Median
Olive oil (ml/d)	15.4 (0.1)	15.1	17.7 (0.2) *	17.5	15.5 (0.2)	15.5	13.5 (0.5) *	13.7
Vegetables (g/d)	117 (1.0)	114	137 (1.7) *	137	128 (1.2)	126	148 (3.3) *	147
Fruit (g/d)	88.7 (2.1)	88.3	122 (2.8) *	121	106 (2.0)	108	147 (6.1) *	147
Pulses (g/d)	12.9 (0.1)	12.8	13.3 (0.2)	13.3	13.2 (0.1)	13.3	13.4 (0.2)	13.5
Fish (g/d)	37.8 (0.3)	37.8	55.2 (0.5) *	55.7	41.9 (0.2)	42.0	80.4 (0.7) *	80.7
Bread (g/d)	95.5 (1.8)	90.9	96.7 (3.1)	97.2	80.8 (1.6)	78.8	79 (4.5)	79.6
Pasta (g/d)	24.7 (0.8)	23.9	23.8 (0.6)	23.9	19.1 (0.2)	19.3	15.5 (0.6)	15.8
Bakery products (g/d)	48.3 (1.3)	46.4	46.1 (2.3)	46.7	41.1 (0.8)	40.4	48.4 (2.4)	48.8
Sugar and sugary products (g/d)	23.8 (0.3)	23.5	20.8 (0.6) *	20.7	24.0 (0.6)	23.4	24.1 (1.8)	24.3
Milk (g/d)	274 (2.8)	267	247 (4.8) *	248	208 (2.6)	211	209 (7.8)	215
Cheese (g/d)	16.0 (0.4)	14.9	17.2 (0.6)	17.1	15.0 (0.4)	14.5	21.9 (0.9) *	21.8
Yoghurt and fermented milk (g/d)	51.8 (1.3)	53.2	73.3 (2.2) *	74.9	50.2 (1.6)	51.8	69.1 (4.8) *	72.2
Meats (g/d)	105 (1.0)	103	117 (1.5) *	116	88.6 (1.2)	88.7	79.4 (2.7) *	79.5
Cold and processed meats (g/d)	59.4 (0.9)	57.3	51.4 (1.6)	51.6	48.7 (0.9)	49.2	50.6 (2.9)	51.9
Water (g/d)	582 (5.2)	578	627 (9.3) *	625	526 (0.8)	527	629 (2.3) *	630
Sugared soft drinks (g/d)	143 (3.8)	138	98.1 (5.2) *	91.4	95.6 (2.9)	95.1	66.8 (6.8) *	50.3
Juices (g/d)	115 (1.9)	115	126 (3.5) *	125	114 (1.9)	111	159 (5.3) *	160
Sauces and dressings (g/d)	15.4 (0.2)	15.2	15.8 (0.4)	15.8	14.0 (0.2)	14.4	15.4 (0.7)	15.7

[a] Unhealthier lifestyle pattern: *Low physical activity-poorer diet*. Healthier lifestyle pattern: *High physical activity, low sedentary behavior, longer sleep duration, healthier diet*. [b] General linear models were used to estimate multivariate means for food consumption and dietary pattern scores across lifestyle patterns adjusted for age and energy intake; * $p < 0.05$.

Table 4. Prevalence ratio (PR) of overweight/obesity in children and adolescents, according to gender, age, family level of education, socioeconomic level and lifestyle pattern [a] in children and in adolescents.

Variables	Children				Adolescents			
	PR	95% C.I.PR		*p*	PR	95% C.I.PR		*p*
		Lower	Upper			Lower	Upper	
Gender								
Girls	1				1			
Boys	1.26	0.70	2.25	NS	1.79	0.85	3.76	NS
Age	0.92	0.72	1.18	NS	0.78	0.62	0.97	0.026
Family Level of education				NS				NS
High	1				1			
Secondary	1.00	0.46	2.19	NS	0.67	0.26	1.17	NS
Primary	1.15	0.49	2.69	NS	0.52	0.19	1.43	NS
SES				NS				NS
Mid-high-High	1				1			
Mid	0.88	0.42	1.87	NS	0.66	0.27	1.59	NS
Mid-low-Low	1.27	0.65	2.50	NS	1.88	0.87	4.06	NS
Lifestyle pattern								
Healthier lifestyle patter					1			
Unhealthier lifestyle pattern	1.07	0.55	2.04	NS	2.00	0.82	4.86	NS

Note: Binary logistic regression models adjusted for age, sex, family SES, family educational level and energy intake. [a] Unhealthier lifestyle pattern: *Low physical activity-poorer diet*. Healthier lifestyle pattern: *High physical activity, low sedentary behavior, longer sleep duration, healthier diet*.

4. Discussion

This study showed that dietary patterns, physical activity behaviors, sedentary behaviors and sleep time on weekdays in Spanish children and adolescents cluster in two different groups. A *low physical activity-poorer diet* lifestyle pattern (Unhealthier lifestyle pattern), which included a higher proportion of girls, and a *high physical activity, low sedentary behavior, longer sleep duration, healthier diet* lifestyle pattern (Healthier lifestyle pattern). Although increased risk of being overweight was not significant, the ORs for the unhealthier lifestyle pattern (*low physical activity-poorer diet*) were >1 in children and in adolescents.

Analysis of dietary patterns has been increasingly used to consider total food intake and the potentially synergistic effects of foods and nutrients [10,18]. Factor analysis and cluster analysis are procedures commonly used for that purpose. In this study factor analysis was used to identify dietary patterns that were later used in cluster analysis. This approach has been used by other authors [37]. Several studies have identified a healthier or traditional DP in children and adolescents, with higher scores on fruits and vegetables and lower scores in energy-dense foods [7,11–17,38,39], such as the Mediterranean like DP identified in this study. A DP high in sandwiches or packed lunches, similar to that identified in this analysis, has also been described in different studies [7,10,40].

The results of cluster analysis in this study are consistent with findings by other authors reporting a healthy energy balance-related behavior pattern that combines a healthier diet with high levels of physical activity and low levels of sedentary behavior, among children and adolescents in different countries [13,22,32,40–45]. Several studies also report the clustering of a combination of sedentary lifestyle with healthy diet [44,45]. A systematic review on the clustering of diet, physical activity, and sedentary behavior among children and adolescents aged 9–21 years, except one study of children aged 5–12 years, found that most children and adolescents in those studies fell into a mixed category of one or more healthy behaviors together with one or more unhealthy behaviors [18]. Te Velde *et al.* also identified a cluster with low physical activity and low sedentary behaviors in 10- to 12-year-old European children, with a higher proportion of girls [46].

In our study, sleep time scored positively in the healthier lifestyle pattern. A long sleep duration-physically inactive lifestyle pattern was identified among European children aged 10–12 years [32]. The same study also identified a short sleep duration-physically inactive lifestyle pattern. Sleep quality is an issue, which deserves further research in addition to sleep duration.

The healthier lifestyle pattern included 23% of children and adolescents in our study and a significantly different gender distribution; this lifestyle pattern characterized by high physical activity and healthier diet had a lower proportion of girls (25%). Several studies have reported that boys score higher than girls on less healthy dietary patterns or poorer diet-sedentary behaviors, such as observations from the KOALA Birth Cohort Study in The Netherlands [23] and the Young Finns Study [11]. Boys have also been reported to cluster into a high physical activity-healthy diet pattern or a high physical activity-high sedentary pattern [44]. In our analysis, Mediterranean like DP factor scores adjusted for age and energy intake were significantly higher in girls in line with findings that report girls to be more likely within a healthy or traditional dietary pattern [47].

Differences between boys and girls in sedentary and physical activity behaviors have been reported by other authors [46,48]. Gender difference in physical activity seems consistent in several studies, girls being less physically active particularly in adolescents [20]. This was also reported in the PERSEO project (Pilot Reference School Program for Health and Physical Actitvity against Obesity)—a school based intervention aimed to foster healthier eating and physical activity behaviors in Primary School children—among Spanish school children [49]. A consistent finding in the review by Leech *et al.* [18] was a higher proportion of boys in the high physical activity lifestyle patterns and more girls in those with low physical activity, as observed in our analysis.

Contradictory results have been reported regarding sedentary behavior [50]. Jago *et al.* [51] suggested that girls engage in sedentary activities that are often not assessed, such as personal care and social interactions.

In this study, the unhealthier lifestyle pattern (*low physical activity-poorer diet*) included a higher proportion of families with a low SES level (22.3%). Leech *et al.* [18] reported in their systematic review a higher proportion of children or adolescents from a low SES in the lifestyle patterns defined by low levels of physical activity. Some evidence has also been found suggesting that children from low SES tend to be in lifestyle patterns defined by high levels of sedentary behaviors. However, some studies have found no association between cluster grouping and SES [44].

An inverse association between parental education and sedentary behavior has been observed in other studies. In their systematic review, Leech *et al.* found that lifestyle patterns characterized by high physical activity or participation in sports were significantly associated with higher levels of parental education, adolescent education, and family income [18]. High sedentary behavior lifestyle patterns were associated with low parental education and low family income levels [17,20]. We found no significant association with family educational level, although a higher proportion of children from lower education families were included in the low physical activity lifestyle pattern.

In this study, increased risk of being overweight was not significant across lifestyle patterns in children or adolescents. Systematic reviews on this issue have concluded that the evidence is inconsistent with respect to a cumulative effect of these behaviors on obesity outcomes; some studies have found a higher prevalence of overweight and obesity in unhealthy lifestyle patterns, whereas others have found no association at all. In the review by Leech *et al.*, five studies, including two longitudinal studies, showed evidence of a possible synergistic effect of multiple unhealthy behaviors on overweight or obesity, two studies found an unexpected inverse association with an unhealthy lifestyle pattern, and seven studies found no association [18]. In those studies that found a possible synergistic effect, lifestyle patterns characterized by either low physical activity or high sedentary behavior were positively associated with overweight [52]. A pattern combining inactivity and sedentary behavior with television viewing during meals was related to increased cross-sectional odds of overweight in boys in the Pro Children study among 10–12 year-old European school children [46]. This inconsistency can likely be attributed to the cross-sectional design of many of these studies, but it also reflects the complexity of energy balance-related behavior, sociodemographic correlates, other determinant factors, and their relationships with obesity. To date, most studies investigating dietary patterns have focused on food consumption but do not consider eating routines, how, when, or where people eat. Several studies have found that determinants of energy balance-related behaviors also cluster, such as parenting practices [10,23].

Strengths of this study include the careful design, protocol, and methodology used in the ANIBES study, conducted among a random representative sample of the Spanish population aged 9–75 years. Food consumption assessment was made using digital tablets and included a thorough quality control process. The use of factor analysis allowed us to identify dietary patterns without any *a priori* defined criteria and their inclusion in cluster analysis together with physical activity, sedentary behaviors, and sleep time provided a broader perspective.

One limitation of this study is the cross-sectional design, which provides evidence for association but not causal relationships, and residual confounding by unobserved and unmeasured factors is likely. Measures of food consumption and physical activity relied on self-reports and were possibly biased, although a careful multistep quality control procedure was implemented to minimize bias. However, misreporting can influence the potential association with overweight. Information on physical activity and sedentary behaviors used in this analysis was self-reported as well. Accelerometers were used to collect data in a subsample and showed modest significant correlations with vigorous physical activity ($r = 0.26$), in line with those observed in validation studies of a modified version of IPAQ for children and adolescents [28]. The validity correlation coefficients from the majority of existing PAQs has been considered poor to moderate and it has been suggested that most PAQs may be valid for ranking individuals' behavior rather than quantifying physical activity. In this analysis we used Z-scores of time spent on physical activity and sedentary behaviors, capturing ranking rather than absolute magnitude. Time spent in physical activities was used to describe cluster characteristics.

In addition, we used factor analysis to identify DPs based on food consumption information collected by three-day food records and one 24-h recall, considering food groups to further collapse dietary intake data and avoid missing data from non-consumers of episodically consumed foods. This procedure has been used by other authors [37], although Food Frequency Questionnaires (FFQ) data has often been used as input source to identify dietary patterns. Similar DPs have been identified in adolescents using food records or FFQ as input data [42]. It has been argued whether food consumption data should be energy adjusted for such analysis. Smith *et al.* [53] did not find obvious differences between the patterns derived by principal component analysis on three-day diet diary data in children using percentage energy or adjusting weight for total energy intake compared to those derived using gram weights.

Finally, both factor analysis and cluster analysis are procedures commonly used to identify DPs and analyze clustering of lifestyles. These procedures rely on several subjective decisions that may influence outcomes regarding the number and type of patterns and clusters identified.

5. Conclusions

Four dietary patterns were identified, one closer to the traditional Mediterranean diet. Cluster analysis classified Spanish children and adolescents in two different groups. A *low physical activity-poorer diet* lifestyle pattern (Unhealthier lifestyle pattern), and *a high physical activity, low sedentary behavior, longer sleep duration, healthier diet* lifestyle pattern (Healthier lifestyle pattern). The prevalence odds ratio for overweight and obesity was not significantly different in children or adolescents allocated into the different clusters, although the ORs for the *low physical activity-poorer diet* lifestyle pattern were >1 in children and in adolescents. Prospective research using larger samples is needed to further examine how lifestyle patterns of energy balance-related behaviors track over time and influence the development of overweight and obesity. These behavior patterns are helpful to identify specific issues and suggest potential intervention strategies.

Supplementary Materials: Supplementary materials can be accessed at: http://www.mdpi.com/2072-6643/8/1/0011/s1.

Acknowledgments: The authors would like to thank Coca-Cola Iberia for its support and technical advice, particularly Rafael Urrialde and Isabel de Julián.

Author Contributions: Carmen Pérez-Rodrigo analyzed the data and drafted the manuscript. Javier Aranceta-Bartrina contributed to the analysis and wrote the manuscript. This author is a member of the Scientific Advisory Board of the ANIBES study and, together with the other members, was responsible for careful review of the protocol, design, and methodology. This author provided continuous scientific advice for the study and for the interpretation of results. Ángel Gil, Marcela González-Gross, RosaM.Ortega., and Lluis Serra-Majem are members of the Scientific Advisory Board of the ANIBES study, and were responsible for careful review of the protocol, design, and methodology. These authors provided continuous scientific advice for the study and for the interpretation of results. These authors also critically reviewed the manuscript. Gregorio Varela-Moreiras, Principal Investigator of the ANIBES study, was responsible for the design, protocol, methodology, and follow-up checks of the study. All authors approved the final version of the manuscript.

Conflicts of Interest: The ANIBES study was financially supported by a grant from Coca-Cola Iberia through an agreement with the Spanish Nutrition Foundation (FEN). The funding sponsor had no role in the design of the study, the collection, analysis, or interpretation of the data, writing of the manuscript, or in the decision to publish the results. The authors declare no conflict of interest.

References

1. Jackson-Leach, R.; Lobstein, T. Estimated burden of paediatric obesity and co-morbidities in Europe. Part 1. The increase in the prevalence of child obesity in Europe is itself increasing. *Int. J. Pediatr. Obes.* **2006**, *1*, 26–32. [CrossRef] [PubMed]

2. Organisation for Economic Co-Operation and Development. OECD Health Statistics 2014. Obesity Update. Available online: http://www.oecd.org/els/health-systems/Obesity-Update-2014.pdf (accessed on 10 June 2015).

3. Kremers, S.P. Theory and practice in the study of influences on energy balance-related behaviors. *Patient Educ. Couns.* **2010**, *79*, 291–298. [CrossRef] [PubMed]

4. Brug, J.; Lien, N.; Klepp, K.I.; van Lenthe, F.J. Exploring overweight, obesity and their behavioural correlates among children and adolescents: Results from the Health-promotion through Obesity Prevention across Europe project. *Public Health Nutr.* **2010**, *13*, 1676–1679. [CrossRef] [PubMed]

5. Pate, R.R.; O'Neill, J.R.; Liese, A.D.; Janz, K.F.; Granberg, E.M.; Colabianchi, N.; Harsha, D.W.; Condrasky, M.M.; O'Neil, P.M.; Lau, E.Y.; *et al.* Factors associated with development of excessive fatness in children and adolescents: A review of prospective studies. *Obes. Rev.* **2013**, *14*, 645–658. [CrossRef] [PubMed]

6. Chen, X.; Beydoun, M.A.; Wang, Y. Is sleep duration associated with childhood obesity? A systematic review and meta-analysis. *Obesity* **2008**, *16*, 265–274. [CrossRef] [PubMed]

7. Smith, A.D.; Emmett, P.M.; Newby, P.K.; Northstone, K. Dietary patterns and changes in body composition in children between 9 and 11 years. *Food Nutr. Res.* **2014**, *58*. [CrossRef] [PubMed]

8. Appannah, G.; Pot, G.K.; Huang, R.C.; Oddy, W.H.; Beilin, L.J.; Mori, T.A.; Jebb, S.A.; Ambrosini, G.L. Identification of a dietary pattern associated with greater cardiometabolic risk in adolescence. *Nutr. Metab. Cardiovasc. Dis.* **2015**, *25*, 643–650. [CrossRef] [PubMed]

9. Ambrosini, G. Childhood dietary patterns and later obesity: A review of the evidence. *Proc. Nutr. Soc.* **2014**, *73*, 137–146. [CrossRef] [PubMed]

10. Gubbels, J.S.; van Assema, P.; Kremers, S.P.J. Physical Activity, Sedentary Behavior, and Dietary Patterns among Children. *Curr. Nutr. Rep.* **2013**, *2*, 105–112. [CrossRef] [PubMed]

11. Mikkilä, V.; Räsänen, L.; Raitakari, O.T.; Pietinen, P.; Viikari, J. Consistent dietary patterns identified from childhood to adulthood: The cardiovascular risk in Young Finns Study. *Br. J. Nutr.* **2005**, *93*, 923–931. [CrossRef] [PubMed]

12. Shin, K.O.; Oh, S.Y.; Park, H.S. Empirically derived major dietary patterns and their associations with overweight in Korean preschool children. *Br. J. Nutr.* **2007**, *98*, 416–421. [CrossRef] [PubMed]

13. Lioret, S.; Touvier, M.; Lafay, L.; Volatier, J.L.; Maire, B. Dietary and physical activity patterns in French children are related to overweight and socioeconomic status. *J. Nutr.* **2008**, *138*, 101–107. [PubMed]

14. Craig, L.C.; McNeill, G.; Macdiarmid, J.I.; Masson, L.F.; Holmes, B.A. Dietary patterns of school-age children in Scotland: Association with socio-economic indicators, physical activity and obesity. *Br. J. Nutr.* **2010**, *103*, 319–334. [CrossRef] [PubMed]
15. Ritchie, L.D.; Spector, P.; Stevens, M.J.; Schmidt, M.M.; Schreiber, G.B.; Striegel-Moore, R.H.; Wang, M.C.; Crawford, P.B. Dietary patterns in adolescence are related to adiposity in young adulthood in black and white females. *J. Nutr.* **2007**, *137*, 399–406. [PubMed]
16. McNaughton, S.A.; Ball, K.; Mishra, G.D.; Crawford, D.A. Dietary patterns of adolescents and risk of obesity and hypertension. *J. Nutr.* **2008**, *138*, 364–370. [PubMed]
17. Aranceta, J.; Perez-Rodrigo, C.; Ribas, L.; Serra-Majem, L. Sociodemographic and lifestyle determinants of food patterns in Spanish children and adolescents: The enKid study. *Eur. J. Clin. Nutr.* **2003**, *57*, S40–S44. [CrossRef] [PubMed]
18. Leech, R.M.; McNaughton, S.A.; Timperio, A. The clustering of diet, physical activity and sedentary behavior in children and adolescents: A review. *Int. J. Behav. Nutr. Phys. Act.* **2014**, *11*, 4. [CrossRef] [PubMed]
19. Pronk, N.P.; Anderson, L.H.; Crain, A.L.; Martinson, B.C.; O'Connor, P.J.; Sherwood, N.E.; Whitebird, R.R. Meeting recommendations for multiple healthy lifestyle factors. Prevalence, clustering, and predictors among adolescent, adult, and senior health plan members. *Am. J. Prev. Med.* **2004**, *27*, 25–33. [CrossRef] [PubMed]
20. Boone-Heinonen, J.; Gordon-Larsen, P.; Adair, L.S. Obesogenic clusters: Multidimensional adolescent obesity-related behaviors in the U.S. *Ann. Behav. Med.* **2008**, *36*, 217–230. [CrossRef] [PubMed]
21. Huh, J.; Riggs, N.R.; Spruijt-Metz, D.; Chou, C.P.; Huang, Z.; Pentz, M. Identifying patterns of eating and physical activity in children: A latent class analysis of obesity risk. *Obesity* **2011**, *19*, 652–658. [CrossRef] [PubMed]
22. Cameron, A.J.; Crawford, D.A.; Salmon, J.; Campbell, K.; McNaughton, S.A.; Mishra, G.D.; Ball, K. Clustering of obesity-related risk behaviors in children and their mothers. *Ann. Epidemiol.* **2011**, *21*, 95–102. [CrossRef] [PubMed]
23. Gubbels, J.S.; Kremers, S.P.; Stafleu, A.; Goldbohm, R.A.; de Vries, N.K.; Thijs, C. Clustering of energy balance-related behaviors in 5-year-old children: Lifestyle patterns and their longitudinal association with weight status development in early childhood. *Int. J. Behav. Nutr. Phys. Act.* **2012**, *9*, 77. [CrossRef] [PubMed]
24. Prochaska, J.J.; Prochaska, J.O. A Review of Multiple Health Behavior Change Interventions for Primary Prevention. *Am. J. Lifestyle Med.* **2011**, *5*. [CrossRef] [PubMed]
25. Ruiz, E.; Ávila, J.M.; Castillo, A.; Valero, T.; del Pozo, S.; Rodriguez, P.; Aranceta Bartrina, J.; Gil, A.; González-Gross, M.; Ortega, R.M.; et al. The ANIBES Study on Energy Balance in Spain: Design, protocol and methodology. *Nutrients* **2015**, *7*, 970–998. [CrossRef] [PubMed]
26. Ruiz, E.; Ávila, J.M.; Valero, T.; del Pozo, S.; Rodriguez, P.; Aranceta-Bartrina, J.; Gil, A.; González-Gross, M.; Ortega, R.M.; Serra-Majem, L.; et al. Energy Intake, Profile, and Dietary Sources in the Spanish Population: Findings of the ANIBES Study. *Nutrients* **2015**, *7*, 4739–4762. [CrossRef] [PubMed]
27. Moreiras, O.; Carbajal, A.; Cabrera, L.; Cuadrado, C. *Tablas de Composición de Alimentos*, 15th ed.; Pirámide: Madrid, Spain, 2011.
28. Hagströmer, M.; Bergman, P.; de Bourdeaudhuij, I.; Ortega, F.B.; Ruiz, J.R.; Manios, Y.; Rey-López, J.P.; Phillipp, K.; von Berlepsch, J.; Sjöström, M.; et al. Concurrent validity of a modified version of the International Physical Activity Questionnaire (IPAQ-A) in European adolescents: The HELENA Study. *Int. J. Obes.* **2008**, *32*, S42–S48. [CrossRef] [PubMed]
29. IPAQ. Guidelines for Data Processing and Analysis of the International Physical Activity Questionnaire (IPAQ)—Short and Long Forms, November 2005. Available online: https://sites.google.com/site/theipaq/scoring-protocol (accessed on 27 October 2015).
30. Bauman, A.; Ainsworth, B.E.; Bull, F.; Craig, C.L.; Hagströmer, M.; Sallis, J.F.; Pratt, M.; Sjöström, M. Progress and Pitfalls in the Use of the International Physical Activity Questionnaire (IPAQ) for Adult Physical Activity Surveillance. *J. Phys. Act. Health* **2009**, *6* (Suppl. 1), S5–S8. [PubMed]
31. Hense, S.; Pohlabeln, H.; de Henauw, S.; Eiben, G.; Molnar, D.; Moreno, L.A.; Barba, G.; Hadjigeorgiou, C.; Veidebaum, T.; Ahrens, W. Sleep duration and overweight in European children: Is the association modified by geographic region? *Sleep* **2011**, *34*, 885–890. [CrossRef] [PubMed]

32. Fernández-Alvira, J.M.; de Bourdeaudhuij, I.; Singh, A.S.; Vik, F.N.; Manios, Y.; Kovacs, E.; Jan, N.; Brug, J.; Moreno, L.A. Clustering of energy balance-related behaviors and parental education in European children: The ENERGY-project. *Int. J. Behav. Nutr. Phys. Act.* **2013**, *10*, 5. [CrossRef] [PubMed]

33. Marfell-Jones, M.; Olds, T.; Stewart, A.; Carter, L. *International Standards for Anthropometric Assessment*; International Society for the Advancement of Kinanthropometry: Potchefstroom, South Africa, 2006; pp. 1–137.

34. Cole, T.J.; Bellizzi, M.C.; Flegal, K.M.; Dietz, W.H. Establishing a standard definition for child overweight and obesity worldwide: International survey. *BMJ* **2000**, *320*, 1240–1243. [CrossRef] [PubMed]

35. Newby, P.K.; Tucker, K.L. Empirically derived eating patterns using factor or cluster analysis: A review. *Nutr. Rev.* **2004**, *62*, 177–203. [CrossRef] [PubMed]

36. Everitt, B.S.; Landau, S.; Leese, M.; Stahl, D. *Cluster Analysis*, 5th ed.; John Wiley & Sons, Ltd.: West Sussex, UK, 2011.

37. Shang, X.; Li, Y.; Liu, A.; Zhang, Q.; Hu, X.; Du, S.; Ma, J.; Xu, G.; Li, Y.; Guo, H.; *et al.* Dietary pattern and its association with the prevalence of obesity and related cardiometabolic risk factors among Chinese children. *PLoS ONE* **2012**, *7*, e43183. [CrossRef] [PubMed]

38. Diethelm, K.; Günther, A.L.; Schulze, M.B.; Standl, M.; Heinrich, J.; Buyken, A.E. Prospective relevance of dietary patterns at the beginning and during the course of primary school to the development of body composition. *Br. J. Nutr.* **2014**, *111*, 1488–1498. [CrossRef] [PubMed]

39. Gubbels, J.; Kremers, S.; Goldbohm, A.; Stafleu, A.; Thijs, C. Energy balance-related behavioral patterns in 5-year-old children and the longitudinal association with weight status development in early childhood. *Public Health Nutr.* **2012**, *15*, 1402–1410. [CrossRef] [PubMed]

40. Ambrosini, G.L.; Emmett, P.M.; Northstone, K.; Howe, L.D.; Tilling, K.; Jebb, S.A. Identification of a dietary pattern prospectively associated with increased adiposity during childhood and adolescence. *Int. J. Obes.* **2012**, *36*, 1299–1305. [CrossRef] [PubMed]

41. Van der Sluis, M.E.; Lien, N.; Twisk, J.W.; Steenhuis, I.H.; Bere, E.; Klepp, K.I.; Wind, M. Longitudinal associations of energy balance-related behaviours and cross-sectional associations of clusters and body mass index in Norwegian adolescents. *Public Health Nutr.* **2011**, *13*, 1716–1721. [CrossRef] [PubMed]

42. Appannah, G.; Pot, G.K.; O'Sullivan, T.A.; Oddy, W.H.; Jebb, S.A.; Ambrosini, G.L. The reliability of an adolescent dietary pattern identified using reduced-rank regression: Comparison of a FFQ and 3 d food record. *Br. J. Nutr.* **2014**, *112*, 609–615. [CrossRef] [PubMed]

43. Yannakoulia, M.; Ntalla, I.; Papoutsakis, C.; Farmaki, A.E.; Dedoussis, G.V. Consumption of vegetables, cooked meals, and eating dinner is negatively associated with overweight status in children. *J. Pediatr.* **2011**, *157*, 815–820. [CrossRef] [PubMed]

44. Sabbe, D.; de Bourdeaudhuij, I.; Legiest, E.; Maes, L. A cluster analytical approach towards physical activity and eating habits among 10-year-old children. *Health Educ. Res.* **2008**, *23*, 753–762. [CrossRef] [PubMed]

45. Ottevaere, C.; Huybrechts, I.; Benser, J.; de Bourdeaudhuij, I.; Cuenca-Garcia, M.; Dallongeville, J.; Zaccaria, M.; Gottrand, F.; Kersting, M.; Rey-López, J.P.; *et al.* Clustering patterns of physical activity, sedentary and dietary behavior among European adolescents: The HELENA study. *BMC Public Health* **2011**, *11*, 328. [CrossRef] [PubMed]

46. Te Velde, S.J.; de Bourdeaudhuij, I.; Thorsdottir, I.; Rasmussen, M.; Hagstromer, M.; Klepp, K.I.; Brug, J. Patterns in sedentary and exercise behaviors and associations with overweight in 9–14-year-old boys and girls—A cross-sectional study. *BMC Public Health* **2007**, *7*, 16. [CrossRef] [PubMed]

47. Seghers, J.; Rutten, C. Clustering of multiple lifestyle behaviours and its relationship with weight status and cardiorespiratory fitness in a sample of Flemish 11- to 12-year-olds. *Public Health Nutr.* **2010**, *13*, 1838–1846. [CrossRef] [PubMed]

48. Marshall, S.J.; Biddle, S.J.H.; Sallis, J.F.; McKenzie, T.L.; Conway, T.L. Clustering of sedentary behaviors and physical activity among youth: A cross-national study. *Pediatr. Exerc. Sci.* **2002**, *14*, 401–417.

49. Aranceta-Bartrina, J.; Pérez-Rodrigo, C.; Santolaya-Jiménez, J.; Juan Gondra Rezola y Grupo Colaborativo Para el Estudio Perseo en Bilbao. El Proyecto PERSEO en Bilbao: Evaluación preliminar. *Rev. Esp. Nutr. Comunitaria* **2013**, *19*, 88–97.

50. Kautiainen, S.; Koivusilta, L.; Lintonen, T.; Virtanen, S.M.; Rimpela, A. Use of information and communication technology and prevalence of overweight and obesity among adolescents. *Int. J. Obes.* **2005**, *29*, 925–933. [CrossRef] [PubMed]
51. Jago, R.; Anderson, C.B.; Baranowski, T.; Watson, K. Adolescent patterns of physical activity: Differences by gender, day, and time of day. *Am. J. Prev. Med.* **2005**, *28*, 447–452. [CrossRef] [PubMed]
52. Spengler, S.; Mess, F.; Schmocker, E.; Woll, A. Longitudinal associations of health-related behavior patterns in adolescence with change of weight status and self-rated health over a period of 6 years: Results of the MoMo longitudinal study. *BMC Pediatr.* **2014**, *14*, 242. [CrossRef] [PubMed]
53. Smith, A.; Emmett, P.; Newby, P.K.; Northstone, K. Dietary patterns obtained through principal components analysis: The effect of input variable quantification. *Br. J. Nutr.* **2013**, *109*, 1881–1891. [CrossRef] [PubMed]

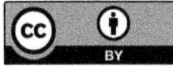

nutrients

MDPI

Article

A *Priori* and *a Posteriori* Dietary Patterns during Pregnancy and Gestational Weight Gain: The Generation R Study

Myrte J. Tielemans [1,2,*], Nicole S. Erler [1,3], Elisabeth T. M. Leermakers [1,2], Marion van den Broek [1], Vincent W. V. Jaddoe [1,2,4], Eric A. P. Steegers [5], Jessica C. Kiefte-de Jong [1,6] and Oscar H. Franco [1]

[1] Department of Epidemiology, Erasmus MC, University Medical Center Rotterdam, P.O. Box 2040, 3000 CA Rotterdam, The Netherlands; n.erler@erasmusmc.nl (N.S.E.); e.leermakers@erasmusmc.nl (E.T.M.L.); marion.vdbroek90@gmail.com (M.V.D.B.); v.jaddoe@erasmusmc.nl (V.W.V.J.); j.c.kiefte-dejong@erasmusmc.nl (J.C.K.-D.J.); o.franco@erasmusmc.nl (O.H.F.)

[2] The Generation R Study Group, Erasmus MC, University Medical Center Rotterdam, P.O. Box 2040, 3000 CA Rotterdam, The Netherlands

[3] Department of Biostatistics, Erasmus MC, University Medical Center Rotterdam, P.O. Box 2040, 3000 CA Rotterdam, The Netherlands

[4] Department of Pediatrics, Erasmus MC, University Medical Center Rotterdam, P.O. Box 2040, 3000 CA Rotterdam, The Netherlands

[5] Department of Obstetrics and Gynecology, Erasmus MC, University Medical Center Rotterdam, P.O. Box 2040, 3000 CA Rotterdam, The Netherlands; e.a.p.steegers@erasmusmc.nl

[6] Department of Global Public Health, Leiden University College the Hague, P.O. Box 13228, 2501 EE the Hague, The Netherlands

* Correspondence: m.tielemans@erasmusmc.nl; Tel.: +31-10-7043351; Fax: +31-10-7044657

Received: 27 August 2015 ; Accepted: 4 November 2015 ; Published: 12 November 2015

Abstract: Abnormal gestational weight gain (GWG) is associated with adverse pregnancy outcomes. We examined whether dietary patterns are associated with GWG. Participants included 3374 pregnant women from a population-based cohort in the Netherlands. Dietary intake during pregnancy was assessed with food-frequency questionnaires. Three *a posteriori*-derived dietary patterns were identified using principal component analysis: a "Vegetable, oil and fish", a "Nuts, high-fiber cereals and soy", and a "Margarine, sugar and snacks" pattern. The *a priori*-defined dietary pattern was based on national dietary recommendations. Weight was repeatedly measured around 13, 20 and 30 weeks of pregnancy; pre-pregnancy and maximum weight were self-reported. Normal weight women with high adherence to the "Vegetable, oil and fish" pattern had higher early-pregnancy GWG than those with low adherence (43 g/week (95% CI 16; 69) for highest *vs.* lowest quartile (Q)). Adherence to the "Margarine, sugar and snacks" pattern was associated with a higher prevalence of excessive GWG (OR 1.45 (95% CI 1.06; 1.99) Q4 *vs.* Q1). Normal weight women with higher scores on the "Nuts, high-fiber cereals and soy" pattern had more moderate GWG than women with lower scores (−0.01 (95% CI −0.02; −0.00) per SD). The *a priori*-defined pattern was not associated with GWG. To conclude, specific dietary patterns may play a role in early pregnancy but are not consistently associated with GWG.

Keywords: pregnancy; gestational weight gain; dietary pattern; maternal diet; cohort

1. Introduction

Abnormal maternal weight gain during pregnancy (*i.e.*, too little or too much) has been associated with unfavorable pregnancy outcomes in both mother and child. Insufficient gestational weight gain

(GWG) is associated with both preterm birth and low birthweight [1], and excessive GWG increases the risk of giving birth to large-for-gestational-age infants [2]. Excessive GWG is also associated with maternal pregnancy complications, including hypertensive disorders [3,4] and gestational diabetes [5], which can increase the risk of the mother developing cardiometabolic diseases after pregnancy [6,7].

Energy intake during pregnancy is associated with GWG [4,8], but literature is scarce on whether GWG could be influenced by dietary composition. Some studies have examined the influence of food groups on GWG [9–11]. These studies found no association of fruit or vegetable intake with GWG [9,11] but unhealthier foods (e.g., sweets and processed foods) were associated with higher prevalence of excessive GWG [9–11]. Weight gain during pregnancy involves both maternal components (e.g., blood volume increase, fat accretion) and fetal components (e.g., weight of the fetus, amniotic fluid) [12]. Therefore, the effect of diet on weight gain may differ between pregnant and non-pregnant women.

Assessing overall diet in relation to GWG has several advantages over studying individual foods or nutrients. First, the intakes of different nutrients are often highly correlated, which complicates the assessment of individual nutrients [13]. Second, possible associations between nutrient intake and GWG might be affected by biological interactions between nutrients [13]. For these reasons, evaluating diet using a dietary pattern approach may improve our understanding of which dietary pattern is most beneficial during pregnancy. Also, this approach can facilitate future food-based dietary guidelines [14].

Only a few studies have focused on the relationship between dietary patterns and GWG [15–18]. However, no study evaluated dietary patterns and longitudinal development of weight during pregnancy. We hypothesized that specific dietary patterns may influence the development of maternal weight during pregnancy. In addition, dietary patterns are likely to differ between countries and populations [13], so it is important to identify country-specific dietary patterns that may be associated with GWG.

Hence, the purpose of our study was to determine whether *a posteriori*-derived and *a priori*-defined dietary patterns are associated with GWG during different phases in pregnancy, adequacy of GWG and weight development during pregnancy in Dutch women participating in a population-based cohort.

2. Experimental Section

2.1. Study Design

This study was embedded in the Generation R Study, a population-based prospective cohort from fetal life onwards in Rotterdam (The Netherlands). Details of this study have been described previously [19]. Briefly, pregnant women with an expected delivery date between April 2002 and January 2006, living in the urban area around Rotterdam were approached to participate. All participants provided written informed consent. The study was conducted according to the World Medical Association Declaration of Helsinki and was approved by the Medical Ethics Committee, Erasmus Medical Center Rotterdam (The Netherlands, MEC 198.782.2001.31).

2.2. Population of Analysis

For the current analysis, we included women of Dutch ancestry who entered the Generation R Study during pregnancy ($n = 4097$). We did not include women of non-Dutch ancestry because the dietary assessment method that we used was designed to evaluate a Dutch diet. We excluded women with missing dietary information ($n = 538$) and restricted our analysis to women with singleton live births ($n = 3479$). We excluded 5 women whose weight was not measured during pregnancy. Finally, we excluded women who were underweight before pregnancy (body mass index (BMI) $< 18.5 \text{ kg/m}^2$; $n = 100$), leaving 3374 women for the current analysis (Figure 1).

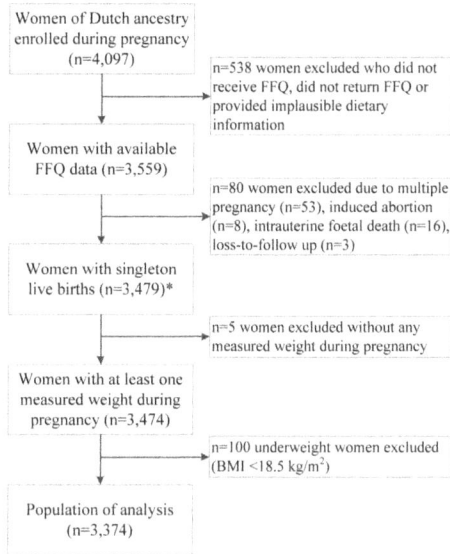

Figure 1. Flow chart of the study population: the Generation R Study (2002–2006). * Population in which the *a posteriori*-derived dietary patterns were determined. Abbreviations: BMI: body mass index; FFQ: food-frequency questionnaire.

2.3. Dietary Assessment

Dietary intake in early pregnancy was assessed at enrolment (median 13.4 weeks of gestation (Inter Quartile Range (IQR) 12.2–15.5)) using a 293-item semi-quantitative food-frequency questionnaire (FFQ) that covered dietary intake over the previous three months. The FFQ contained questions regarding foods that are frequently consumed in a traditionally Dutch diet, their consumption frequency, portion size [20], preparation methods, and additions to foods. The average daily intake of energy and nutrients was calculated using the Dutch food-composition table (2006) [21]. The FFQ was designed for and validated in an elderly population [22], and has additionally been validated against three 24-h dietary recalls in 71 Dutch pregnant women who visited a midwifery in Rotterdam. The intra-class correlation coefficients for energy-adjusted macronutrients ranged between 0.48 and 0.68.

2.3.1. A Posteriori-Derived Dietary Patterns

We used principal component analysis (PCA) with Varimax rotation to identify *a posteriori*-derived dietary patterns [13,23]. Our dietary patterns have been described in detail previously [24]. Briefly, the 293 individual food items from the FFQ were aggregated into 23 food groups (Table S1). Subsequently, we extracted those factors (*i.e.*, dietary patterns) of the PCA that had an Eigenvalue of ⩾1.5 [25]. The factor loadings, which described how strong the association between the food groups and each of the extracted patterns is, are presented in Table 1. Finally, we determined factor scores (*i.e.*, adherence scores) for each participant and each pattern, by calculating the individual sum of the intake of the food groups, weighted with their factor loadings and standardizing those weighted sums to have mean zero and standard deviation one (standard deviation score). A higher factor score indicated that a woman's diet was closer to that dietary pattern.

Three *a posteriori*-derived dietary patterns were identified, namely a "Vegetable, oil and fish" pattern, a "Nuts, high-fiber cereals and soy" pattern and a "Margarine, sugar and snacks" pattern, together explaining 25.8% of the variance in maternal dietary intake (Table 1).

Table 1. Factor loadings food groups in *a posteriori*-derived dietary patterns [1].

Food Group	"Vegetable, Oil and Fish" Dietary Pattern	"Nuts, High-Fiber Cereals and Soy" Dietary Pattern	"Margarine, Sugar and Snacks" Dietary Pattern
Potatoes and other tubers	0.05	−0.53	0.21
Vegetables	0.78 *	0.17	−0.03
Fruits	0.13	0.37	0.02
Dairy products—high fat	0.26	−0.26	0.29
Dairy products—low fat	−0.15	0.29	0.16
Cereals—high fiber	0.24	0.43 *	0.36
Cereals—low fiber	0.23	−0.16	0.25
Meat and meat products	0.08	−0.54	0.33
Fish and shellfish	0.45 *	0.24	−0.11
Eggs and egg products	0.27	0.05	0.19
Vegetable oils	0.74 *	0.08	−0.12
Margarine and butter	−0.06	−0.03	0.61 *
Sugar and confectionary and cakes	−0.11	0.13	0.56 *
Snacks	0.05	0.08	0.40 *
Coffee and tea	0.28	0.34	0.10
Sugar-containing beverages	−0.14	−0.28	0.29
Light soft drinks	0.13	0.28	0.02
Alcoholic beverages	0.35	−0.00	−0.04
Condiments and sauces	0.05	−0.09	0.39
Soups and bouillon	0.19	−0.02	0.15
Nuts, seeds and olives	0.03	0.64 *	0.30
Soy products	0.01	0.39 *	−0.10
Legumes	0.44	−0.02	0.07

[1] Reprinted with permission from van den Broek *et al.* [24]. The food groups that are considered to have a strong association with a dietary pattern (factor loading ⩾0.2 or ⩽−0.2) are shown in bold. The three factor loadings with the highest positive factor loading are used to name the dietary pattern and are presented with an asterisk (*). The three dietary patterns together explained 25.8% of the total variance in maternal dietary intake.

2.3.2. A Priori-Defined Dietary Pattern

The *a priori*-defined dietary pattern was based on the Dutch Healthy Diet Index [26]. This index was developed to measure adherence to the Dutch guidelines for a healthy diet [27] and consisted of ten components: physical activity, vegetable, fruit, dietary fiber, fish, saturated fatty acids, trans-fatty acids, consumption of acidic drinks and foods, sodium, and alcohol. We omitted the components physical activity, trans-fatty acids, and the consumption of acidic drinks and foods because this information had not been collected. Furthermore, we did not include the alcohol component because alcohol abstinence is recommended during pregnancy. The score of each component ranged between 0 and 10 points, resulting in a total score ranging from 0 to 60 points (Table S2). A higher score on the Dutch Healthy Diet Index corresponds with a higher adherence to the 2006 Dutch healthy diet guidelines and thus reflects a healthier diet. Finally, to facilitate comparison between all dietary patterns, we standardized the "Dutch Healthy Diet Index" pattern to a standard deviation score.

2.4. Maternal Weight Gain

Information on pre-pregnancy weight was collected at enrollment using a questionnaire and was used to calculate a pre-pregnancy BMI (kg/m^2). Women visited our research center three times at median (IQR) gestational ages of 12.9 (12.1–14.4) weeks (*first visit*), 20.4 (19.9–21.1) weeks (*second visit*), and 30.2 (29.9–30.8) weeks (*third visit*). During each visit, maternal height and weight were measured without shoes and heavy clothing. Six weeks after childbirth, women were asked to report their highest weight during pregnancy using a questionnaire, which we used as maximum weight in pregnancy.

Pre-pregnancy weight was highly correlated with weight measured during *the first visit* ($R = 0.96$, *p*-value < 0.001, *n* = 2425), and there was no indication for systematic measurement error (Figure S1).

Also, a high correlation was found between weight during *the third visit* and maximum weight in pregnancy ($R = 0.89$, *p*-value < 0.001, $n = 2177$) without an indication for systematic measurement error (Figure S1). To evaluate long-term maternal weight gain, we measured maternal weight at our research center six years after childbirth.

2.4.1. Gestational Weight Gain during Different Phases in Pregnancy

GWG in different phases of pregnancy was calculated for three consecutive periods, namely early-pregnancy GWG (calculated as weight at *the first visit* minus pre-pregnancy weight, divided by follow-up duration (g/week), $n = 2425$), mid-pregnancy GWG (calculated as weight at *the second visit* minus weight *the first visit*, divided by follow-up duration (g/week), $n = 2748$), and late-pregnancy GWG (calculated as weight at *the third visit* minus weight at *the second visit*, divided by follow-up duration (g/week), $n = 3158$). GWG until early-third trimester was calculated as weight at *the third visit* minus pre-pregnancy weight, divided by follow up duration (g/week, $n = 2815$).

2.4.2. Adequacy of Gestational Weight Gain

Women's total GWG (calculated as maximum weight in pregnancy minus pre-pregnancy weight, $n = 1917$) was used to classify their GWG into inadequate, adequate, or excessive GWG. Cut-off values of GWG adequacy were based on recommendations published by the US Institute of Medicine (2009) and were BMI-specific [28]. Normal weight women (BMI 18.5–24.9 kg/m^2) were categorized as having an adequate GWG with a GWG between 11.5 and 16 kg, overweight women (BMI 25–29.9 kg/m^2) were classified as adequate GWG with GWG between 7 and 11.5 kg, and adequate GWG for obese women (BMI $\geqslant$ 30 kg/m^2) was between 5 and 9 kg.

2.5. Covariates

Several maternal sociodemographic and lifestyle characteristics were considered as potential confounders. We obtained information from prenatal questionnaires that were sent in different trimesters regarding maternal age, educational level [29], household income ($\leqslant$2200 *vs.* >2200 Euro/month), parity (no child *vs.* $\geqslant$1 child), pre-pregnancy weight, pre-existing comorbidities, vomiting, smoking or alcohol consumption (both categorized as never during pregnancy, stopped when pregnancy was known, or continued throughout pregnancy), folic acid supplementation (started periconceptionally, started first 10 weeks, or no supplementation), energy intake, and stress during pregnancy (using the Global Severity Index [30]). To calculate pre-pregnancy BMI, height was measured at enrollment. Gestational age was determined based on ultrasound examination, and during *the third visit* an ultrasound was performed to estimate fetal weight. Information on fetal sex was obtained from delivery reports.

2.6. Statistical Analyses

We considered two sets of possible confounders in the analysis. *Model 1* was adjusted for median gestational age at follow-up and pre-pregnancy BMI. *Model 2* was further adjusted for age, educational level, household income, parity, smoking during pregnancy, alcohol consumption during pregnancy, stress during pregnancy, and fetal sex. The selection of potential confounders was based on factors found in the literature and on a change of at least 10% in effect estimate in a preliminary analysis assessing the association of dietary patterns with GWG until early-third trimester. As GWG is related to BMI [28] and the preliminary analysis showed significant interaction terms for the "Vegetable, oil and fish" pattern (*p*-value < 0.01) and the "Nuts, high-fiber cereals and soy" pattern (*p*-value $= 0.01$) with pre-pregnancy BMI, we stratified all analyses on the basis of weight status (normal weight (BMI < 25 kg/m^2) and overweight (BMI $\geqslant$ 25 kg/m^2)).

In order to adequately estimate the relationship between diet and trajectories of gestational weight in the presence of incomplete covariates, we performed a longitudinal analysis using linear mixed modelling in the Bayesian framework. This method has been described in detail previously [31]. Briefly, by modelling the joint distribution of exposure, outcome and covariates, all available information is used to impute the missing values and estimate the parameters of interest simultaneously.

In the Bayesian linear mixed model, all main effects from *Model 2*, interaction terms between the dietary pattern variables (as derived by PCA) and a linear and quadratic effect for gestational age were included in the fixed effects structure. The correlation between the weight measurements within an individual was modelled by including random effects for the intercept and slope (for gestational age) into the model. No additional correlation structure was assumed for the error terms. For this analysis, the reported parameter estimates and 95% credible intervals were obtained by taking the mean and 2.5% and 97.5% quantiles of the posterior sample of the respective parameters.

To analyze the association of the *a priori*-defined and *a posteriori*-derived dietary patterns with GWG during different phases in pregnancy, GWG until early third trimester and maximal GWG, we performed multivariable linear regression analysis. Missing covariate values were multiply imputed by randomly drawing ten values from the posterior samples of each incomplete covariate derived in the Bayesian analysis. Missing observations of gestational weight were not imputed. The reported results from the cross-sectional models were pooled over all ten completed datasets. Separate models were fitted with the dietary patterns discretized in quartiles, with the lowest quartile (quartile 1) as a reference category, as well as continuously per SD score. Quartiles were constructed separately for normal weight and overweight women; each of these analyses was done for *Model 1* and *Model 2*. To identify cases that have an influence on the regression models we calculated Cook's distance [32].

Because GWG is a physiological process in pregnancy and resulting in weight gain in almost all women during pregnancy [28], we also evaluated the associations between dietary patterns and GWG adequacy (inadequate, adequate *vs.* excessive GWG) using multinomial regression models. We included all covariates from *Model 2* and used "adequate GWG" as a reference category.

Sensitivity Analyses

To test the stability of our results, we performed four sensitivity analyses in *Model 2* for the association between dietary patterns and GWG until early-third trimester. First, because energy intake may be an intermediate factor in the association of maternal diet with GWG, we further adjusted for energy intake (kcal/day). Second, we further adjusted for estimated fetal weight in the early-third trimester to evaluate whether higher GWG could be explained by greater fetal growth because we previously found that specific dietary patterns may be associated with fetal weight [33]. Third, we excluded women with pre-existing comorbidities ($n = 182$) and women with hypertensive complications in pregnancy [34] or gestational diabetes ($n = 272$) since these conditions may influence both dietary intake and GWG. Fourth, we excluded women who reported vomiting more than once per week during the three months prior to enrolment ($n = 421$), since this might alter dietary intake and GWG. Also, we explored effect modification of the association between dietary patterns and GWG with educational level and household income.

Additionally, we evaluated whether the associations of dietary patterns with GWG would markedly change when using self-reported maximum weight during pregnancy instead of measured weight at *the third visit* ($n = 1917$). Furthermore, we evaluated whether the associations found between the dietary patterns and adequacy of weekly GWG (between *the first* and *the third visit*) were similar to those with adequacy of total GWG ($n = 2745$), because some measurement error was found in the self-reported weights (Figure S1). The cut-off values of adequate weekly GWG were 0.35–0.50 kg/week for normal weight women, 0.23–0.33 kg/week of overweight women, and 0.17–0.27 kg/week for obese women [28]. In addition, we explored long-term maternal weight gain and evaluated whether this long-term weight gain differed in women with inadequate, adequate or excessive GWG using Analysis of Variance (ANOVA). Finally, we calculated the correlation between weight at *the third visit* and weight 6 years after childbirth.

All statistical analyses were performed in SPSS version 21.0 (IBM Corp., Armonk, NY, USA), R version 3.2.1 (R Foundation for Statistical Computing, Vienna, Austria) and JAGS version 3.4.0 [35].

3. Results

3.1. Study Population

Baseline characteristics for normal weight women (*n* = 2544; 75%) and overweight women (*n* = 830; 25%) are presented in Table 2. The mean score ±SD on the Dutch Healthy Diet Index was 32 ± 8 and ranged from 8 to 59. Overall, 43% of women had excessive GWG (*n* = 826); excessive GWG was found in 37% of the normal weight women (*n* = 557) and in 63% of the overweight women (*n* = 269).

We did not identify women with large influence on the effect estimates of the association between dietary patterns and GWG (all Cook's distances were <1).

Table 2. Subject characteristics (*n* = 3374), the Generation R Study (2002–2006) [1].

Subject Characteristics	Normal Weight Women (*n* = 2544)	Overweight Women (*n* = 830)
Age (years)	31.6 ± 4.3	31.0 ± 4.4
Educational level, *n* (%)		
Low and midlow	307 (12.1)	201 (24.2)
Midhigh	1283 (50.4)	436 (52.5)
High	954 (37.5)	193 (23.3)
Household income, *n* (%)		
<2200 Euro/month	620 (24.4)	266 (32.1)
⩾2200 Euro/month	1924 (75.6)	564 (67.9)
Parity, *n* (%)		
0	1554 (61.1)	465 (56.0)
⩾1	990 (38.9)	365 (44.0)
Pre-pregnancy BMI (kg/m^2)	21.6 (20.4–23.0)	27.7 (26.0–30.5)
Smoking during pregnancy, *n* (%)		
Never during pregnancy	1911 (75.1)	612 (73.7)
Until pregnancy was known	233 (9.2)	61 (7.3)
Continued throughout pregnancy	400 (15.7)	157 (19.0)
Alcohol consumption during pregnancy, *n* (%)		
Never during pregnancy	764 (30.0)	359 (43.2)
Until pregnancy was known	416 (16.4)	138 (16.6)
Continued throughout pregnancy	1364 (53.6)	334 (40.2)
Stress during pregnancy (score 0–4)	0.12 (0.06–0.24)	0.13 (0.06–0.26)
Energy intake (kcal/day)	2162 ± 507	2090 ± 514
Dutch Healthy Diet Index (score 0–60)	32 ± 8	30 ± 8
Fetal sex, *n* (%)		
Male	1287 (50.6)	415 (50.0)
Female	1257 (49.4)	415 (50.0)
Gestational weight gain (kg)	14.7 ± 7.3	12.9 ± 7.7
Adequacy of gestational weight gain, *n* (%)		
Inadequate	370 (24.8)	89 (20.9)
Adequate	565 (37.9)	67 (15.8)
Excessive	557 (37.3)	269 (63.3)

[1] Values represent *n* (%) for categorical variables, and for continuous variables they represent mean ± SD or median (interquartile range). Missing data: educational level (1.3%), household income (10.3%), parity (0.2%), pre-pregnancy BMI (14.2%), smoking during pregnancy (7.4%), alcohol consumption during pregnancy (8.1%), stress during pregnancy (12.0%), gestational weight gain (43.2%), adequacy of gestational weight gain (43.2%). No missing data for maternal age, energy intake, Dutch Healthy Diet Index or fetal sex. Numbers may not add up to total due to rounding after imputation.

3.2. Dietary Patterns and Gestational Weight Gain in Different Phases in Pregnancy

Normal weight women in the highest quartile of the "Vegetable, oil and fish" pattern had a 43 g/week (95% CI 16; 69) greater early-pregnancy GWG than women in the lowest quartile, independent of lifestyle and sociodemographic variables. We observed no such association in overweight women (Table 3). The "Nuts, high-fiber cereals and soy" pattern was associated with a lower early-pregnancy GWG in *Model 1* in both normal weight and overweight women. However, after additional adjustment (*Model 2*) this pattern was no longer significantly associated with early-pregnancy GWG. Neither the "Margarine, sugar and snacks" pattern nor the "Dutch Healthy Diet Index" pattern was associated with early-pregnancy GWG.

Table 3. Association of dietary patterns with gestational weight gain in early pregnancy (*n* = 2425) [1].

Quartiles of the Dietary Patterns	Early-Pregnancy Weight Gain (g/Week)			
	Normal Weight Women (*n* = 1849)		Overweight Women (*n* = 576)	
	Model 1	*Model 2*	*Model 1*	*Model 2*
"Vegetable, Oil And Fish" Pattern				
Q1 (low)	Reference	Reference	Reference	Reference
Q2	−8 (−34; 17)	−3 (−28; 23)	18 (−44; 80)	29 (−34; 91)
Q3	−14 (−40; 11)	−4 (−30; 22)	59 (−3; 121)	**77 (14; 141)**
Q4 (high)	**38 (12; 63) ***	**43 (16; 69) ***	4 (−58; 66)	31 (−37; 99)
Per SD	*p* < 0.01 *	*p* < 0.01 *	*p* = 0.63	*p* = 0.24
"Nuts, High-Fiber Cereals and Soy" Pattern				
Q1 (low)	Reference	Reference	Reference	Reference
Q2	−10 (−36; 15)	5 (−21; 30)	−19 (−81; 43)	−17 (−79; 45)
Q3	**−26 (−52; −1)**	−4 (−31; 23)	−54 (−117; 10)	−44 (−109; 21)
Q4 (high)	**−31 (−57; −6)**	−10 (−37; 18)	−64 (−128; 1)	−52 (−120; 15)
Per SD	*p* < 0.01 *	*p* = 0.22	*p* = 0.02	*p* = 0.06
"Margarine, Sugar and Snacks" Pattern				
Q1 (low)	Reference	Reference	Reference	Reference
Q2	3 (−22; 29)	2 (−23; 27)	33 (−28; 94)	28 (−32; 88)
Q3	5 (−21; 30)	−1 (−26; 24)	35 (−29; 98)	41 (−22; 103)
Q4 (high)	20 (−6; 46)	13 (−12; 39)	52 (−9; 114)	45 (−17; 106)
Per SD	*p* = 0.11	*p* = 0.36	*p* = 0.20	*p* = 0.24
"Dutch Healthy Diet Index" Pattern				
Q1 (low)	Reference	Reference	Reference	Reference
Q2	0 (−25; 26)	−2 (−27; 23)	4 (−58; 65)	3 (−58; 64)
Q3	16 (−10; 42)	7 (−19; 32)	48 (−14; 110)	38 (−23; 100)
Q4 (high)	3 (−22; 29)	−14 (−40; 12)	34 (−28; 96)	11 (−54; 75)
Per SD	*p* = 0.86	*p* = 0.17	*p* = 0.32	*p* = 0.86

[1] Results from multivariable linear regression analyses, based on imputed data. Values (regression coefficients with 95%-confidence interval) reflect the difference in early-pregnancy weight gain (g/week) for quartile 2 until 4 relative to quartile 1. *p*-Values correspond to the effect of 1SD increase in dietary pattern score. *Model 1*: adjusted for pre-pregnancy BMI and median gestational age at follow-up. *Model 2*: *Model 1* further adjusted for age, educational level, household income, parity, smoking during pregnancy, alcohol consumption during pregnancy, stress during pregnancy, and fetal sex. *p* For interaction between dietary patterns and pre-pregnancy BMI was <0.10 for the "Vegetable, oil and fish" pattern and for the other patterns >0.10. Significant results are presented in bold (*p*-value < 0.05) and results with a *p*-value < 0.0125 with an asterisk (*). Abbreviations: BMI: body mass index; Q: quartile; SD: standard deviation.

No significant associations were found for any of the dietary patterns with mid-pregnancy GWG in normal weight or overweight women (Table 4). Table 5 shows that in normal weight women, only the "Nuts, high-fiber cereals and soy" pattern was inversely associated with late-pregnancy GWG in *Model 1* (*p*-value for 1SD increase < 0.01), but these results largely attenuated after adjustment for sociodemographic and lifestyle factors (*p*-value = 0.48). In overweight women, none of the dietary patterns were significantly associated with late-pregnancy GWG.

Table 4. Association of dietary patterns with gestational weight gain in mid-pregnancy (*n* = 2748) [1].

Quartiles of the Dietary Patterns	Mid-Pregnancy Weight Gain (g/Week)			
	Normal Weight Women (*n* = 2079)		Overweight Women (*n* = 669)	
	Model 1	*Model 2*	*Model 1*	*Model 2*
"Vegetable, Oil and Fish" Pattern				
Q1 (low)	Reference	Reference	Reference	Reference
Q2	−0 (−39; 38)	6 (−33; 45)	37 (−42; 115)	17 (−64; 97)
Q3	2 (−36; 39)	12 (−27; 51)	21 (−59; 101)	7 (−76; 90)
Q4 (high)	−13 (−52; 25)	−4 (−44; 36)	23 (−56; 103)	−19 (−105; 68)
Per SD	*p* = 0.48	*p* = 0.72	*p* = 0.36	*p* = 0.92
"Nuts, High-Fiber Cereals and Soy" Pattern				
Q1 (low)	Reference	Reference	Reference	Reference
Q2	22 (−16; 60)	25 (−14; 64)	28 (−52; 107)	8 (−73; 89)
Q3	−7 (−46; 31)	−2 (−42; 39)	47 (−33; 128)	19 (−65; 102)
Q4 (high)	25 (−13; 64)	30 (−11; 70)	62 (−19; 142)	17 (−68; 103)
Per SD	*p* = 0.38	*p* = 0.32	*p* = 0.14	*p* = 0.72
"Margarine, Sugar and Snacks" Pattern				
Q1 (low)	Reference	Reference	Reference	Reference
Q2	31 (−7; 68)	31 (−6; 69)	25 (−53; 102)	30 (−47; 107)
Q3	15 (−23; 53)	18 (−21; 56)	8 (−71; 87)	17 (−62; 96)
Q4 (high)	16 (−22; 54)	18 (−20; 57)	14 (−64; 92)	24 (−54; 103)
Per SD	*p* = 0.44	*p* = 0.40	*p* = 0.65	*p* = 0.48
"Dutch Healthy Diet Index" Pattern				
Q1 (low)	Reference	Reference	Reference	Reference
Q2	−15 (−53; 23)	−14 (−52; 24)	−36 (−113; 41)	−31 (−109; 47)
Q3	−0 (−38; 37)	−1 (−39; 36)	−23 (−101; 54)	−4 (−81; 74)
Q4 (high)	−7 (−46; 31)	−10 (−49; 30)	−9 (−89; 70)	27 (−56; 109)
Per SD	*p* = 0.66	*p* = 0.76	*p* = 0.43	*p* = 0.88

[1] Results from multivariable linear regression analyses, based on imputed data. Values (regression coefficients with 95%-confidence interval) reflect the difference in mid-pregnancy weight gain (g/week) for quartile 2 until 4 relative to quartile 1. *p*-Values correspond to the effect of 1SD increase in dietary pattern score. *Model 1*: adjusted for pre-pregnancy BMI and median gestational age at follow-up. *Model 2*: *Model 1* further adjusted for age, educational level, household income, parity, smoking during pregnancy, alcohol consumption during pregnancy, stress during pregnancy, and fetal sex. *p* For interaction between dietary patterns and pre-pregnancy BMI was <0.10 for the "Dutch Healthy Diet Index" pattern and for the other patterns >0.10. Abbreviations: BMI: body mass index; Q: quartile; SD: standard deviation.

Table 5. Association of dietary patterns with gestational weight gain in late pregnancy (*n* = 3158) [1].

Quartiles of the Dietary Patterns	Late-Pregnancy Weight Gain (g/week)			
	Normal Weight Women (*n* = 2384)		Overweight Women (*n* = 774)	
	Model 1	*Model 2*	*Model 1*	*Model 2*
"Vegetable, Oil and Fish" Pattern				
Q1 (low)	Reference	Reference	Reference	Reference
Q2	−3 (−32; 26)	10 (−20; 39)	21 (−35; 78)	36 (−21; 93)
Q3	−18 (−47; 10)	−4 (−33; 26)	−3 (−60; 55)	21 (−38; 80)
Q4 (high)	−19 (−47; 10)	−0 (−31; 30)	−8 (−64; 49)	24 (−38; 86)
Per SD	*p* = 0.09	*p* = 0.54	*p* = 0.42	*p* = 0.82

Table 5. *Cont.*

Quartiles of the Dietary Patterns	Late-Pregnancy Weight Gain (g/week)			
	Normal Weight Women (*n* = 2384)		Overweight Women (*n* = 774)	
	Model 1	*Model 2*	*Model 1*	*Model 2*
"Nuts, High-Fiber Cereals and Soy" Pattern				
Q1 (low)	Reference	Reference	Reference	Reference
Q2	−2 (−30; 27)	14 (−15; 44)	4 (−54; 62)	18 (−41; 77)
Q3	−16 (−45; 12)	8 (−22; 38)	−3 (−60; 55)	15 (−45; 74)
Q4 (high)	−37 (−65; −8)	−13 (−43; 18)	3 (−55; 61)	21 (−41; 83)
Per SD	*p* < 0.01 *	*p* = 0.48	*p* = 0.91	*p* = 0.66
"Margarine, Sugar and Snacks" Pattern				
Q1 (low)	Reference	Reference	Reference	Reference
Q2	−21 (−49; 8)	−20 (−48; 8)	−8 (−65; 49)	−7 (−63; 50)
Q3	−12 (−41; 16)	−12 (−40; 17)	7 (−49; 64)	17 (−40; 74)
Q4 (high)	−5 (−34; 24)	−6 (−35; 23)	8 (−49; 65)	10 (−48; 68)
Per SD	*p* = 0.86	*p* = 0.76	*p* = 0.64	*p* = 0.66
"Dutch Healthy Diet Index" Pattern				
Q1 (low)	Reference	Reference	Reference	Reference
Q2	−14 (−43; 14)	−13 (−41;15)	46 (−10; 102)	51 (−5; 108)
Q3	−2 (−31; 27)	−10 (−39; 18)	23 (−34; 81)	25 (−33; 82)
Q4 (high)	−3 (−31; 26)	−14 (−43; 15)	33 (−24; 90)	28 (−31; 88)
Per SD	*p* = 0.61	*p* = 0.57	*p* = 0.46	*p* = 0.58

[1] Results from multivariable linear regression analyses, based on imputed data. Values (regression coefficients with 95%-confidence interval) reflect the difference in late-pregnancy weight gain (g/week) for quartile 2 until 4 relative to quartile 1. *p*-Values correspond to the effect of 1SD increase in dietary pattern score. *Model 1*: adjusted for pre-pregnancy BMI and median gestational age at follow-up. *Model 2*: *Model 1* further adjusted for age, educational level, household income, parity, smoking during pregnancy, alcohol consumption during pregnancy, stress during pregnancy, and fetal sex. *p* For interaction between dietary patterns and pre-pregnancy BMI was >0.10 for the "Nuts, high-fiber cereals and soy" and the "Dutch Healthy Diet Index" pattern, but <0.10 for the "Vegetable, oil and fish" and the "Margarine, sugar and snacks" pattern. Significant results are presented in bold (*p*-value < 0.05) and results with a *p*-value < 0.0125 with an asterisk (*). Abbreviations: BMI: body mass index, Q: quartile, SD: standard deviation.

In line with the results from early-pregnancy GWG, normal weight women in the highest quartile of the "Vegetable, oil and fish" pattern had higher GWG by 25 g/week (95% CI 9; 42) until the early-third trimester than women in the lowest quartile (Table S3), whereas no association was found in overweight women (Table S4). The other dietary patterns were not associated with GWG until the early-third trimester.

3.3. Dietary Patterns and Gestational Weight Gain Adequacy

Higher adherence to the dietary patterns was not associated with the prevalence of inadequate GWG (Table 6). The "Vegetable, oil and fish", the "Nuts, high-fiber cereals and soy" and the "Dutch Healthy Diet Index" pattern were also not associated with prevalence of excessive GWG. Yet, women with higher scores on the "Margarine, sugar and snacks" pattern had a higher prevalence of excessive GWG than women in the lowest quartile (ORs Q2: 1.40 (95% CI 1.04; 1.90), Q3: 1.37 (95% CI 1.00; 1.87), and Q4: 1.45 (95% CI 1.06; 1.99)).

Table 6. Association of dietary patterns with gestational weight gain adequacy (*n* = 1917) [1].

Quartiles of the Dietary Patterns	Inadequate GWG (*n* = 459)	Adequate GWG (*n* = 632)	Excessive GWG (*n* = 826)
	OR (95% CI)		OR (95% CI)
"Vegetable, Oil and Fish" Pattern			
Q1 (low)	Reference	Reference	Reference
Q2	0.85 (0.60; 1.22)	Reference	1.08 (0.79; 1.48)
Q3	0.86 (0.60; 1.23)	Reference	1.05 (0.76; 1.46)
Q4 (high)	0.84 (0.58; 1.22)	Reference	1.06 (0.76; 1.48)
Per SD	*p* = 0.21		*p* = 0.91
"Nuts, High-Fiber Cereals and Soy" Pattern			
Q1 (low)	Reference	Reference	Reference
Q2	0.77 (0.53; 1.13)	Reference	1.16 (0.82; 1.62)
Q3	0.86 (0.59; 1.25)	Reference	1.26 (0.89; 1.77)
Q4 (high)	0.85 (0.58; 1.24)	Reference	1.09 (0.77; 1.53)
Per SD	*p* = 0.76		*p* = 0.46
"Margarine, Sugar and Snacks" Pattern			
Q1 (low)	Reference	Reference	Reference
Q2	0.97 (0.69; 1.36)	Reference	**1.40 (1.04; 1.90)**
Q3	0.93 (0.66; 1.32)	Reference	**1.37 (1.00; 1.87)**
Q4 (high)	0.98 (0.69; 1.40)	Reference	**1.45 (1.06; 1.99)**
Per SD	*p* = 0.73		*p* = 0.09
"Dutch Healthy Diet Index" Pattern			
Q1 (low)	Reference	Reference	Reference
Q2	1.04 (0.74; 1.45)	Reference	0.92 (0.69; 1.24)
Q3	0.84 (0.59; 1.20)	Reference	0.95 (0.70; 1.27)
Q4 (high)	1.32 (0.92; 1.90)	Reference	1.11 (0.80; 1.53)
Per SD	*p* = 0.07		*p* = 0.66

[1] Results (OR with 95%-confidence interval) from multivariable multinomial logistic regression analyses, based on imputed data. Low dietary pattern adherence (Q1) is the reference category for diet and adequate GWG is the reference category for adequacy of GWG in the multinomial regression model. *p*-Values correspond to the effect of 1SD increase in dietary pattern score. Adjusted for pre-pregnancy BMI, age, educational level, household income, parity, smoking during pregnancy, alcohol consumption during pregnancy, stress during pregnancy, and fetal sex. Abbreviations: GWG: gestational weight gain; OR: odds ratio; Q: quartile, SD: standard deviation.

3.4. Dietary Patterns and trajectories of Gestational Weight

Figure S2 shows the longitudinal relationship between the *a posteriori*-derived dietary patterns with trajectories of maternal weight during pregnancy, as the difference in weight (kg) between the 12.5% quantile ("quartile 1") and the 37.5%, 62.5% and 87.5% quantiles ("quartiles" 2, 3 and 4, respectively) of adherence to the dietary pattern in normal weight women. Corresponding results for overweight women are displayed in Figure S3. In both normal weight and overweight women, most of the main effects of diet as well as the interaction terms with gestational age were not significant (Table S5). Only the "Margarine, sugar and snacks" pattern was significantly associated with higher weight in normal weight women (0.30 (95% CI 0.07; 0.52)) throughout pregnancy and the "Nuts, high-fiber cereals and soy" pattern was associated with slightly slower weight gain in normal weight women (−0.01 (95% CI −0.02; −0.00)).

3.5. Sensitivity Analyses

The results of the sensitivity analyses are presented in Table S3 for normal weight women and in Table S4 for overweight women. Additional adjustment for energy intake resulted in little attenuation of the effect estimate of the "Vegetable, oil and fish" pattern with GWG until early-third trimester, however the association remained statistically significant. Further adjustment of estimated fetal weight did not change the effect estimates of any dietary pattern with GWG in normal weight or overweight women. The results did not alter greatly after exclusion of women who vomited more than once per week, or exclusion of women with pre-existing comorbidities or pregnancy complications. The evaluation of maximum GWG showed that normal weight women with high adherence to the "Vegetable, oil and fish" pattern had 29 g/week (95% CI 2; 57) higher maximal GWG than women with low adherence. In addition, normal weight women in the highest quartile of the "Dutch Healthy Diet Index" had a 28 g/week (95% CI −55; −1) lower maximal GWG than women in quartile 1. The association between dietary patterns and GWG was not modified by educational level. For household income, women with higher household income (≥2200 Euro/month) and higher scores on the "Dutch Healthy Diet Index" pattern had lower GWG (p-value = 0.01 per 1SD score) than women with higher income and lower scores on this dietary pattern, whereas no association was found in women with lower household income (p-value = 0.11).

Evaluating adequacy of GWG using weekly GWG instead of total GWG resulted in a higher percentage women being classified as having "excessive GWG" (57% *vs.* 43%). However, also with this different definition a high adherence to the "Margarine, sugar and snacks" pattern was associated with a higher prevalence excessive weekly GWG. Nonetheless, high adherence to this pattern was also associated with higher prevalence of inadequate weekly GWG, although without dose-response association (Table S6).

Six years after childbirth, women had gained on average 3.4 kg (IQR: 0.4; 7.0) compared to their pre-pregnancy weight (n = 2247). The median (IQR) long-term weight gain was significantly different between the categories of GWG adequacy: women with inadequate GWG gained 2.2 kg (−0.6; 5.2), those with adequate GWG gained on average 2.6 kg (0.2; 5.2), and women with excessive GWG were 4.6 kg (1.4; 8.8) heavier (*F*-test 27.5, p-value < 0.001). The weight 6 years after childbirth was highly correlated with the weight at *the third visit* in pregnancy (R = 0.85; p-value < 0.001).

4. Discussion

4.1. Summary of Main Findings

Our results from a population-based Dutch cohort suggest that specific *a posteriori*-derived dietary patterns have a limited influence in early-pregnancy GWG, the prevalence of excessive GWG, and weight development in pregnancy. We found neither consistent associations of any dietary pattern with the prevalence of inadequate GWG, nor was the *a priori*-defined dietary pattern associated with GWG.

4.2. Interpretation and Comparison with Other Studies

The association of dietary patterns during pregnancy with GWG has been evaluated previously in a few studies [15–18], but these studies did not evaluate longitudinal development of gestational weight and were conducted in different populations. Uusitalo *et al.*, found that higher adherence to an *a posteriori*-derived dietary pattern characterized by high intake of sweets, fast food and snacks was associated with higher weekly GWG [15]. In line with these results [15], we found that higher adherence to the unhealthy "Margarine, sugar and snacks" pattern was associated with higher prevalence of excessive GWG. Additionally, Uusitalo *et al.*, reported that a pattern that was high in vegetables, fish and fruits was not associated with GWG [15]. In contrast, we found that the "Vegetable, oil and fish" pattern, a relatively healthy pattern, was associated with higher GWG, particularly in early pregnancy.

In our study, the *a priori*-defined "Dutch Healthy Diet Index" pattern was not consistently associated with any measure of GWG. This result was in accordance with two studies showing no relationship between the *a priori*-defined "US healthy eating index of 2005" (HEI-2005) and the "Alternate Healthy Eating Index, slightly modified for pregnancy" (AHEI-P) with the prevalence of inadequate or excessive GWG [16,17]. Nevertheless, a large population-based cohort study of over 66,000 participants found that high adherence to the *a priori*-defined "New Nordic Diet score" was associated with a 7% lower prevalence of excessive GWG in normal weight women, compared with low adherence [18]. The inconsistent significant associations between the *a priori*-defined dietary patterns may be due to different items that were included in the diet scores, whereas the "New Nordic Diet score" contained items on meal patterns and the type of beverages consumed, among others [18]; these items were not evaluated in our Dutch Healthy Diet Index, nor in other *a priori*-defined dietary patterns [16,17].

The association of *a posteriori*-derived dietary patterns with weight trajectories over pregnancy has not been evaluated previously, to our knowledge. Studying this association longitudinally has the advantage that all available weight measurements can be used, and takes into account the correlation between these measurements. In addition, weekly GWG is not constant over pregnancy and differs considerably by individual [28,36], which complicates cross-sectional comparisons of GWG. Our longitudinal analysis showed that women with higher adherence to the "Nuts, high-fiber and soy" pattern had a more moderate increase in weight during pregnancy than did women with low adherence to this dietary pattern, although absolute differences were small.

Results from both observational and interventional studies indicated that women with higher energy intake had higher GWG compared with women who have lower energy intake [8], results that were also found in our cohort [4]. In our analyses, the association of the "Vegetable, oil and fish" pattern remained significantly associated with GWG after additional adjustment for energy intake. This may indicate that dietary patterns are associated with GWG beyond energy intake.

Evaluating weight gain in pregnancy is important because GWG has been associated with many adverse pregnancy and birth outcomes. Gaining excessive weight during pregnancy can have short-term consequences such as delivery complications, and giving birth to a child that is large for its gestational age [3,4,28]. Additionally, it has been associated with long-term health consequences including post-partum obesity of the mother [37] due to retaining their excess fat mass, and childhood obesity [4]. Indeed, in our population, six years after childbirth women had gained on average 3.4 kg from their pre-pregnancy weight.

Weight gain during pregnancy consists of several maternal and fetal components that contribute differently to GWG over time [12]. For example, during the first half of pregnancy, maternal fat gain is a major contributor of GWG [38,39], and most of the fat gain that takes place during pregnancy is in that period [40]. In our study, the higher GWG in women with high adherence to the "Vegetable, oil and fish" pattern could not be explained by fetal growth and was mainly found in early pregnancy, meaning this higher GWG is likely due to maternal components, e.g., fat mass.

Our results for normal weight women differed from those for overweight women, particularly for the "Vegetable, oil and fish" pattern and for the "Nuts, high-fiber cereals and soy" pattern. Similarly, Hillesund *et al.* reported differential associations for women below and above a BMI of 25 kg/m^2 [18]. These differential findings may be explained by different reporting of dietary intake [41] or by differing contribution of the individual components of GWG for normal weight and overweight women [42]. In addition, our longitudinal analyses showed that over the whole course of pregnancy, normal weight women with higher adherence to the "Margarine, sugar and snacks" pattern tend to be heavier than women with lower adherence.

4.3. Strengths and Limitations

A strength of our study is that we used a comprehensive approach to analyze the relation between diet and GWG by evaluating the associations of dietary patterns with (1) GWG during different phases in pregnancy, (2) adequacy of GWG, and (3) trajectories of gestational weight. Another strength is the use of two distinct methods to define dietary patterns, which enabled us to evaluate the effects of dietary patterns derived by a data-driven and by a hypothesis-driven approach. Dietary patterns represent the combined effects of all foods consumed [13], which may lead to a more powerful effect than the effects of the individual components, although it may also have led to a dilution of the effects of individual components that are associated with GWG [43]. For example, the food groups of vegetables and high-fat dairy products were strongly associated with the "Vegetable, oil and fish" dietary pattern.

Yet, higher intake of fruits and vegetables has been associated with lower GWG [44], whereas dairy products were associated with higher GWG [9,10]. Consequently, this may result in an overall null effect of the dietary pattern. Furthermore, imputing the missing covariate values in the Bayesian framework allowed us to use all available information in the imputation. Especially in settings with a longitudinal outcome, imputation methods that are available in standard software and, hence, are more commonly used, often fail to appropriately include the outcome into the imputation procedure which may lead to severely biased results [31]. Other strengths of our study are its population-based design, the collection of numerous covariates, and that the population was restricted to women of Dutch ancestry. We excluded women with other ethnicities to minimize measurement error, since the FFQ was designed to evaluate a Dutch diet. However, this restriction may have reduced the generalizability of our results to other ethnicities.

Our study also has some limitations. First, maternal weight before pregnancy as well as maximum weight were obtained using questionnaires, which may have resulted in a larger measurement error. Although we found no indication of systematic measurement error, random error may have resulted in loss of precision in GWG assessment. Furthermore, we were not able to calculate GWG per trimester because we did not have weight measurements at the required time points and the available data was insufficient for imputing those values. Another limitation is the lack of information on the separate components of GWG, in particular maternal fat mass, and the lack of information on postpartum maternal weight. Future studies should collect detailed information on maternal body composition during pregnancy or measure the participants' weight a few weeks postpartum to evaluate associations with the different components of GWG. Also, we could not use information on absolute dietary intake because dietary information collected using an FFQ does not provide this information. However, FFQs have been shown to be accurate in ranking participants according to their dietary intake [45]. Furthermore, we assessed maternal diet only once during pregnancy and were therefore not able to account for changes in dietary intake. Nevertheless, dietary patterns and macronutrient composition may not change largely during pregnancy despite an increased energy intake [46,47]. Additionally, we found that our results did not change after excluding women who may have altered their dietary intake due to illness or vomiting. Finally, the numerous statistical analyses performed may have resulted in chance findings (*type I error*). However, our results for weight trajectories and early-pregnancy GWG remained statistically significant when a more stringent alpha-level was used (alpha-level 0.05/4 = 0.0125).

4.4. Conclusions and Implications

In conclusion, our results suggest that dietary composition during pregnancy may play a role in GWG in early pregnancy but has limited influence on total GWG in a population of Dutch women. The strength of the associations between dietary patterns and GWG differs for different definitions of dietary patterns and GWG. This suggests that the relationship between dietary patterns and GWG may be complex and may need further elucidation in order to facilitate the development of dietary guidelines during pregnancy and to adequately advise pregnant women on their diet.

Supplementary Materials: The following are available online at www.mdpi.com/2072-6643/7/11/5476/s1, Figure S1: Bland Altman plots for self-reported pre-pregnancy weight and maximum weight in pregnancy. (A) Bland-Altman plot for pre-pregnancy weight and weight during the *first visit* (n = 2425); (B) Bland-Altman plot for maximum weight in pregnancy and weight during the *third visit* (n = 2177), Figure S2: Trajectories of gestational weight in normal weight women (n = 2564). The figure shows the development of weight during pregnancy in normal weight women as estimated by the linear mixed model. Trends are plotted for 37.5%, 62.5%, and 87.5% quantiles (denoted as quartiles 2 until 4) as compared with the 12.5% quantile (denoted as quartile 1). Adjusted for gestational age at measurements, age, educational level, household income, parity, smoking during pregnancy, alcohol consumption during pregnancy, stress during pregnancy, and fetal sex. Panel A displays effect estimates with 95% CI. Panel B zooms in on the effect estimates, Figure S3: Trajectories of gestational weight in overweight women (n = 810). The figure shows the development of weight during pregnancy in overweight women as estimated by the linear mixed model. Trends are plotted for 37.5%, 62.5%, and 87.5% quantiles (denoted as quartiles 2 until 4) as compared with the 12.5% quantile (denoted quartile 1). Adjusted for gestational age at measurements, age, educational level, household income, parity, smoking during pregnancy, alcohol consumption during pregnancy, stress during pregnancy, and fetal sex. Panel A displays effect estimates with 95% CI. Panel B zooms in on the effect estimates, Table S1: Food groups and its food components, Table S2: Modified version of the Dutch Healthy Diet-index, Table S3: Sensitivity analyses in normal weight women (n = 2141), Table S4: Sensitivity analyses in overweight women (n = 674), Table S5: Gestational weight trajectories in normal weight and overweight women (n = 3374), Table S6: Association of dietary patterns with adequacy of weekly gestational weight gain (n = 2745).

Acknowledgments: The Generation R Study was conducted by the Erasmus Medical Center in close collaboration with the School of Law and Faculty of Social Sciences of the Erasmus University Rotterdam, the Municipal Health Service Rotterdam Metropolitan Area, the Rotterdam Homecare Foundation, and the Stichting Trombosedienst & Artsenlaboratorium Rijnmond, Rotterdam. The authors gratefully acknowledge the contributions of children and parents, general practitioners, hospitals and midwives in Rotterdam. The general design of the Generation R Study was made possible by financial support from the Erasmus MC, University Medical Centre Rotterdam; the Erasmus University, Rotterdam; the Dutch Ministry of Health, Welfare and Sport; and the Netherlands Organization for Health Research and Development (ZonMw). V.W.V.J. received an additional grant from the Netherlands Organization for Health Research and Development (ZonMW VIDI: 016.136.361). M.J.T., N.S.E., E.T.M.L., J.C.K.-D.J. and O.H.F. work in ErasmusAGE, a center for aging research across the life course funded by Nestlé Nutrition (Nestec Ltd., Vevey, Switzerland) and Metagenics Inc. (Aliso Viejo, CA, USA). Nestlé Nutrition and Metagenics Inc. had no role in design and conduct of the study; collection, management, analysis, and interpretation of the data; or preparation, review or approval of the manuscript.

Author Contributions: The authors' contributions to this study were as follows: M.J.T., J.C.K.-D.J., and O.H.F. designed the research project; V.W.V.J. and E.A.P.S. were involved in the design and planning of the study and data collection; N.S.E., M.J.T., E.T.M.L., and M.V.D.B. conducted the analyses; N.S.E., J.C.K.-D.J., E.T.M.L., and O.H.F. provided consultation regarding the analyses and interpretation of the data; N.S.E. assisted with writing the paper; M.J.T. and J.C.K.-D.J. wrote the paper; M.J.T. and O.H.F. had primary responsibility for the final content. All authors critically reviewed and approved the final manuscript.

Conflicts of Interest: The authors declare no conflict of interest.

References

1. Han, Z.; Lutsiv, O.; Mulla, S.; Rosen, A.; Beyene, J.; McDonald, S.D.; Synthesis, G.K. Low gestational weight gain and the risk of preterm birth and low birthweight: A systematic review and meta-analyses. *Acta Obstet. Gynecol. Scand.* **2011**, *90*, 935–954. [CrossRef] [PubMed]
2. Kim, S.Y.; Sharma, A.J.; Sappenfield, W.; Wilson, H.G.; Salihu, H.M. Association of maternal body mass index, excessive weight gain, and gestational diabetes mellitus with large-for-gestational-age births. *Obstet. Gynecol.* **2014**, *123*, 737–744. [CrossRef] [PubMed]
3. Johnson, J.; Clifton, R.G.; Roberts, J.M.; Myatt, L.; Hauth, J.C.; Spong, C.Y.; Varner, M.W.; Wapner, R.J.; Thorp, J.M., Jr.; Mercer, B.M.; *et al.* Pregnancy outcomes with weight gain above or below the 2009 Institute of Medicine guidelines. *Obstet. Gynecol.* **2013**, *121*, 969–975. [CrossRef] [PubMed]
4. Gaillard, R.; Durmus, B.; Hofman, A.; Mackenbach, J.P.; Steegers, E.A.; Jaddoe, V.W. Risk factors and outcomes of maternal obesity and excessive weight gain during pregnancy. *Obesity* **2013**, *21*, 1046–1055. [CrossRef] [PubMed]
5. Hedderson, M.M.; Gunderson, E.P.; Ferrara, A. Gestational weight gain and risk of gestational diabetes mellitus. *Obstet. Gynecol.* **2010**, *115*, 597–604. [CrossRef] [PubMed]
6. Brown, M.C.; Best, K.E.; Pearce, M.S.; Waugh, J.; Robson, S.C.; Bell, R. Cardiovascular disease risk in women with pre-eclampsia: Systematic review and meta-analysis. *Eur. J. Epidemiol.* **2013**, *28*, 1–19. [CrossRef] [PubMed]
7. Bellamy, L.; Casas, J.P.; Hingorani, A.D.; Williams, D. Type 2 diabetes mellitus after gestational diabetes: A systematic review and meta-analysis. *Lancet* **2009**, *373*, 1773–1779. [CrossRef]
8. Streuling, I.; Beyerlein, A.; Rosenfeld, E.; Schukat, B.; von Kries, R. Weight gain and dietary intake during pregnancy in industrialized countries—A systematic review of observational studies. *J. Perinat. Med.* **2011**, *39*, 123–129. [CrossRef] [PubMed]
9. Stuebe, A.M.; Oken, E.; Gillman, M.W. Associations of diet and physical activity during pregnancy with risk for excessive gestational weight gain. *Am. J. Obstet. Gynecol.* **2009**, *201*. [CrossRef] [PubMed]
10. Olafsdottir, A.S.; Skuladottir, G.V.; Thorsdottir, I.; Hauksson, A.; Steingrimsdottir, L. Maternal diet in early and late pregnancy in relation to weight gain. *Int. J. Obes. (Lond.)* **2006**, *30*, 492–499. [CrossRef] [PubMed]
11. Martins, A.P.B.; Benicio, M.H.D. Influence of dietary intake during gestation on postpartum weight retention. *Rev. Saude Publica* **2011**, *45*, 870–877. [CrossRef] [PubMed]

12. Pitkin, R.M. Nutritional support in obstetrics and gynecology. *Clin. Obstet. Gynecol.* **1976**, *19*, 489–513. [CrossRef] [PubMed]

13. Hu, F.B. Dietary pattern analysis: A new direction in nutritional epidemiology. *Curr. Opin. Lipidol.* **2002**, *13*, 3–9. [CrossRef] [PubMed]

14. World Health Organization (WHO). *Preparation and Use of Food-Based Dietary Guidelines: Report of a Joint Fao/Who Consultation*; WHO: Geneva, Switzerland, 1998.

15. Uusitalo, U.; Arkkola, T.; Ovaskainen, M.L.; Kronberg-Kippila, C.; Kenward, M.G.; Veijola, R.; Simell, O.; Knip, M.; Virtanen, S.M. Unhealthy dietary patterns are associated with weight gain during pregnancy among Finnish women. *Public Health Nutr.* **2009**, *12*, 2392–2399. [CrossRef] [PubMed]

16. Shin, D.; Bianchi, L.; Chung, H.; Weatherspoon, L.; Song, W.O. Is gestational weight gain associated with diet quality during pregnancy? *Matern. Child Health J.* **2014**, *18*, 1433–1443. [CrossRef] [PubMed]

17. Rifas-Shiman, S.L.; Rich-Edwards, J.W.; Kleinman, K.P.; Oken, E.; Gillman, M.W. Dietary quality during pregnancy varies by maternal characteristics in Project Viva: A US cohort. *J Am. Diet. Assoc.* **2009**, *109*, 1004–1011. [CrossRef] [PubMed]

18. Hillesund, E.R.; Bere, E.; Haugen, M.; Overby, N.C. Development of a new nordic diet score and its association with gestational weight gain and fetal growth—A study performed in the Norwegian mother and child cohort study (MoBa). *Public Health Nutr.* **2014**, *17*, 1909–1918. [CrossRef] [PubMed]

19. Kruithof, C.J.; Kooijman, M.N.; van Duijn, C.M.; Franco, O.H.; de Jongste, J.C.; Klaver, C.C.; Mackenbach, J.P.; Moll, H.A.; Raat, H.; Rings, E.H.; *et al.* The generation R study: Biobank update 2015. *Eur. J. Epidemiol.* **2014**, *29*, 911–927. [CrossRef] [PubMed]

20. Donders-Engelen, M.; van der Heijden, L. *Maten, Gewichten en Codenummers 2003 (Measures, Weights and Code Numbers 2003)*; Wageningen UR, Vakgroep Humane Voeding Wageningen and TNO Voeding: Zeist, The Netherlands, 2003.

21. Netherlands-Nutrition-Centre. *Dutch Food Composition Database 2006*; Nevo: Hague, The Netherlands, 2006.

22. Klipstein-Grobusch, K.; den Breeijen, J.H.; Goldbohm, R.A.; Geleijnse, J.M.; Hofman, A.; Grobbee, D.E.; Witteman, J.C. Dietary assessment in the elderly: Validation of a semiquantitative food frequency questionnaire. *Eur. J. Clin. Nutr.* **1998**, *52*, 588–596. [CrossRef] [PubMed]

23. Kaiser, H. The varimax criterion for analytic rotation in factor analysis. *Psychometrika* **1958**, *23*, 187–200. [CrossRef]

24. Van den Broek, M.; Leermakers, E.T.; Jaddoe, V.W.; Steegers, E.A.; Rivadeneira, F.; Raat, H.; Hofman, A.; Franco, O.H.; Kiefte-de Jong, J.C. Maternal dietary patterns during pregnancy and body composition of the child at age 6 y: The generation R study. *Am. J. Clin. Nutr.* **2015**, *102*, 873–880. [CrossRef] [PubMed]

25. Jolliffe, I. Principal component analysis. In *International Encyclopedia of Statistical Science*; Springer: Berlin/Heidelberg, Germany, 2011; pp. 1094–1096. Available online: http://dx.doi.org/10.1007/978-3-642-04898-2_455 (accessed on 16 July 2015).

26. Van Lee, L.; Geelen, A.; van Huysduynen, E.J.; de Vries, J.H.; van't Veer, P.; Feskens, E.J. The Dutch healthy diet index (DHD-index): An instrument to measure adherence to the Dutch guidelines for a healthy diet. *Nutr. J.* **2012**, *11*. [CrossRef] [PubMed]

27. Health Council of the Netherlands. *Guidelines for a Healthy Diet 2006*; Health Council of the Netherlands: Hague, The Netherlands, 2006.

28. Rasmussen, K.M.; Yaktine, A.L.; Editors Committee to Reexamine IOM Pregnancy Weight Guidelines; Institute of Medicine; National Research Council. *Weight Gain during Pregnancy: Reexamining the Guidelines*; National Academies Press (US): Washington, DC, USA, 2009.

29. Van Rossem, L.; Oenema, A.; Steegers, E.A.; Moll, H.A.; Jaddoe, V.W.; Hofman, A.; Mackenbach, J.P.; Raat, H. Are starting and continuing breastfeeding related to educational background? The generation R study. *Pediatrics* **2009**, *123*, e1017–e1027. [CrossRef] [PubMed]

30. Derogatis, L.R.; Spencer, P.M. *Brief Symptom Inventory: BSI*; Pearson: Upper Saddle River, NJ, USA, 1993.

31. Erler, N.S.; Rizopoulos, D.; van Rosmalen, J.; Jaddoe, V.W.; Franco, O.H.; Lesaffre, E.M. Dealing with missing covariates in epidemiologic studies. A comparison between multiple imputation and a full Bayesian approach. *Stat. Med.* **2015**, submitted.

32. Cook, R.D. Detection of influential observation in linear regression. *Technometrics* **1977**, *19*, 15–18. [CrossRef]

33. Timmermans, S.; Steegers-Theunissen, R.P.; Vujkovic, M.; den Breeijen, H.; Russcher, H.; Lindemans, J.; Mackenbach, J.; Hofman, A.; Lesaffre, E.E.; Jaddoe, V.V.; *et al.* The mediterranean diet and fetal size parameters: The generation R study. *Br. J. Nutr.* **2012**, *108*, 1399–1409. [CrossRef] [PubMed]

34. Coolman, M.; de Groot, C.J.; Jaddoe, V.W.; Hofman, A.; Raat, H.; Steegers, E.A. Medical record validation of maternally reported history of preeclampsia. *J. Clin. Epidemiol.* **2010**, *63*, 932–937. [CrossRef] [PubMed]

35. Plummer, M. JAGS: A Program for Analysis of Bayesian Graphical Models Using Gibbs Sampling. In Proceedings of the 3rd International Workshop on Distributed Statistical Computing, Wien, Austria, 20–22 March 2003; Technische Universit at Wien: Wien, Austria, 2003; p. 125.

36. Carmichael, S.; Abrams, B.; Selvin, S. The pattern of maternal weight gain in women with good pregnancy outcomes. *Am. J. Public Health* **1997**, *87*, 1984–1988. [CrossRef] [PubMed]

37. Nehring, I.; Schmoll, S.; Beyerlein, A.; Hauner, H.; von Kries, R. Gestational weight gain and long-term postpartum weight retention: A meta-analysis. *Am. J. Clin. Nutr.* **2011**, *94*, 1225–1231. [CrossRef] [PubMed]

38. Clapp, J.F., 3rd; Seaward, B.L.; Sleamaker, R.H.; Hiser, J. Maternal physiologic adaptations to early human pregnancy. *Am. J. Obstet. Gynecol.* **1988**, *159*, 1456–1460. [CrossRef]

39. Kopp-Hoolihan, L.E.; van Loan, M.D.; Wong, W.W.; King, J.C. Fat mass deposition during pregnancy using a four-component model. *J. Appl. Physiol.* **1999**, *87*, 196–202.

40. Forsum, E.; Sadurskis, A.; Wager, J. Resting metabolic rate and body composition of healthy Swedish women during pregnancy. *Am. J. Clin. Nutr.* **1988**, *47*, 942–947. [PubMed]

41. Freisling, H.; van Bakel, M.M.; Biessy, C.; May, A.M.; Byrnes, G.; Norat, T.; Rinaldi, S.; de Magistris, M.S.; Grioni, S.; Bueno-de-Mesquita, H.B.; *et al.* Dietary reporting errors on 24 h recalls and dietary questionnaires are associated with BMI across six European countries as evaluated with recovery biomarkers for protein and potassium intake. *Br. J. Nutr.* **2012**, *107*, 910–920. [CrossRef] [PubMed]

42. Butte, N.F.; Ellis, K.J.; Wong, W.W.; Hopkinson, J.M.; Smith, E.O. Composition of gestational weight gain impacts maternal fat retention and infant birth weight. *Am. J. Obstet. Gynecol.* **2003**, *189*, 1423–1432. [CrossRef]

43. Willett, W. *Nutritional Epidemiology*, 3rd ed.; Oxford University Press: New York, NY, USA, 2012.

44. Olson, C.M.; Strawderman, M.S. Modifiable behavioral factors in a biopsychosocial model predict inadequate and excessive gestational weight gain. *J. Am. Diet. Assoc.* **2003**, *103*, 48–54. [CrossRef] [PubMed]

45. Kipnis, V.; Subar, A.F.; Midthune, D.; Freedman, L.S.; Ballard-Barbash, R.; Troiano, R.P.; Bingham, S.; Schoeller, D.A.; Schatzkin, A.; Carroll, R.J. Structure of dietary measurement error: Results of the open biomarker study. *Am. J. Epidemiol.* **2003**, *158*, 14–21. [CrossRef] [PubMed]

46. Crozier, S.R.; Robinson, S.M.; Godfrey, K.M.; Cooper, C.; Inskip, H.M. Women's dietary patterns change little from before to during pregnancy. *J. Nutr.* **2009**, *139*, 1956–1963. [CrossRef] [PubMed]

47. Rad, N.T.; Ritterath, C.; Siegmund, T.; Wascher, C.; Siebert, G.; Henrich, W.; Buhling, K.J. Longitudinal analysis of changes in energy intake and macronutrient composition during pregnancy and 6 weeks post-partum. *Arch. Gynecol. Obstet.* **2011**, *283*, 185–190.

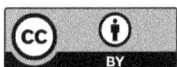

nutrients

MDPI

Article

Analysis of Dietary Pattern Impact on Weight Status for Personalised Nutrition through On-Line Advice: The Food4Me Spanish Cohort

Rodrigo San-Cristobal [1,†], Santiago Navas-Carretero [1,2,†], Carlos Celis-Morales [3], Lorraine Brennan [4], Marianne Walsh [4], Julie A. Lovegrove [5], Hannelore Daniel [6], Wim H. M. Saris [7], Iwonna Traczyk [8], Yannis Manios [9], Eileen R. Gibney [4], Michael J. Gibney [4], John C. Mathers [3] and J. Alfredo Martinez [1,2,10,*]

[1] Department of Nutrition, Food Science and Physiology, Centre for Nutrition Research, University of Navarra, Pamplona 31008, Spain; rsan.1@alumni.unav.es (R.S.-C.); snavas@unav.es (S.N.-C.)
[2] CIBER Fisiopatología Obesidad y Nutrición (CIBERobn), Instituto de Salud Carlos III, Madrid 28029, Spain
[3] Human Nutrition Research Centre, Institute of Cellular Medicine, Newcastle University, Campus for Ageing and Vitality, Newcastle Upon Tyne NE1 7RU, UK; carlos.celis@glasgow.ac.uk (C.C.-M.); john.mathers@newcastle.ac.uk (J.C.M.)
[4] UCD Institute of Food and Health, University College Dublin, Belfield, Dublin 4, Ireland; lorraine.brennan@ucd.ie (L.B.); marianne.walsh@ucd.ie (M.W.); eileen.gibney@ucd.ie (E.R.G.); mike.gibney@ucd.ie (M.J.G.)
[5] Hugh Sinclair Unit of Human Nutrition and Institute for Cardiovascular and Metabolic Research, University of Reading, Reading RG6 6AA, UK; j.a.lovegrove@reading.ac.uk
[6] Biochemistry Unit, ZIEL Research Center of Nutrition and Food Sciences, Technische Universität München, Munich 85354, Germany; hannelore.daniel@tum.de
[7] Department of Human Biology, NUTRIM, School for Nutrition and Translational Research in Metabolism, Maastricht University Medical Centre, Maastricht 6200MD, The Netherlands; w.saris@hb.unimaas.nl
[8] National Food & Nutrition Institute (IZZ), Warsaw 02-903, Poland; itraczyk@izz.waw.pl
[9] Department of Nutrition and Dietetics, Harokopio University, Athens 17671, Greece; manios@hua.gr
[10] Instituto de Investigación Sanitaria de Navarra (IdiSNA), Pamplona 31008, Spain
[*] Correspondence: jalfmtz@unav.es; Tel.: +34-948-425-740 (ext. 806424); Fax: +34-948-425-600
[†] These authors contributed equally to this work.

Received: 10 September 2015 ; Accepted: 3 November 2015 ; Published: 17 November 2015

Abstract: Obesity prevalence is increasing. The management of this condition requires a detailed analysis of the global risk factors in order to develop personalised advice. This study is aimed to identify current dietary patterns and habits in Spanish population interested in personalised nutrition and investigate associations with weight status. Self-reported dietary and anthropometrical data from the Spanish participants in the Food4Me study, were used in a multidimensional exploratory analysis to define specific dietary profiles. Two opposing factors were obtained according to food groups' intake: Factor 1 characterised by a more frequent consumption of traditionally considered unhealthy foods; and Factor 2, where the consumption of "Mediterranean diet" foods was prevalent. Factor 1 showed a direct relationship with BMI ($\beta = 0.226$; $r^2 = 0.259$; $p < 0.001$), while the association with Factor 2 was inverse ($\beta = -0.037$; $r^2 = 0.230$; $p = 0.348$). A total of four categories were defined (Prudent, Healthy, Western, and Compensatory) through classification of the sample in higher or lower adherence to each factor and combining the possibilities. Western and Compensatory dietary patterns, which were characterized by high-density foods consumption, showed positive associations with overweight prevalence. Further analysis showed that prevention of overweight must focus on limiting the intake of known deleterious foods rather than exclusively enhance healthy products.

Keywords: dietary pattern; dietary habits; obesity; personalised nutrition

Nutrients **2015**, *7*, 9523–9537

1. Introduction

Obesity, which is defined by an excessive body fat mass accumulation, is one of the most important public health problems worldwide [1]. The continuous increase in obesity prevalence has been repeatedly found to be a key factor associated with the onset of important chronic diseases [2]. Classical nutritional studies have attempted to find the relationship between the differences in the consumption of single nutritional compounds and anthropometric or biochemical markers [3]. However, the current epidemiological trends are helping to identify potential causes of obesity and accompanying comorbidities through the study of phenotypical features associated with global dietary patterns and lifestyle habits as well as the role of food exposures and their interactions [4–6].

Lifestyle and eating attitudes cannot be easily evaluated directly in target populations. For this reason, *a priori* dietary pattern determination (scores or indices) are used to evaluate the adherence to already known beneficial diets [7–9] or the adequacy/adherence to national guidelines [10], with focus on preventing metabolic disorders. On the other hand, *a posteriori* dietary pattern determinations through statistical analyses, such as principal component, factor analysis or clustering analysis, from food frequency questionnaires, allow researchers to explore the similarities of habitual food choices in specific populations and health outcomes. Subsequent post-estimation approaches can be carried out to find characteristics related to the risk of developing different non-communicable diseases as a result of long-term consumption of these patterns [11]. The study of the diversity in dietary patterns and habits also enable the inclusion of synergetic or cumulative effects of foods in association with the prevalence of obesity and its related diseases [12]. The validity of statistical determinations has been studied thoroughly in order to interpret and improve traditional dietary patterns of specific populations as well as to evaluate the biological interactions of nutrients and health [13].

The identification of dietary food patterns in large populations may contribute to identify different combinations of food choices, to assess the quality of food intake and to evaluate the effects of dietary changes for the prevention of obesity onset and the associated complications.

In this context, this research aimed to examine the lifestyle habits and dietary patterns in a Spanish cohort with interest in Personalised Nutrition (PN) by participating in the Food4Me European study, and to analyse the association with overweight and obesity prevalence. This approach tries to derive a preventative dietary pattern for obesity management and for understanding body weight regulation.

2. Experimental Section

2.1. Study Population

The subjects were selected from the Food4Me project (Trial registration: NCT01530139 http://clinicaltrials.gov/show/NCT01530139). This trial was a web-based randomised controlled intervention carried out to bring about a Personalised Nutrition assessment in seven European countries [14]. All participants that signed up on the Spanish webpage (http://www.food4me.org/es/) from November 2013 to February 2014 (*n* = 1839 individuals) were selected as potential participants for the Food4Me project. To be included in the study, the volunteers had to complete two screening questionnaires, the first of them about their socio-demographic characteristics, while the second one included also medication, habits and a Food Frequency Questionnaire (FFQ). If the participants met the inclusion criteria, two consent forms were given to sign in order to proceed [14]. The criteria to be eligible to participate in the Food4Me study were the following: participants had to be more than 18 years-old, not having followed a prescribed diet within the three months prior to the study, to have access to the internet, and not to suffer any physiological condition (pregnancy) or chronic metabolic disease (Diabetes, Crohn's disease, thyroid disorders, *etc.*). Afterwards, to ensure the validity of data collection, all the volunteers that could be considered misreporting based on the energy intake (over-reporting and under-reporting) were excluded according to the Goldberg cut-offs as updated by Black [15]. Finally the study was carried out in 617 volunteers meeting the mentioned inclusion criteria (Figure 1).

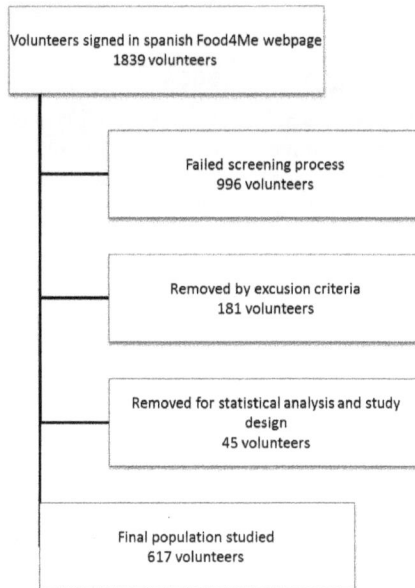

Figure 1. Flowchart of selection of sample.

2.2. Dietary Assessment

The Food4Me Food Frequency Questionnaire (FFQ) was developed to assess the food and nutritional intakes of the volunteers. This survey was an online, semi-quantitative food frequency questionnaire (developed by University College Dublin and Crème Software Ltd.), based on the EPIC-Norfolk FFQ with 157 food items divided in 11 categories [16]. Validity and reproducibility of Food4Me FFQ was tested for the population studied by comparing with a four-day weighed food record [17]. To complete the FFQ the volunteers had to log-in to the website and answer the questionnaire with the average amount of the food consumed in the previous month. The volunteers received specific instructions to complete the FFQ and pictures were available to best estimate the portion size of each food item.

A priori dietary patterns analyses were used to compare the food intake with the adherence to healthy dietary patterns previously described. Thus, a Mediterranean-Diet Scale (MDScale) [7,11] and the Alternative Healthy Eating Index (AHEI) [18] were applied to find out similarities with the dietary patterns obtained by factor analysis. Energy intake was also reported to the basal metabolic rate ratio (EIR:BMR ratio), was calculated and analysed to avoid biases in estimation of nutrient intake [15].

2.3. Anthropometric Measurements

Health and anthropometric data were collected from the second screening questionnaire [14]. These data included self-reported measurements as required of the volunteers in order to select the potential participants in the study.

The validity of self-reported weight and height collected in the second screening questionnaire was examined and compared to the measurements carried out with the standardised instructions [14] by the participants. A validation study of self-reported measurements has been already carried out to ensure the reliability of data collection through the internet [19].

2.4. Statistical Analyses

Statistical analyses were performed using STATA statistical software (Stata IC version 12.0, StataCorp, College Station, TX, USA).

Dietary patterns were identified using factor analysis. This approach allows identification of similarities in food intakes among a large number of subjects [13], facilitating a primary classification depending on determined exposures and by reducing the number of variables introduced in the analysis. Thus, a total of 157 food items were gathered in 24 foods groups according to their nutritional value and their similar nature in order to minimize within-person variations for specific food intake (Supplementary Table S1). Subsequently, factor analysis of principal components was performed to set up the existence of one or more dietary patterns. From the statistical solution, two factors were considered to further carry out analyses taking into account the eigenvalue (greater than 2), the inflexion point on the screeplot and variance explanation of each pattern solution. Also Kaiser-Meyer-Olkin measure of sampling adequacy of overall variables was performed (greater than 0.6) to warrant the fit of factor analysis. For the factors arisen, food groups which received loading factors higher than 0.3, in absolute values, were considered as representative contributors to each dietary pattern.

In order to elucidate the relative influence of specific food groups (loading factors and absolute intakes of food) to each factor, a score was developed through a linear regression model to assess the adherence of every volunteer to both factors. A higher score indicated greater adherence to the specific pattern.

These scores were used to categorize the sample and to carry out the statistical analysis of differences in macronutrient intake, energy intake and body mass index; as well as to feature the association, through multiple linear regression, between each pattern adherence and weight status adjusting by the biological, behavioural and environmental factors. Wald tests were carried out to explore interaction effects in each level of adherence to factors. Prevalence ratio of obesity (BMI > 30 kg/m^2) was estimated using a robust regression model. Power calculations on the analysis of differences in categories according to factors' adherence, gave a statistical power ranging from 90% to 100% ($\beta = 0.9093$ to $\beta = 1.000$).

Subjects showing opposed adherence to each factor were categorised, in order to prevent possible deviations in the study of the resulting dietary patterns, triggered by the effects between factors.

Normal distributions were graphically verified, assuming the central limit theorem, given that the sample size was sufficiently large and the statistical distribution tests for this sample size had low power. Also homogeneity of variances, homokedasticity and absence of colinearity were checked to ensure the adequacy of the test for differences and association, respectively.

3. Results

3.1. Baseline Characteristics

The mean age of the sample was 38.0 years and 56% were females (Table 1). Significant differences in BMI and physical activity factor were found when the sample was categorised by gender and also by age (divided by the median age, 37 years). Females and younger volunteers exhibited lower BMI (24.9–27.1 and 24.7–26.9 kg/m^2 respectively), showing females were more sedentary than males (1.48–1.52), and younger participants slightly more actives than older volunteers (1.51–1.48). Concerning macronutrient distribution, males reported higher energy, alcohol and salt intake, while females presented greater percentages in fat (total, saturated, monounsaturated and omega 3), sugar and fibre intakes. Female participants reported higher energy consumption when this was adjusted by the estimated basal metabolic rate (EIR:BMR ratio), while differences were not significant when the sample was categorised by age (1.82–1.61 and 1.74–1.73, respectively).

Table 1. Baseline characteristics of Spanish Food4Me volunteers included in the study.

Variable		Categorized by Gender			Categorized by Age		
		Female	Male	p¹	≤37 years	>37 years	p¹
n	617	368	249	-	315	304	-
Age (years)	38.3 ± 9.6	37.9 ± 9.5	38.9 ± 9.8	-	30.7 ± 4.5	46.1 ± 7.0	-
BMI (kg/m²)	25.8 ± 4.5	24.9 ± 4.7	27.1 ± 3.7	***	24.7 ± 4.2	26.9 ± 4.4	***
BMI status (% of n)							
Normal weight	48.8%	59.8%	32.5%		61.2%	36.0%	
Overweight	35.0%	25.5%	49.0%	***³	29.0%	41.3%	***³
Obese	16.2%	14.7%	18.5%		9.9%	22.8%	**
Physical activity factor	1.50 ± 4.47	1.48 ± 0.08	1.52 ± 0.11	***	1.51 ± 0.10	1.48 ± 0.09	
Energy (kcal)	2651 ± 796	2472 ± 759	2916 ± 777	***	2632 ± 798	2670 ± 795	
EIR:BMR ratio²	1.74 ± 0.50	1.82 ± 0.53	1.61 ± 0.42	***	1.74 ± 0.50	1.73 ± 0.49	
Fat (% of energy)	35.7 ± 6.4	36.3 ± 6.2	34.8 ± 6.6	**	35.7 ± 6.0	35.7 ± 6.7	
Saturated fat (% of energy)	13.1 ± 2.8	13.3 ± 2.7	12.8 ± 2.9	*	13.2 ± 2.8	13.0 ± 2.8	
Monounsaturated fat (% of energy)	14.8 ± 3.7	15.2 ± 3.8	14.3 ± 3.4	**	14.8 ± 3.5	14.9 ± 3.9	
Polyunsaturated fat (% of energy)	5.3 ± 1.3	5.4 ± 1.4	5.2 ± 1.3		5.3 ± 1.3	5.3 ± 1.4	
Omega 3 acids (% of energy)	0.82 ± 0.24	0.84 ± 0.25	0.78 ± 0.23	**	0.81 ± 0.24	0.82 ± 0.24	
Protein (% of energy)	19.2 ± 4.0	19.4 ± 4.1	19.0 ± 3.7		19.5 ± 4.0	19.0 ± 3.9	
Carbohydrate (% of energy)	44.7 ± 8.5	44.7 ± 8.4	44.7 ± 8.7		44.4 ± 7.8	45.0 ± 9.2	
Sugar (% of energy)	21.2 ± 6.8	21.9 ± 7.1	20.1 ± 6.3	**	21.2 ± 6.3	21.1 ± 7.4	
Alcohol (% of energy)	3.0 ± 3.8	2.1 ± 2.6	4.2 ± 4.8	***	2.8 ± 3.7	3.1 ± 3.9	
Salt (g)	7.7 ± 3.0	7.1 ± 2.8	8.6 ± 3.2	***	7.6 ± 3.0	7.8 ± 3.0	
Dietary fibre (g/1000 kcal)	10.6 ± 3.7	11.0 ± 3.8	10.0 ± 3.3	***	10.4 ± 3.6	10.8 ± 3.7	
Disease prevalence (% of n)⁴	54.5%	57.1%	50.6%	³	49.0%	60.1%	**³
Prescribed medication (% of n)	29.0%	31.8%	24.9%	³	23.6%	34.7%	**³
Supplement user (% of n)	21.2%	25.3%	15.3%	**³	21.0%	21.5%	³
Smoke (% of n)	16.9%	16.6%	17.3%	³	20.4%	13.2%	*³

[1] p values for *t*-test analysis: * for p < 0.05; ** for p < 0.01 *** for p < 0.001. [2] EIR:BMR, Energy Intake Reported to Basal Metabolic Rate ratio. [3] p values for chi square analisys. [4] Disease prevalence refers to the participant's self-reporting in the online questionnaire of suffering from any non-communicable disease (e.g., hypertension, dyslipidaemia, osteoporosis . . .)

Nutrients **2015**, *7*, 9523–9537

3.2. Factor Scores: Association and Effects with BMI

The factor analysis enabled to define two main factors (Table 2). The first one was characterised by a higher consumption of fast and processed food, potatoes, red meat, refined grains, snacks, and white meat and low intake of fruits, and vegetables. The second dietary pattern featured a higher consumption of eggs, fish products, legumes, low calorie beverages, nuts, oils, oily fruits, vegetables, and white meat.

Table 2. Factor loading of pattern matrix.

Variable	Factor 1	Factor 2
Alcoholic beverages		
Eggs		0.3606
Fast and processed food	0.6578	
Fat and spreads		
Fish products		0.4804
Fruits	−0.3904	
Full fat dairy products		
High fat dairy products		
Legumes		0.458
Low calorie beverages		0.3206
Nuts		0.3022
Oils		0.3305
Oily fruits		0.5014
Potatoes	0.3221	
Red meat	0.6336	
Reduced fat dairy products		
Refined grains	0.4483	
Snacks	0.6094	
Soup and sauces		
Sweets		
Sweets beverages		
Vegetables	−0.3582	0.6345
White meat	0.4622	0.3023
Whole grains		

Blanks represent absolute loading <0.3.

Association analyses including all volunteers for each factor score showed a relationship with BMI separately and no interactions were found between factors (Figure 2a,b). The score Factor 1 showed a direct association ($\beta = 0.226$; $r^2 = 0.259$; $p < 0.001$), while score Factor 2 presented a non-statistically significant inverse association ($\beta = -0.037$; $r^2 = 0.230$; $p = 0.348$) with BMI when adjusted for age, gender, physical activity, smoking habits and use of supplements.

The sample was categorized according to the adherence (scores) to each factor (Supplementary Table S2). Analyses for the differences between scores did not show statistical significant outcomes due to the wide variances, resulting in opposite scores for both factors (*i.e.*, High adherence Factor 1 + High adherence Factor 2). Consequently, analyses of interaction between high and low adherence for each factor were performed, studying the effects in the slopes for BMI relationship (Figure 3a,b). Adherence to Factor 1, presented a significant fixed effect on Factor 2 ($F = 9.54$, $p < 0.001$ for joint effect) increasing for those volunteers who had high adherence for Factor 1 ($F = 15.89$, $p < 0.001$). In the opposite analysis, slight effects were found for volunteers that presented high adherence to Factor 2 ($F = 4.18$, $p = 0.041$).

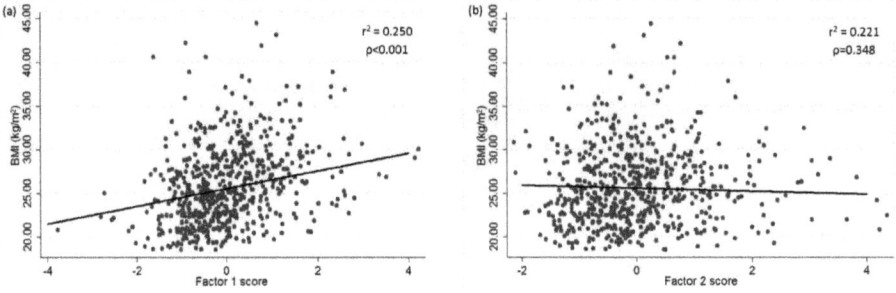

Figure 2. (a) Regression representation of BMI for Factor 1 adjusted for age, gender, energy intake, physical activity, supplement user, and smoking habit; (b) Regression representation of BMI for Factor 2 adjusted for age, gender, energy intake, physical activity, smoking habit, and supplement user.

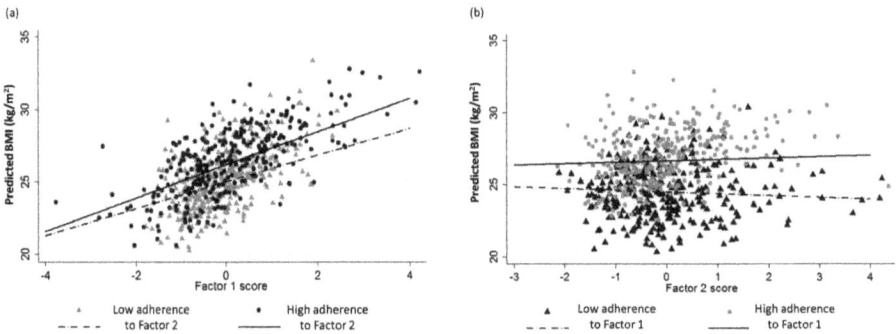

Figure 3. (a) Regression plotting of predicted BMI for Factor 1 adjusted for age, gender, energy intake, physical activity, supplement user, and smoking habit categorized by adherence to Factor 2; (b) Regression plotting of predicted BMI for Factor 2 adjusted for age, gender, energy intake, physical activity, smoking habit, and supplement user categorized by adherence to Factor 1.

3.3. Dietary Patterns: Obesity Prevalence

The categorisation of volunteers depending on the adherence to Factor 1 and 2, resulted in four differentiated groups of volunteers with well-defined dietary patterns, which were denominated as "Prudent" dietary pattern for the volunteers with low adherence to both factors ($n = 162$, 126 being females), "Healthy" dietary patterns for volunteers that showed lower adherence to Factor 1 and higher adherence to Factor 2 ($n = 147$, being females 105), "Western" dietary pattern for volunteers who presented higher adherence to Factor 1 and lower adherence to Factor 2 ($n = 147$, being females 67), and "Compensatory" dietary pattern for those who had high adherence to both factors ($n = 161$, being females 70).

The trend for prevalence of overweight ($p < 0.001$) and obesity ($p < 0.01$) increased in those dietary patterns with high adherence to Factor 1 (Western and Compensatory), while the Healthy pattern showed a reduction in obesity prevalence compared to the Prudent dietary pattern. Statistical increased odds ratio for obesity (BMI > 30 kg/m^2) was found (Figure 4) when comparing the Healthy dietary pattern to the Western (OR = 2.66, CI: 1.22–5.81) and Compensatory (OR = 3.16, CI: 1.46–6.83) patterns, but not to the Prudent pattern (OR = 1.85, CI: 0.84–4.07).

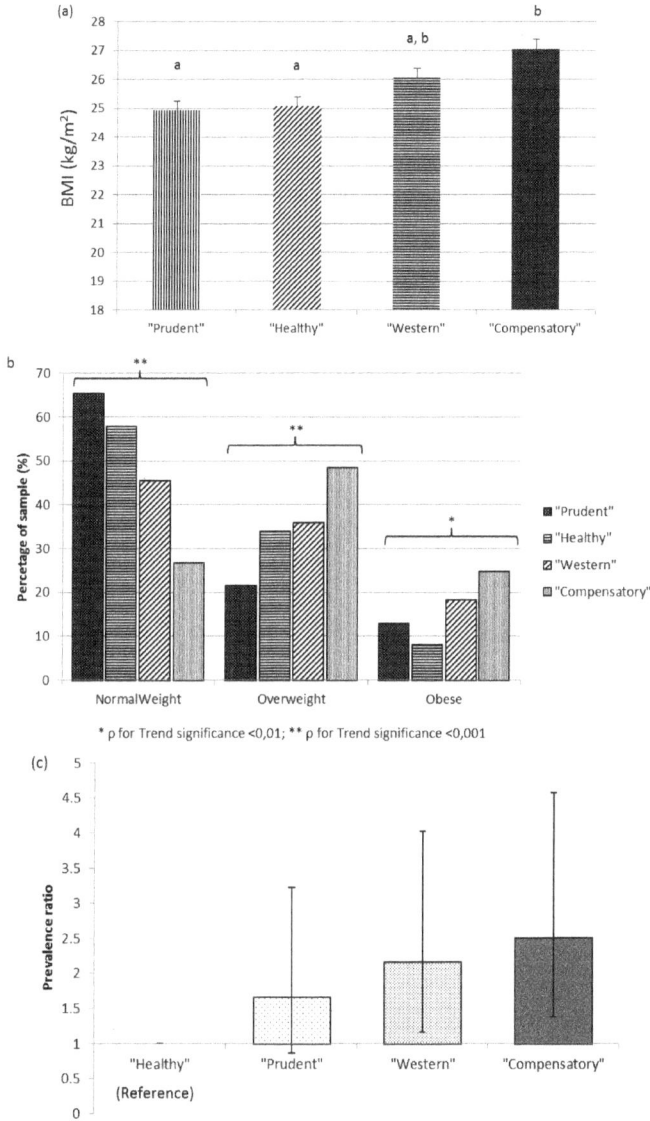

Figure 4. (**a**) Least square means of BMI for each dietary pattern. Values are adjusted for age, gender, energy intake reported, physical activity factor, smoking habit, and supplement user; (**b**) Prevalence of normal weight, overweight and obesity by dietary pattern; (**c**) Prevalence ratio and confidence interval (95%) for obesity (BMI $\geq$ 30 kg/m^2).

Volunteers adhering to the "Prudent" dietary pattern showed a good fit between energy intake reported and basal metabolic rate (EIR:BMR ratio), although they did not provide any characterised dietary pattern (Supplementary Table S3), while the "Healthy" dietary pattern showed higher energy intake and an intake profile similar to Mediterranean diet (Supplementary Table S4), with a higher score on the MDScale and AHEI. Volunteers ascribed to the "Western" dietary pattern presented an energy intake reported as high as "Healthy" but with lower scores for both dietary indexes (AHEI and

MDScale). Finally, volunteers that presented the "Compensatory" dietary pattern exhibited the highest energy intake, but with a slightly higher score than "Western". According to the nutritional profile of the dietary patterns, differences for all the nutrients were observed, highlighting greatest intakes of omega 3 and dietary fibre in the Healthy dietary pattern, and highest consumption of salt in the Compensatory dietary pattern.

Differences in BMI were also observed between the dietary patterns, being "Compensatory" higher than "Prudent" and "Healthy". Concurring to the obesity prevalence, a significantly increased obesity presence was observed among the volunteers adhering to the "Western" and "Compensatory" patterns.

3.4. Habits and Attitude towards Feeding

To appraise the dietary habits and attitudes of volunteers towards feeding, some questions were included in the survey. The analysis of frequencies in responses exhibited (Supplementary Figure S1) that the time preparing main meal was an important factor in the selections of recipes for the volunteers with "Western" and "Compensatory" patterns. The volunteers who reported dedicating less time to prepare the main meal and skipping meals by replacing them with snacks, were the volunteers with the "Western" pattern. These same volunteers, along with the "Compensatory" pattern subjects, presented a greater frequency in the intake of fried food, including almost one portion per week in half of the subjects of each group. Regarding the questions on how healthy was their feeding, and if this healthy eating was deliberate, "Prudent" and "Healthy" patterns exposed higher feeling to adhere to healthy habits, and these two groups reported to have those habits without having consciously to think about them.

4. Discussion

4.1. Personalised Nutrition (PN) Seekers Status

The participants were individuals interested in receiving PN through a web-based platform, and presented a similar age (40 ± 5 years) to other web-based programs for the modification of dietary and behavioural habits [20–28]. Concerning gender distribution, although there were wide variations in the percentage, female participants were generally found to be in higher proportion [20–26,29], as it occurs in the present work; only one study showed higher rates of males [28]. Concerning the BMI, the present study showed slight discrepancies in the number of overweight/obese individuals participating, compared to similar programmes [25,28] that were not specifically focused on weight-loss or directed to overweight or obese individuals. Indeed, matching our sample with the National Health Survey of 2013 [30], the weight distribution exhibited representative outcomes for Spanish population, with around 17% of obese individuals and more than half of the population exhibiting overweight or obesity [30]. Nevertheless, and despite the similarities in weight distribution, the generalization of the current outcomes to the overall Spanish population should be made with caution. The sample analysed in the present study were frequent internet users, with a specific interest on improving their health and nutritional status. The identification of a potentially interested population will be useful in order to develop further research on the predisposition for specific diseases, and prepare more tailored and targeted advice.

4.2. Adherence to Dietary Patterns and Obesity

The self-reported measurements used in the Food4Me study have already been validated through the assessment of the precision and the authenticity of measures [19]. In addition, the reproducibility and accuracy for the Food4Me Food Frequency Questionnaire has been also tested [16,17] as well as the study of the presence of misreporting (under and over reporting volunteers) [15], which contributes to ensure that there are no measurement errors. In addition, total energy, smoking, supplements consumption and physical activity level adjustments have been used to reduce inter-individual variance and to control for confounding factors in the prediction of dietary intake [31,32].

The multidimensional exploratory analysis from a matrix of foods sheds light on synergistic and additive effects of nutrients contained in food [4]. However, the reproducibility of this type of analyses may turn into a too laborious work, taking into account the variety of foods in the different regions worldwide [13]. Nevertheless, dietary patterns seem to be stable across demographical variances in other studied populations [33], and dietary patterns based on foods or food groups consumption probably have an easier interpretation and thus implementation in nutritional assessment [34].

The number of dietary patterns obtained from other studies varied from two to eight [35], and food-groups or food items included in each pattern differed [35,36]. However, it has been shown that there is a direct association between food content within the different dietary patterns, and the increase of body weight. Thus, Sun *et al.* [37] established that adults with a Western dietary pattern have a higher waist-hip ratio, BMI and relative risk of obesity hypertension, metabolic syndrome, and dyslipidaemia in adults. Also, Newby *et al.* [38] found in a prospective study that the individuals following a dietary pattern characterised by greater energy contributions from fruits, high-fibre cereal, and reduced fat dairy, with smaller contributions from fast food, non-diet soda, and salty snacks were associated with smaller gains in BMI and waist circumference. In this context, Flores *et al.* [39] showed an increase in the odds ratio to be obese in subjects that had higher energy intake from alcohol, soft drinks, white bread, fast food, sweets and candies, and salty snacks, and lowest contribution from maize and the highest proportion of whole-fat dairy, rice and pasta, meat, poultry, eggs, saturated fat, fruits, and vegetables, compared to a traditional dietary pattern with main intake resulting from maize foods.

There are also other studies that have established a connection between dietary patterns with overlapping food groups and the variance on body composition in children and adolescents [40, 41], changes in the risk of metabolic syndrome [42–44] or other relevant chronic diseases [45,46]. Therefore, the evidence found in the present study contributes to confirm these previous findings.

Additional epidemiological studies suggest that the current Spanish dietary pattern is in transition [47], as it has been observed in other Mediterranean and European countries [48], from a traditional Mediterranean lifestyle to imported Western habits [49]. Migrations, socioeconomical factors and larger variety of food availability promotes the evolution of traditional dietary patterns [50], and seems to cause "Westernization".

In this context, the Compensatory dietary pattern, established in the current research, may be identified in those volunteers who have adopted western dietary habits, but try to "*compensate*" this unhealthy pattern by increasing the consumption of "*healthy food*" or "*healthy snacks*" in addition to current intake [51–54]. This attempt of improvement leads to an overconsumption of energy with the subsequent weight gain [55,56]. These findings could help to explain the existing hypothesis of Mediterranean paradox [57].

Following this concept, the study of the Mediterranean paradox may be studied through the statistical analysis of dietary habits proposed in this study, which would allow the identification of the current clusters of diets and their evolution, preventing potential confounders [58], and not limiting the classification of individuals to a specific adherence.

In addition to dietary patterns, the study of attitudes towards diet and food may be considered an important tool for profiling individuals, and estimating the most suitable advice to obtain the most effective response in weight loss programs. Variables such as the advice provider (whose profession is delivering dietary advice), or concerns on how the information provided is held [59,60] can affect the acceptance of personalised nutrition advice.

However, it is important to take into account other synergistic conditions for overweight and obesity, such as genetic factors [61]. Although diet and lifestyle are triggers to maintain or increase body weight and fat mass, the success of prescribed dietary programs may also rely on the presence of determined SNPs related with the metabolism of different nutrients [62]. In addition, those dietary habits may modulate epigenetic marks in earlier life-stages that could alter the disease risk and may also modify the response to futures dietary interventions [63].

4.3. Tailoring the Advice Based on Prediction of Dietary Behaviours

Based on the results obtained in the current analyses, and taking into account the previously discussed Mediterranean paradox [57], it seems of major importance to enhance Public Health Advice with the use of feasible and relatively simple tools to diagnose and predict specific targets for specific dietary patterns [64].

If a patient shows a "Compensatory" eating behaviour, the advice on increasing omega-3, shall be led to a secondary scenario, and the reduction of Factor 1 foods may be more effective to prevent future diseases. Furthermore, overconsumption of energy, with an important component of oils and snacks, may be a major contributor of this inflammation, which would revert more rapidly than increasing omega-3 intake. Nevertheless, sensible and evidence-based nutritional advice should always prevail [61]; it may be proposed to further explore changes in the priority of the advice, depending on subjects' behaviours.

5. Conclusions

The results obtained in the present study suggest that statistical analyses of dietary intake from populations help to describe current dietary patterns, which facilitate the targeting of nutritional objectives to tailor dietary management. Furthermore, prevention of overweight may not be reached by only encouraging the inclusion of healthy choices, but also by a specific stress on limiting deleterious foods.

Supplementary Materials: Supplementary materials can be accessed at: http://www.mdpi.com/2072-6643/7/11/5482/s1.

Acknowledgments: The Food4Me study is supported by the European Commission under the Food, Agriculture, Fisheries and Biotechnology Theme of the 7th Framework Programme for Research and Technological Development, Grant Number 265494. The authors want to thank all the volunteers who took part in the study, as well as Maria Hernández Ruiz de Eguilaz, Salomé Perez-Diez and Blanca Martínez de Morentin for technical and laboratory support. Rodrigo San-Cristóbal is thankful for the scholarship of the University of Navarra (Asociación de Amigos—ADA). Johanna Bolinder (St. Mary's University) is gratefully acknowledged for careful reading of the final version of the manuscript.

Author Contributions: Author responsibilities were as follows: R.S.-C. and S.N.-C. wrote the paper and performed the statistical analysis for the manuscript. R.S.-C. and S.N.-C. are joint first authors. J.A.M. was the responsible of Spanish centre of intervention. C.C.-M., L.B., M.W., J.A.L., H.D., W.H.M.S., I.T., Y.M., E.R.G., M.J.G., J.C.M. and J.A.M. contributed to the research design. All authors contributed to a critical review of the manuscript during the writing process. All authors approved the final version to be published.

Conflicts of Interest: The authors declare no conflict of interest.

References

1. Margetts, B. Feedback on WHO/FAO global report on diet, nutrition and prevention of chronic diseases(NCD). *Public Health Nutr.* **2003**, *6*, 423–424. [CrossRef] [PubMed]
2. Nishida, C.; Uauy, R.; Kumanyika, S.; Shetty, P. The joint WHO/FAO expert consultation on diet, nutrition and the prevention of chronic diseases: Process, product and policy implications. *Public Health Nutr.* **2004**, *7*, 245–250. [CrossRef] [PubMed]
3. Tonstad, S.; Malik, N.; Haddad, E. A high-fibre bean-rich diet *versus* a low-carbohydrate diet for obesity. *J. Hum. Nutr. Diet.* **2014**, *27*, 109–116. [CrossRef] [PubMed]
4. Barkoukis, H. Importance of understanding food consumption patterns. *J. Am. Diet. Assoc.* **2007**, *107*, 234–236. [CrossRef] [PubMed]
5. Jebb, S.A. Carbohydrates and obesity: From evidence to policy in the UK. *Proc. Nutr. Soc.* **2015**, *74*, 215–220. [CrossRef] [PubMed]
6. Te Morenga, L.; Mallard, S.; Mann, J. Dietary sugars and body weight: Systematic review and meta-analyses of randomised controlled trials and cohort studies. *BMJ* **2013**, *346*, e7492. [CrossRef] [PubMed]
7. Trichopoulou, A.; Costacou, T.; Bamia, C.; Trichopoulos, D. Adherence to a mediterranean diet and survival in a Greek population. *N. Engl. J. Med.* **2003**, *348*, 2599–2608. [CrossRef] [PubMed]

8. Sleiman, D.; Al-Badri, M.R.; Azar, S.T. Effect of mediterranean diet in diabetes control and cardiovascular risk modification: A systematic review. *Front. Public Health* **2015**, *3*, 69. [CrossRef] [PubMed]

9. Hong, X.; Xu, F.; Wang, Z.; Liang, Y.; Li, J. Dietary patterns and the incidence of hyperglyacemia in China. *Public Health Nutr.* **2015**. [CrossRef] [PubMed]

10. Guenther, P.M.; Casavale, K.O.; Reedy, J.; Kirkpatrick, S.I.; Hiza, H.A.; Kuczynski, K.J.; Kahle, L.L.; Krebs-Smith, S.M. Update of the healthy eating index: HEI-2010. *J. Acad. Nutr. Diet.* **2013**, *113*, 569–580. [CrossRef] [PubMed]

11. Trichopoulou, A.; Kourisblazos, A.; Wahlqvist, M.L.; Gnardellis, C.; Lagiou, P.; Polychronopoulos, E.; Vassilakou, T.; Lipworth, L.; Trichopoulos, D. Diet and overall survival in elderly people. *BMJ* **1995**, *311*, 1457–1460. [CrossRef] [PubMed]

12. Wirfalt, A.K.; Jeffery, R.W. Using cluster analysis to examine dietary patterns: Nutrient intakes, gender, and weight status differ across food pattern clusters. *J. Am. Diet. Assoc.* **1997**, *97*, 272–279. [CrossRef]

13. Moeller, S.M.; Reedy, J.; Millen, A.E.; Dixon, L.B.; Newby, P.K.; Tucker, K.L.; Krebs-Smith, S.M.; Guenther, P.M. Dietary patterns: Challenges and opportunities in dietary patterns research an Experimental Biology workshop, April 1, 2006. *J. Am. Diet. Assoc.* **2007**, *107*, 1233–1239. [CrossRef] [PubMed]

14. Celis-Morales, C.; Livingstone, K.M.; Marsaux, C.F.; Forster, H.; O'Donovan, C.B.; Woolhead, C.; Macready, A.L.; Fallaize, R.; Navas-Carretero, S.; San-Cristobal, R.; *et al.* Design and baseline characteristics of the Food4Me study: A web-based randomised controlled trial of personalised nutrition in seven European countries. *Genes Nutr.* **2015**, *10*, 450. [CrossRef] [PubMed]

15. Black, A.E. Critical evaluation of energy intake using the goldberg cut-off for energy intake: Basal metabolic rate. A practical guide to its calculation, use and limitations. *Int. J. Obes. Relat. Metab. Disord.* **2000**, *24*, 1119–1130. [CrossRef] [PubMed]

16. Forster, H.; Fallaize, R.; Gallagher, C.; O'Donovan, C.B.; Woolhead, C.; Walsh, M.C.; Macready, A.L.; Lovegrove, J.A.; Mathers, J.C.; Gibney, M.J.; *et al.* Online dietary intake estimation: The Food4Me food frequency questionnaire. *J. Med. Int. Res.* **2014**, *16*, e150. [CrossRef] [PubMed]

17. Fallaize, R.; Forster, H.; Macready, A.L.; Walsh, M.C.; Mathers, J.C.; Brennan, L.; Gibney, E.R.; Gibney, M.J.; Lovegrove, J.A. Online dietary intake estimation: Reproducibility and validity of the Food4Me food frequency questionnaire against a 4-day weighed food record. *J. Med. Internet Res.* **2014**, *16*, e190. [CrossRef] [PubMed]

18. Chiuve, S.E.; Fung, T.T.; Rimm, E.B.; Hu, F.B.; McCullough, M.L.; Wang, M.; Stampfer, M.J.; Willett, W.C. Alternative dietary indices both strongly predict risk of chronic disease. *J. Nutr.* **2012**, *142*, 1009–1018. [CrossRef] [PubMed]

19. Celis-Morales, C.; Livingstone, K.; Woolhead, C.; Forster, H.; O'Donovan, C.; Macready, A.; Fallaize, R.; Marsaux, C.M.; Tsirigoti, L.; Efstathopoulou, E.; *et al.* How reliable is internet-based self-reported identity, socio-demographic and obesity measures in european adults? *Genes Nutr.* **2015**, *10*, 1–10. [CrossRef] [PubMed]

20. Svensson, M.; Hult, M.; van der Mark, M.; Grotta, A.; Jonasson, J.; von Hausswolff-Juhlin, Y.; Rossner, S.; Lagerros, Y.T. The change in eating behaviors in a web-based weight loss program: A longitudinal analysis of study completers. *J. Med. Internet Res.* **2014**, *16*, e234. [CrossRef] [PubMed]

21. Collins, C.E.; Morgan, P.J.; Hutchesson, M.J.; Callister, R. Efficacy of standard *versus* enhanced features in a Web-based commercial weight-loss program for obese adults, part 2: Randomized controlled trial. *J. Med. Internet Res.* **2013**, *15*, e140. [CrossRef] [PubMed]

22. Brindal, E.; Freyne, J.; Saunders, I.; Berkovsky, S.; Smith, G.; Noakes, M. Features predicting weight loss in overweight or obese participants in a web-based intervention: Randomized trial. *J. Med. Internet Res.* **2012**, *14*, e173. [CrossRef] [PubMed]

23. O'Brien, K.M.; Hutchesson, M.J.; Jensen, M.; Morgan, P.; Callister, R.; Collins, C.E. Participants in an online weight loss program can improve diet quality during weight loss: A randomized controlled trial. *Nutr. J.* **2014**, *13*, 82. [CrossRef] [PubMed]

24. Postrach, E.; Aspalter, R.; Elbelt, U.; Koller, M.; Longin, R.; Schulzke, J.D.; Valentini, L. Determinants of successful weight loss after using a commercial web-based weight reduction program for six months: Cohort study. *J. Med. Internet Res.* **2013**, *15*, e219. [CrossRef] [PubMed]

25. Kaipainen, K.; Payne, C.R.; Wansink, B. Mindless eating challenge: Retention, weight outcomes, and barriers for changes in a public web-based healthy eating and weight loss program. *J. Med. Internet Res.* **2012**, *14*, e168. [CrossRef] [PubMed]

26. Springvloet, L.; Lechner, L.; de Vries, H.; Oenema, A. Long-term efficacy of a Web-based computer-tailored nutrition education intervention for adults including cognitive and environmental feedback: A randomized controlled trial. *BMC Public Health* **2015**, *15*, 372. [CrossRef] [PubMed]

27. Ashwell, M.; Howarth, E.; Chesters, D.; Allan, P.; Hoyland, A.; Walton, J. A web-based weight loss programme including breakfast cereals results in greater loss of body mass than a standardised web-based programme in a randomised controlled trial. *Obes. Facts* **2014**, *7*, 361–375. [CrossRef] [PubMed]

28. Spittaels, H.; de Bourdeaudhuij, I.; Brug, J.; Vandelanotte, C. Effectiveness of an online computer-tailored physical activity intervention in a real-life setting. *Health Educ. Res.* **2007**, *22*, 385–396. [CrossRef] [PubMed]

29. Hutchesson, M.J.; Collins, C.E.; Morgan, P.J.; Watson, J.F.; Guest, M.; Callister, R. Changes to dietary intake during a 12-week commercial web-based weight loss program: A randomized controlled trial. *Eur. J. Clin. Nutr.* **2014**, *68*, 64–70. [CrossRef] [PubMed]

30. De Sanidad, S.; Estadística, S.E. Encuesta Nacional de Salud 2011–2012. Available online: http://www.ine.es/prensa/np770.pdf (accessed on 10 November 2015).

31. Willett, W.C.; Howe, G.R.; Kushi, L.H. Adjustment for total energy intake in epidemiologic studies. *Am. J. Clin. Nutr.* **1997**, *65*, 1220S–1228S. [PubMed]

32. Northstone, K.; Ness, A.R.; Emmett, P.M.; Rogers, I.S. Adjusting for energy intake in dietary pattern investigations using principal components analysis. *Eur. J. Clin. Nutr.* **2008**, *62*, 931–938. [CrossRef] [PubMed]

33. Judd, S.E.; Letter, A.J.; Shikany, J.M.; Roth, D.L.; Newby, P.K. Dietary patterns derived using exploratory and confirmatory factor analysis are stable and generalizable across race, region, and gender subgroups in the regards study. *Front. Nutr.* **2014**, *1*, 29. [CrossRef] [PubMed]

34. Smith, A.D.; Emmett, P.M.; Newby, P.K.; Northstone, K. Dietary patterns obtained through principal components analysis: The effect of input variable quantification. *Br. J. Nutr.* **2013**, *109*, 1881–1891. [CrossRef] [PubMed]

35. Newby, P.K.; Tucker, K.L. Empirically derived eating patterns using factor or cluster analysis: A review. *Nutr. Rev.* **2004**, *62*, 177–203. [CrossRef] [PubMed]

36. Devlin, U.M.; McNulty, B.A.; Nugent, A.P.; Gibney, M.J. The use of cluster analysis to derive dietary patterns: Methodological considerations, reproducibility, validity and the effect of energy mis-reporting. *Proc. Nutr. Soc.* **2012**, *71*, 599–609. [CrossRef] [PubMed]

37. Sun, J.; Buys, N.J.; Hills, A.P. Dietary pattern and its association with the prevalence of obesity, hypertension and other cardiovascular risk factors among chinese older adults. *Int. J. Environ. Res. Public Health* **2014**, *11*, 3956–3971. [CrossRef] [PubMed]

38. Newby, P.K.; Muller, D.; Hallfrisch, J.; Qiao, N.; Andres, R.; Tucker, K.L. Dietary patterns and changes in body mass index and waist circumference in adults. *Am. J. Clin. Nutr.* **2003**, *77*, 1417–1425. [PubMed]

39. Flores, M.; Macias, N.; Rivera, M.; Lozada, A.; Barquera, S.; Rivera-Dommarco, J.; Tucker, K.L. Dietary patterns in mexican adults are associated with risk of being overweight or obese. *J. Nutr.* **2010**, *140*, 1869–1873. [CrossRef] [PubMed]

40. Howe, A.S.; Black, K.E.; Wong, J.E.; Parnell, W.R.; Skidmore, P.M. Dieting status influences associations between dietary patterns and body composition in adolescents: A cross-sectional study. *Nutr. J.* **2013**, *12*, 51. [CrossRef] [PubMed]

41. Ambrosini, G.L. Childhood dietary patterns and later obesity: A review of the evidence. *Proc. Nutr. Soc.* **2014**, *73*, 137–146. [CrossRef] [PubMed]

42. He, Y.; Li, Y.; Lai, J.; Wang, D.; Zhang, J.; Fu, P.; Yang, X.; Qi, L. Dietary patterns as compared with physical activity in relation to metabolic syndrome among chinese adults. *Nutr. Metab. Cardiovasc. Dis.* **2013**, *23*, 920–928. [CrossRef] [PubMed]

43. Hong, S.; Song, Y.; Lee, K.H.; Lee, H.S.; Lee, M.; Jee, S.H.; Joung, H. A fruit and dairy dietary pattern is associated with a reduced risk of metabolic syndrome. *Metabolism* **2012**, *61*, 883–890. [CrossRef] [PubMed]

44. Garduno-Diaz, S.D.; Khokhar, S. South asian dietary patterns and their association with risk factors for the metabolic syndrome. *J. Hum. Nutr. Diet.* **2013**, *26*, 145–155. [CrossRef] [PubMed]

Nutrients **2015**, *7*, 9523–9537

45. Hu, F.B.; Rimm, E.B.; Stampfer, M.J.; Ascherio, A.; Spiegelman, D.; Willett, W.C. Prospective study of major dietary patterns and risk of coronary heart disease in men. *Am. J. Clin. Nutr.* **2000**, *72*, 912–921. [PubMed]
46. Mente, A.; de Koning, L.; Shannon, H.S.; Anand, S.S. A systematic review of the evidence supporting a causal link between dietary factors and coronary heart disease. *Arch. Intern. Med.* **2009**, *169*, 659–669. [CrossRef] [PubMed]
47. Varela-Moreiras, G.; Avila, J.M.; Cuadrado, C.; del Pozo, S.; Ruiz, E.; Moreiras, O. Evaluation of food consumption and dietary patterns in spain by the food consumption survey: Updated information. *Eur. J. Clin. Nutr.* **2010**, *64*, S37–S43. [CrossRef] [PubMed]
48. Da Silva, R.; Bach-Faig, A.; Raido Quintana, B.; Buckland, G.; vaz de Almeida, M.D.; Serra-Majem, L. Worldwide variation of adherence to the mediterranean diet, in 1961–1965 and 2000–2003. *Public Health Nutr.* **2009**, *12*, 1676–1684. [CrossRef] [PubMed]
49. Kyriacou, A.; Evans, J.M.; Economides, N. Adherence to the Mediterranean diet by the Greek and Cypriot population: A systematic review. *Eur. J. Public Health* **2015**. [CrossRef]
50. Dernini, S.; Berry, E.M. Mediterranean diet: From a healthy diet to a sustainable dietary pattern. *Front. Nutr.* **2015**, *2*, 15. [CrossRef] [PubMed]
51. De Vet, E.; de Wit, J.B.; Luszczynska, A.; Stok, F.M.; Gaspar, T.; Pratt, M.; Wardle, J.; de Ridder, D.T. Access to excess: How do adolescents deal with unhealthy foods in their environment? *Eur. J. Public Health* **2013**, *23*, 752–756. [CrossRef] [PubMed]
52. De Graaf, C. Effects of snacks on energy intake: An evolutionary perspective. *Appetite* **2006**, *47*, 18–23. [CrossRef] [PubMed]
53. Barnes, T.L.; French, S.A.; Harnack, L.J.; Mitchell, N.R.; Wolfson, J. Snacking behaviors, diet quality, and body mass index in a community sample of working adults. *J. Acad. Nutr. Diet.* **2015**, *115*, 1117–1123. [CrossRef] [PubMed]
54. Berteus Forslund, H.; Torgerson, J.S.; Sjostrom, L.; Lindroos, A.K. Snacking frequency in relation to energy intake and food choices in obese men and women compared to a reference population. *Int. J. Obes.* **2005**, *29*, 711–719. [CrossRef] [PubMed]
55. Bellisle, F. Meals and snacking, diet quality and energy balance. *Physiol. Behav.* **2014**, *134*, 38–43. [CrossRef] [PubMed]
56. Chapelot, D. The role of snacking in energy balance: A biobehavioral approach. *J. Nutr.* **2011**, *141*, 158–162. [CrossRef] [PubMed]
57. Soriguer, F.; Garcia-Escobar, E.; Morcillo, S.; Garcia-Fuentes, E.; de Fonseca, F.; Olveira, G.; Rojo-Martinez, G. Mediterranean diet and the spanish paradox. A hypothesis. *Med. Hypotheses* **2013**, *80*, 150–155. [CrossRef] [PubMed]
58. Panagiotakos, D.B.; Chrysohoou, C.; Pitsavos, C.; Stefanadis, C. Association between the prevalence of obesity and adherence to the mediterranean diet: The ATTICA study. *Nutrition* **2006**, *22*, 449–456. [CrossRef] [PubMed]
59. San-Cristobal, R.; Milagro, F.I.; Martinez, J.A. Future challenges and present ethical considerations in the use of personalized nutrition based on genetic advice. *J. Acad. Nutr. Diet.* **2013**, *113*, 1447–1454. [CrossRef] [PubMed]
60. Stewart-Knox, B.; Kuznesof, S.; Robinson, J.; Rankin, A.; Orr, K.; Duffy, M.; Poinhos, R.; de Almeida, M.D.; Macready, A.; Gallagher, C.; *et al.* Factors influencing european consumer uptake of personalised nutrition. Results of a qualitative analysis. *Appetite* **2013**, *66*, 67–74. [CrossRef] [PubMed]
61. Martinez, J.A.; Navas-Carretero, S.; Saris, W.H.; Astrup, A. Personalized weight loss strategies-the role of macronutrient distribution. *Nat. Rev. Endocrinol.* **2014**, *10*, 749–760. [CrossRef] [PubMed]
62. Martinez, J.A.; Milagro, F.I. Genetics of weight loss: A basis for personalized obesity management. *Trends Food Sci. Technol.* **2015**, *42*, 97–115. [CrossRef]

63. Milagro, F.I.; Mansego, M.L.; de Miguel, C.; Martinez, J.A. Dietary factors, epigenetic modifications and obesity outcomes: Progresses and perspectives. *Mol. Aspects Med.* **2013**, *34*, 782–812. [CrossRef] [PubMed]

64. Friedl, K.E.; Rowe, S.; Bellows, L.L.; Johnson, S.L.; Hetherington, M.M.; de Froidmont-Gortz, I.; Lammens, V.; Hubbard, V.S. Report of an EU-US symposium on understanding nutrition-related consumer behavior: Strategies to promote a lifetime of healthy food choices. *J. Nutr. Educ. Behav.* **2014**, *46*, 445–450. [CrossRef] [PubMed]

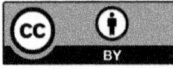

nutrients

MDPI

Article

Nutrient Patterns and Their Association with Socio-Demographic, Lifestyle Factors and Obesity Risk in Rural South African Adolescents

Pedro T. Pisa [1],*, Titilola M. Pedro [1], Kathleen Kahn [2,3,4], Stephen M. Tollman [2,3,4], John M. Pettifor [1] and Shane A. Norris [1]

[1]   MRC/Wits Developmental Pathways for Health Research Unit, Department of Paediatrics, Faculty of Health Sciences, University of the Witwatersrand, Johannesburg 2193 South Africa; titilolapedro@gmail.com (T.M.P.); John.Pettifor@wits.ac.za (J.M.P.); Shane.Norris@wits.ac.za (S.A.N.)
[2]   MRC/Wits Rural Public Health and Health Transitions Research Unit (Agincourt), School of Public Health, Faculty of Health Sciences, University of the Witwatersrand, Johannesburg 2193, South Africa; Kathleen.Kahn@wits.ac.za (K.K.); Stephen.Tollman@wits.ac.za (S.-M.T.)
[3]   Centre for Global Health Research, Umeå University, Umeå SE-901 87, Sweden
[4]   INDEPTH Network: Network of Demographic Surveillance Sites-www.indepth-network.org, Accra, Ghana
*   Author to whom correspondence should be addressed; Pedro.Pisa@wits.ac.za or pppedropissa@gmail.com; Tel.: +27-(0)73-703-2436 or +27-(0)11-717-72383.

Received: 20 March 2015; Accepted: 14 April 2015; Published: 12 May 2015

Abstract: The aim of this study was to identify and describe the diversity of nutrient patterns and how they associate with socio-demographic and lifestyle factors including body mass index in rural black South African adolescents. Nutrient patterns were identified from quantified food frequency questionnaires (QFFQ) in 388 rural South African adolescents between the ages of 11–15 years from the Agincourt Health and Socio-demographic Surveillance System (AHDSS). Principle Component Analysis (PCA) was applied to 25 nutrients derived from QFFQs. Multiple linear regression and partial R^2 models were fitted and computed respectively for each of the retained principal component (PC) scores on socio-demographic and lifestyle characteristics including body mass index (BMI) for age Z scores. Four nutrient patterns explaining 79% of the total variance were identified: PCI (26%) was characterized by animal derived nutrients; PC2 (21%) by vitamins, fibre and vegetable oil nutrients; PC3 (19%) by both animal and plant derived nutrients (mixed diet driven nutrients); and PC4 (13%) by starch and folate. A positive and significant association was observed with BMI for age Z scores per 1 standard deviation (SD) increase in PC1 (0.13 (0.02; 0.24); $p = 0.02$) and PC4 (0.10 (−0.01; 0.21); $p = 0.05$) scores only. We confirmed variability in nutrient patterns that were significantly associated with various lifestyle factors including obesity.

Keywords: nutrient patterns; adolescents; rural; South Africa; transition; Agincourt health and demographic surveillance system

---

1. Introduction

The assessment of food and/or nutrient patterns and their relation with non-communicable diseases (NCDs) and obesity is an alternative to the traditional approach focusing on single foods or nutrients. The traditional approach is limited in its ability to demonstrate the impact of nutrient intakes on NCD outcomes because of difficulties in explaining interactions between nutrients and in the lack of ability to detect small effects from single nutrients [1]. Identifying food or nutrient patterns is less complex methodologically and more relevant from a biological and physiological point of view as they allow the analysis of a small number of patterns rather than an array of individual foods and intakes of nutrients that are usually inter-correlated [2,3]. Thus this approach offers a strong complementary strategy to capture the intrinsic complexity of diet, the inter-relationships between different components and the heterogeneity in food and nutrient patterns existing within and between populations [1,4].

Both food and nutrient pattern analyses have been conducted on usual food consumption derived from quantitative food frequency questionnaires using exploratory dimension reduction methods (*i.e.*, principal component analysis) to empirically derive patterns. These multivariate approaches aim to summarize a large number of correlated dietary variables (foods, food groups, nutrients or biomarkers) into fewer independent components (the so called "patterns") explaining most of the dietary variability despite large within and between variations [1,5–7]. In contrast to food patterns, limited work has been done on nutrient patterns analysis to date, [3,8–22] with no data available for either approach in Africa.

South Africa, a country undergoing a rapid health transition, characterized by a triple burden of disease including infectious-related under-nutrition illnesses, HIV/AIDs and tuberculosis, and emerging NCDs [23–25], has evidence suggesting that the black rural South African population, who were once protected in terms of chronic diseases and obesity, are increasingly susceptible [24]. This could in part be attributed to shifting from traditional prudent diets to high energy, high fat diets, to increasing exposure to less-nutrient-dense foods, and to increasing sedentary behaviour [23,25–27]. Such evidence in African adolescence is scarce and deserves further attention. The few data available suggest increases of childhood and adolescent obesity levels [28–31]. Adolescence, a critical phase characterized by increased vulnerability and exposure to inappropriate diets, could be a major determinant of obesity or developing NCDs in later adulthood [32,33]. To date, no information is available in Africa, characterizing either food or nutrient patterns and associating them with various outcomes including obesity. In this paper, we aim to identify and describe the diversity of nutrient patterns and how depicted patterns associate with socio-demographic and lifestyle factors including body mass index (BMI) in rural black South African adolescents.

2. Materials and Methods

2.1. Study Population and Design

This cross-sectional study was nested within the Agincourt Health and Socio-demographic Surveillance System (AHDSS), which has been described in detail previously [34,35]. Participants were recruited in 2009 and a sub-sample of 600 participants between the ages of 7–15 years were randomly selected from 3511 children and adolescents who had participated in a 2007 growth survey in the Agincourt sub-district of Mpumalanga Province in South Africa [31]. The original 2007growth study randomly selected children and adolescents between the ages of 1 and 20 years (~100 boys and 100 girls for each year of age) who had lived in the study area at least 80% of the time since birth, or since 1992 when enrolment into the Agincourt HDSS had begun. A random sample of children was drawn from each age-sex-village stratum in proportion to the population size of the village. For this present analysis 388 participants aged 11–15 years (Boys: N = 193; mean age 13.53; Girls: N = 195; mean age 13.60) on whom dietary data were collected, were included. To ensure that this sub-sample was representative of the larger 2007 study sample [36] we compared various socio-economic status (SES) parameters between the samples, and found no differences (data not shown). Comprehensive details of the methods of recruitment and design have been published elsewhere [34,35].

2.2. Ethical Approval

Ethical approval was granted by the University of the Witwatersrand Committee for Research on Human Subjects (Ethics number: M090212), and from the Mpumalanga Provincial Government's Department of Health. Parental consent and participant assent were secured after full explanation of the study objectives and testing procedures.

2.3. Measurement of Diet, Lifestyle Factors, Anthropometric Indicators and Socio-Demographic Information

Diet: Usual diet was assessed for each adolescent using an interviewer-administered quantitative food frequency questionnaire (QFFQ) developed for use in South Africa (SA) [37]. The interview took on average 40 minutes to complete and the QFFQ includes a total of 214 commonly eaten foods [37]. Analyses of 11 dietary surveys conducted in rural and urban SA since 1983 were used to derive these food items, and the list includes all foods eaten by at least 3% of the population [38]. To cater for illiteracy and to improve recall ability, this QFFQ utilizes food flash cards (high quality photographs) of all the food items [39].

Data were collected on the previous week's (7 day) dietary intake, including convenience food products, in order to estimate habitual intake for each participant. Participants were asked to separate the food flash cards into a series of piles: firstly, they went through each food card and created a pile of food items they 'rarely/never' ate or drank. Thereafter, the remaining food cards were divided into a pile of food items they eat/drink less frequently ('occasional'), and a pile they eat regularly and in the past seven days. The participant was then prompted for information on the frequency and amounts of the regular food items in their diet consumed, the details of which were recorded on the QFFQ [37].

Portion sizes were estimated using household measures and a combination of two-dimensional life-size drawings of foods and utensils, and three-dimensional food models as described and validated by Steyn *et al.* [40]. Items eaten occasionally or rarely/never were also recorded. Coding involved the conversion of the household measures (for example one cup/one serving spoon/one slice) to grams so that an average intake over the previous seven days could be calculated. The quantity and frequency of all consumed foods were recorded and expressed in g/day. Nutrient composition of foods was calculated and all conversions were based on the South African food composition tables [41].

Anthropometry: Height (in mm) was measured using a stadiometer (Holtain, UK) and converted to metres (m), and weight was measured to the nearest 0.1 kg using an electronic bathroom scale. All participants were measured wearing light clothing and without shoes. BMI was calculated as weight in kilograms (kg) divided by height (m)^2. BMI for age Z-scores were generated using WHO 2007 growth reference standards [42] for children aged 5 to 19 years and obesity is defined as a score above 2SD. Waist circumference was measured using an inelastic tape measure midway between the tenth rib and the iliac crest. Hip circumference was measured at the level of maximum width of the buttocks with the participant standing. Waist-to-hip ratio was calculated by dividing waist (cm) by hip (cm) circumference and waist-to-height ratio was calculated by dividing waist circumference (cm) by height (cm).

Pubertal staging: Pubertal staging was assessed using the Tanner 5-point pubertal self-rating scale which has been validated previously for black South Africans [43]. Genital development in boys and breast development in girls were used to define pubertal stages. Participants were classified as early-puberty ($\leq$Tanner stage 2), and mid-puberty (Tanner stage > 2) [43].

Physical activity: A questionnaire quantifying total physical activity (PA) for the previous 12 months was administered via interview. The questionnaire was developed to be appropriate for South African children, and has been used [44] and validated on urban South African children [45]. Reported frequency and duration of all physical activities (physical education, extra-mural school and club sport, informal physical activity, and walking to and from school) and sedentary activities were recorded. The most reliable (and most complete data) proxy for attaining one's physical activity level was the total time in minutes spent walking to and from school per week [46] and this parameter was used as a covariate in the present analysis.

Socio-demographics: A variety of socio-demographic and other related data were included from the growth survey conducted two years previously. These included data on the participants' mothers (age, education level, marital/union status and whether she resides with the participant or not) and SES. These variables and others have been described in detail previously [31].

2.4. Data Analysis

Data were analyzed using SPSS statistics software version 20. Principal Component Analysis (PCA) was used to depict nutrient patterns [47] based on the QFFQ derived intake of 25 nutrients. Total fat was divided into monounsaturated, polyunsaturated, saturated fatty acids and cholesterol, whilst total available carbohydrates were divided into starch and sugars (monosaccharides and disaccharides). Total proteins were additionally divided into animal and plant proteins. Alcohol consumption was considered as a main lifestyle factor and was not included in the list of variables to derive nutrient patterns. Additionally alcohol intakes in this adolescent population were negligible 0.02 (+/−0.28) g day^{-1}).

Variables were log transformed (natural log) after comparing various analysis options with regard to proportion of variance captured. Log transformation provides an advantage as it renders the variances and covariances independent of scale. PCA was applied with the covariance matrix, rather than the correlation matrix. Variance was based on rotated sums of squared loadings and the Varimax with Kaiser Normalization was used as the orthogonal rotation method, as it maximizes the loading of each variable on one of the extracted factors whilst minimizing the loading on all other factors. In order to capture variability of nutrient intakes independently from variation in energy intake, nutrients (log variables) were adjusted for log total energy intake when applying PCA using the multivariate (standard) method [48]. PCA were conducted on both sexes combined and separated. As comparable patterns were observed in both sexes in PCA the final results are presented for both sexes combined.

The number of retained principal components (PC) or "patterns" was determined taking into account several criteria which included the interpretation of the patterns, the percentage of total variance explained and the visual inflections in the scree-plots of eigen-values (Figure 1) [47]. Nutrients with absolute loadings greater or equal to +/−0.40 on a given PC were used to name the retained PC and provide a nutritional interpretation (Figure 2). The loadings represent covariance between the nutrients and the patterns. Nutrients with positive loadings were positively associated with a nutrient pattern while negative loadings were inversely associated. PCA was the most appropriate multivariate reduction technique to apply in this sample as demonstrated statistically by a Kaiser-Meyer-Olkin measure of sampling adequacy of 0.9 and Bartlett's test of sphericity significant at $p < 0.001$.

Multiple linear regression models were fitted for each of the PC scores on the following socio-demographic and lifestyle characteristics: Sex (by category: males, females), age of adolescent (continuous), BMI (continuous), log of total energy intake (continuous), physical activity (continuous: total minutes to and from school per week), maternal educational level (by category: none, primary school, secondary and higher), Tanner stage (by category: early, mid), marital status of mother (by category: ever in union current, ever in union never, ever in union ended), maternal age (by category: 15–24, 25–34, 35–49, >50 years), maternal SES (by category: lowest tertile (third), middle tertile, highest tertile). Regression coefficients and their standard errors are presented. Partial R^2 were calculated to express the proportion of variance of PC scores explained by each of the measured lifestyle variables. The retained principal components were further divided into tertiles, based on individual PC scores. Analysis of variance (ANOVA) (continuous variables) and chi-squared test (categorical variables) were used to compare differences across tertiles for socio-demographic, anthropometric and dietary intakes.

Multiple linear regression models were computed for each of the PC scores with BMI for age Z scores as an outcome (dependent variable-continuous). Regression coefficients for 1SD increase in PC scores for each depicted nutrient pattern were computed for three models M1: (crude), M2: (adjusted for M1 plus physical activity), M3: (adjusted for M2 plus SES of mother) and M4: (adjusted for M3 plus educational level of the mother). Mutually adjusting for all PCs did not affect the above mentioned models. All statistical significance were defined using a 2-sided p-value < 0.05.

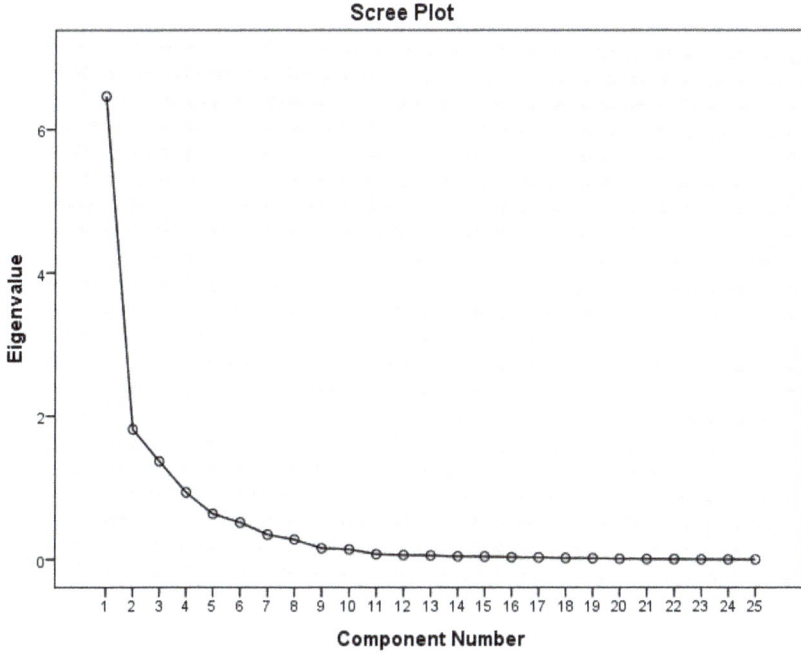

Figure 1. Scree plot of Eigen values after Principal Components Analysis.

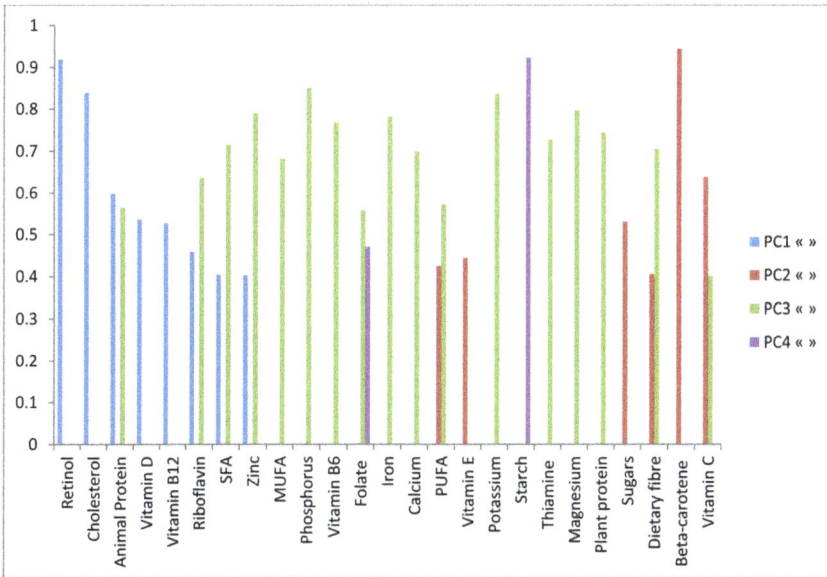

Figure 2. Plotted loadings (all > 0.4) for principal components(1–4).

3. Results

3.1. Identification and Description of Depicted Nutrient Patterns (PC)

Four nutrient patterns, which explained about 79% of the total variance (total nutrient variability), were retained by the overall PCA (N = 388) (Table 1). The 1st PC retained had largest positive loadings on animal protein, saturated fat, cholesterol, riboflavin, vitamin B12, retinol, vitamin D and zinc (nutrients mainly of animal origin). Because of these positive loadings this PC was named *"Animal driven nutrients"*. This pattern accounted for 26% of the variance in nutrient intakes. The 2nd PC had the greatest positive loadings on the following vitamins: vitamin C, beta-carotene, and vitamin E. Additionally, dietary fibre, PUFA and sugars also had strong positive loadings. Because of these loadings this PC was named *"Vitamins, fibre and vegetable oil nutrients"*. This pattern accounted for 21% of the variance in nutrient intakes and is distinctively different from PC1. The 3rd PC was named *"mixed diet driven nutrients"* because of its heterogeneous nature in that both animal and plant derived nutrients had large positive loadings on the matrix. The greatest positive loadings were on the following (i) vitamins and minerals: thiamine, riboflavin, vitamin B12, vitamin B6, folate, vitamin C, calcium, phosphorus, iron, potassium, magnesium and zinc and; (ii) other nutrients: animal protein, plant protein, saturated fat, MUFA, PUFA and dietary fibre. This pattern accounted for 19% of the variance in nutrient intakes. The 4th and last PC retained accounted for 13% of the variance in nutrient intakes. This PC had the largest loadings on starch and folate and was termed the *"Starch and folate driven pattern"*.

Table 1. Principal Components (PC) loading matrix and explained variances for the first four nutrient patterns identified by PCA in rural black South African adolescents: Agincourt.

Nutrients	PC1 (Animal Driven Nutrients)	PC2 (Vitamins, Fibre and Vegetable Oil Nutrients)	PC3 (Mixed Diet Driven Nutrients)	PC4 (Starch and Folate Driven)
Animal Protein	0.599	−0.032	0.565	−0.019
Plant protein	0.127	0.255	0.744	0.249
SFA	0.404	0.205	0.716	0.179
MUFA	0.356	0.326	0.682	0.191
PUFA	0.298	0.425	0.573	0.25
Cholesterol	0.839	−0.005	0.371	0.115
Starch	0.207	0.235	0.165	0.923
Sugars	0.12	0.531	0.276	0.364
Dietary fibre	0.115	0.406	0.705	0.152
Thiamine	0.184	0.053	0.727	0.002
Riboflavin	0.459	0.105	0.636	0.058
Vitamin B$_6$	0.344	0.261	0.768	0.174
Folate	0.316	0.329	0.558	0.471
Vitamin B$_{12}$	0.528	0.059	0.27	0.089
Vitamin C	0.04	0.638	0.402	0.089
Beta-carotene	0.083	0.944	0.136	0.081
Retinol	0.919	0.211	-0.007	0.157
Vitamin E	0.243	0.444	0.381	0.277
Vitamin D	0.537	0.205	0.359	0.148
Calcium	0.307	0.33	0.699	0.118
Phosphorus	0.349	0.163	0.851	0.092
Iron	0.31	0.253	0.782	0.116
Potassium	0.239	0.323	0.837	0.172
Magnesium	0.128	0.308	0.797	0.043
Zinc	0.403	0.172	0.79	0.129
Explained variance (%)	26	21	19	13
Cumulative explained variance (%)	26	47	66	79

Principle Component Analysis (PCA) on 25 log-transformed nutrients adjusted for total energy intake (equivalent to alcohol-free energy in this adolescent sample). PCA, Saturated Fatty Acids (SFA), Monounsaturated Fatty Acids (MUFA), Polyunsaturated Fatty Acids (PUFA). Variance based on rotated Sums of Squared Loadings; Rotation method: Varimax with Kaiser Normalisation.

3.2. Dietary, Lifestyle, Anthropometric and Socio-Demographic Variables Associated with Identified Nutrient Patterns

Tables 2 and 3 show regression coefficients and partial R-squared of individual PC scores for each of the four patterns retained for energy, anthropometric, lifestyle and socio-demographic variables. Energy intake (log) was positively and significantly associated with all four patterns ($p < 0.0001$). Being female, never in union as marital status of mother of the adolescent, and maternal age between 35 and 49 years were positively and significantly associated with PC1 *"Animal driven nutrients"* ($p \leq 0.05$), whilst being in the lowest SES status tertile was negatively associated with the same PC ($p \leq 0.05$). Being in mid-puberty was positively and significantly associated with PC2 *"Vitamins, fibre and vegetable oil nutrients"* ($p \leq 0.05$). Physical activity (walking to and from school) and being in the lowest SES status tertile were positively associated with PC3 *"mixed diet driven nutrients"* ($p \leq 0.05$). PC4 was negatively associated with physical activity (walking to and from school) ($p \leq 0.05$) (Table 2). Variability explained by socio-demographic, anthropometric, lifestyle factors and energy intake for the four PCs is presented in Table 3. Energy intake significantly explained the most variability with 6.5%, 6%, 66.6%, and 6.7% for PC1, PC2, PC3 and PC4 respectively ($p < 0.0001$). Sex (2.6%: $p < 0.0001$), maternal education (5.9%: $p < 0.001$), BMI (1.3%: $p \leq 0.03$) and SES of mother (1.3%: $p \leq 0.04$) significantly contributed to the variability in PC1 *"Animal driven nutrients"*. Tanner stage significantly contributed to the variability (1.1%: $p \leq 0.04$) in PC2 *"Vitamins, fibre and vegetable oil nutrients"*, whilst physical activity (minutes walking to and from school per week) significantly contributed to the variability (1.3%: $p \leq 0.04$) in PC4 *"Starch and folate driven pattern"*.

Table 2. Multiple regression derived coefficients (β) and standard errors (SE) of specified predictors for the four nutrient pattern scores.

Variables	PC1 (Animal Driven Nutrients)			PC2 (Vitamins, Fibre and Vegetable Oil Nutrients)			PC3 (Mixed Diet Driven Nutrients)			PC4 (Starch and Folate Driven)		
	β	SE	p-Value	β	SE	p-Value	β	SE	p-Value	β	SE	p-Value
Age (years) of adolescent	-0.027	0.036	0.46	-0.046	0.036	0.21	0.033	0.022	0.14	0.007	0.037	0.84
BMI	0.024	0.016	0.15	-0.009	0.016	0.58	-0.005	0.1	0.64	0.001	0.017	0.98
Log (Energy)	0.607	0.132	<0.0001	0.601	0.132	<0.0001	2.127	0.08	<0.0001	0.665	0.135	<0.0001
Sex												
Female	0.235	0.11	0.03	-0.052	0.11	0.64	-0.046	0.067	0.5	0.147	0.112	0.19
Male (Ref)												
Maternal Education level												
Primary school	-0.041	0.13	0.75	0.09	0.131	0.49	-0.07	0.079	0.38	-0.16	0.133	0.24
Secondary and higher education	-0.147	0.138	0.29	0.171	0.138	0.22	-0.109	0.084	0.2	-0.57	0.141	0.69
None (Ref)												
Physical activity of adolescent												
Walking to and from school (min week⁻¹)	<0.0001	<0.0001	0.62	<0.0001	<0.0001	0.74	0.001	0.001	0.01	-0.001	0.001	0.05
Tanner stage												
Mid	-0.067	0.151	0.66	0.343	0.151	0.02	-0.045	0.092	0.62	0.014	0.154	0.93
Early (Ref)												
Marital Status of mother												
Never in union	0.231	0.121	0.05	0.196	0.121	0.11	-0.108	0.703	0.14	0.106	0.124	0.4
Ever in union ended	0.017	0.183	0.93	0.104	0.183	0.57	0.051	0.11	0.65	0.001	0.187	0.99
Ever in union current (Ref)												
Maternal age (years)												
15-24	0.289	0.975	0.77	0.966	0.978	0.32	-0.257	0.59	0.66	0.406	0.996	0.68
25-34 (Ref)												
35-49	0.264	0.115	0.02	0.007	0.115	0.95	-0.09	0.07	0.2	0.048	0.117	0.68
>50	-0.251	0.178	0.161	0.188	0.179	0.29	0.117	0.108	0.28	0.076	0.182	0.68
SES status of mother (based on SES Wealth Index)												
lowest tertile	-0.336	0.134	0.01	-0.098	0.134	0.46	0.166	0.081	0.04	-0.06	0.136	0.67
middle tertile	-0.11	0.132	0.4	-0.207	0.133	0.12	0.071	0.08	0.39	-0.07	0.135	0.62
highest tertile (Ref)												

PC scores had means of 0 but standardized to unit variance; PC scores calculated from QFF derived intake of 25 nutrients, *n* = 388; SES, socio-economic status socio-economic status; BMI, body mass index; Ref, reference group in the regression after creating dummy variables (categorical coding in regression analysis).

Table 3. p-Values of F-test on type III sum of squares estimate.

Variable	DF#	PC1 (Animal Driven Nutrients)			PC2 (Vitamins, Fibre and Vegetable Oil Nutrients)			PC3 (Mixed Diet Driven Nutrients)			PC4 (Starch and Folate Driven)		
		Partial R^2	%	p-value	Partial R^2	%	p-value	Partial R^2	%	p-value	Partial R^2	%	p-value
Age	1	0.001	0.1	0.57	0.001	0.1	0.48	0.009	0.9	0.06	0.001	0.1	0.51
BMI	1	0.013	1.3	0.03	0.001	0.1	0.64	0.003	0.3	0.28	0.006	0.6	0.12
Log(Energy)	1	0.065	6.5	<0.0001	0.06	6	<0.0001	0.666	66.6	<0.0001	0.067	6.7	<0.0001
Sex	1	0.026	2.6	<0.0001	0	0	0.85	0.005	0.5	0.17	0.004	0.4	0.23
Maternal education	2	0.059	5.9	<0.0001	0.006	0.6	0.2	0.002	0.2	0.51	0	0	0.84
Physical activity (Walking to and from school (min week^{-1})	1	0.005	0.5	0.17	0.001	0.1	0.5	0	0	0.96	0.013	1.3	0.02
Tanner Stage	1	0.001	0.1	0.65	0.011	1.1	0.04	0.002	0.2	0.33	0.002	0.2	0.41
Marital status of mother	2	0.001	0.1	0.51	0.008	0.8	0.1	0.001	0.1	0.57	0.001	0.1	0.61
Maternal age	3	0.002	0.2	0.4	0.001	0.1	0.55	0.001	0.1	0.59	0.001	0.1	0.6
SES status of mother (based on SES Wealth Index)	2	0.013	1.3	0.04	0.01	1	0.07	0	0	0.84	0.005	0.5	0.23

PC scores had means of 0 but standardized to unit variance; PC scores calculated from QFF derived intake of 25 nutrients, n = 388, # degrees of freedom; socio-economic status socio-economic status.

Table 4. Regression coefficients for BMI for Age Z scores for 1 SD increase in PC 1 (Animal driven nutrients) and PC 4 (Starch and folate driven) scores in rural black South African adolescents.

Nutrient pattern	M1		M2		M3		M4	
	B (95% CI)	p value	B (95% CI)	p value	B (95% CI)	p value	B (95% CI)	p value
PC1	0.129 (0.018–0.239)	0.02	0.137 (0.025; 0.248)	0.02	0.118 (0.005; 0.230)	0.04	0.120 (−0.005; 0.245)	0.06
Physical activity			2.191×10^{-5} (−0.001; 0.001)	0.95	0.0 (−0.001; 0.001)	0.78	6.67×10^{-5} (−0.001; 0.001)	0.87
Socio-economic status								
low tertile					−0.331 (−0.601; −0.060)	0.02	−0.346 (−0.672; −0.020)	0.04
middle tertile					0.009 (−0.262; 0.280)	0.95	0.144 (−0.172; 0.46)	0.37
highest tertile (ref)								
Maternal education								
Total number of years of schooling							0.026 (0.0; 0.053)	0.05
PC4	0.103 (−0.008; 0.213)	0.05	0.092 (−0.022; 0.206)	0.12	0.087 (−0.026; 0.201)	0.13	0.011 (−0.117; 0.138)	0.87
Physical activity			2.74×10^{-5} (−0.001; 0.001)	0.94	0.0 (−0.001; 0.001)	0.75	7.59×10^{-6} (−0.001; 0.001)	0.99
Socio-economic status								
low tertile					−0.361 (−0.629; −0.092)	0.01	−0.407 (−0.729; −0.085)	0.01
middle tertile					0.002 (−0.269; 0.273)	0.98	0.103 (−0.212; 0.418)	0.52
highest tertile (ref)								
Maternal education								
Total number of years of schooling							0.028 (0.002; 0.05)	0.04
R2 values of each model	0.009		0.007		0.029		0.063	

M1: (crude); M2: (adjusted for physical activity); M3: (adjusted for M2 plus socio-economic status of mother); M4: (adjusted for M3 plus educational level of mother); M1, model 1; M2, model 2; M3, model 3; M4 model 4. Ref, reference group in the regression after creating dummy variables (categorical coding in regression analysis).

Differences across tertiles for each retained PC for dietary, anthropometric, lifestyle and socio-demographic factors are presented in supplementary Table 1. BMI for age Z scores were used as a proxy or indicator of obesity status. Table 4 presents the adjusted increase in BMI for age Z scores per 1 SD increase in each retained PC score. For PC1, a positive significant association was observed with BMI for age Z scores in M1 (0.13 (0.02; 0.24); $p = 0.02$), M2 (0.14 (0.03; 0.25); $p = 0.02$) and M3 (0.12 (0.01; 0.24); $p = 0.04$). Comparable results were observed for PC4 in that a positive association was observed as well with BMI for age Z scores for M1 (0.10 (−0.01; 0.21); $p = 0.05$). No significant associations with BMI for age Z scores were observed for PC2 and PC3 and thus not presented.

4. Discussion

This is the first study to our knowledge to identify and describe nutrient patterns and how they relate to various variables/outcomes including obesity in rural black South African adolescents. The PCA technique used for the present analysis has several advantages especially in comparison to the generic factor analysis. PCs retained are generated sequentially, meaning the variance explained by the first factor is removed, and the second factor is then generated to maximally explain the remaining variance in the matrix (this is continuous with successive components [3,4,49]. The definition of each component is independent of the number of components retained [3]. This is useful in identifying various combinations of nutrients that could reflect possible biological mechanisms especially in association with various other health outcomes. Limitations related to PCA include the subjective decisions on how to interpret and name patterns, choice of variables to include in the matrix, whether to transform or standardize data, the number of components to retain, and the threshold for factor loadings to be used in naming patterns (*i.e.*, |+/−0.40| in this analysis) [47]. Furthermore, PCA derived patterns can be used as a standard approach to describe dietary habits of populations but the use of these patterns in examining diet–disease relationships has a minor limitation in that although PCA aims to maximize the fraction of variance explained by a weight linear combination of original variables, this however does not necessarily increase the ability to discriminate between subjects with disease or not.

We identified four nutrient patterns explaining 79% of the total variance in nutrient intakes: PC1 (26%) was characterized by animal derived nutrients; PC2 (21%) was characterized by *vitamins, fibre and vegetable oils*; PC3 (19%) was characterized by both animal and plant derived nutrients (*mixed diet driven nutrients*) and; PC4 (13%) was characterized by starch and folate. All studies published so far on nutrient patterns have been conducted in non-African regions and populations. PC1 is consistent and comparable to patterns depicted in previous studies labelled as "meat" [14,15], "high meat" [12,21], "animal products" [8,9,50,51] which were similarly characterized by high positive loadings of nutrients from animal derived sources. This additionally illustrates the adoption of westernized diets as PC1 explains most of the variance in this rural setting. PC2 which had high loadings for vitamins, fibre and vegetable oils nutrients is comparable to patterns reported in previous studies labelled as "fibre and vitamins" [8–11,16,22,50,51], "vitamin rich" [20], and "antioxidant vitamins and fibre" [17]. PC3 had a high heterogeneous contribution of both animal and plant derived nutrients, characterizing both a "Mediterranean nutrient pattern" and a "Western-like pattern". This two-in-one combination has been shown elsewhere [2,52]. PC4 is unique to this study and has not been reported elsewhere.

With PC1 and PC4, a positive and significant association was observed with BMI for age Z scores whilst no significant associations were observed for either PC2 or PC3. Observed positive associations between PC1 "animal driven nutrients" and BMI for age Z scores are consistent and comparable to those observed for western driven patterns reported in the literature [53–56]. Associations observed for PC4 with BMI for age Z scores are the first to be reported in the present study and are attributed to high starch and folate loadings. It should be noted that PC4 was not associated with BMI for age Z scores after full adjustment. In this rural setting, these associations could be explained in that we seem to be observing at household level that improved education status is positively driving household

SES. Rural households' diets differ with changing SES; improved SES is characterised by less physical activity and increased obesity risk (Table 4).

Though to the best of our knowledge, the food list of the QFFQ used to assess usual diet in this study is known to be comprehensive as reported elsewhere [38–40], we cannot ignore the inherent limitations around measurement errors and the complexity of assessing dietary intake in all nutritional epidemiological studies using self-reported diet. The use of dietary supplements was not included in the calculations of nutrient pattern scores, though these were unlikely to be used to any extent by adolescents in rural South African settings. Energy intake as expected was the most important factor explaining variability in PC scores, despite adjusting for it in the present analysis. Normalization for total energy helps to remove variation due to body size and metabolic rates and contributes to reducing measurement error in reported dietary intakes. Due to the cross sectional nature of the data presented here, the associations observed between the retained PCs and socio-demographic, lifestyle factors, and obesity risk cannot infer causality (problem of reverse causation should be noted) thus longitudinal data are required to do this.

Compared with food patterns, studying nutrient patterns have several advantages including that nutrients are universal, functionally not exchangeable, and in contrast to food patterns may characterize specific nutritional profiles in an easier way for comparison to other populations. Additionally, nutrients, unlike foods, show a limited number of non-consumers, and this approach could better mirror a combination of bioactive nutrients in complex biological mechanisms associated with diseases and obesity as compared to food patterns. From a public health perspective, since, in contrast to foods, nutrients are universal, this allows and supports the development or adaptation of existing food based dietary guidelines (FBDGs) using a variety of different interchangeable foods and/or food groups that mimic each other in nutrients. Different foods can have the same nutrient densities yet they are not equally and easily accessible to all geographic regions in a country (substitution with a food containing more or less the same nutrients should be stressed in FDBGs).

5. Conclusions

The present analysis confirmed a large variability in nutrient intakes but we were able to retain four nutrient patterns that were related to various socio-demographic and lifestyle factors, including BMI. Both poorer households and those with improving socio-economic status are placing adolescents at risk of obesity given the concomitant nutrient patterns and lifestyle behaviors. It is critical that intervention programs constructively address the consequences of the economic and nutrition transition underway in South Africa by assisting healthier diet choices around reduced carbohydrate intake, increasing food diversity, and promoting active lifestyles.

Acknowledgments: The study was funded by a National Research Foundation Niche grant (Grant No: 62496). The Agincourt Health and Socio-demographic Surveillance System is funded by the Welcome Trust, UK (Grants 058893/Z/99/A; 069683/Z/02/Z; 085477/Z/08/Z) and the University of the Witwatersrand and Medical Research Council, South Africa. We thank study participants and the communities within the Agincourt study site.

Author Contributions: PTP performed all the statistical analysis and drafted the manuscript; TMP collected and coded the dietary data for the study; KK and ST are responsible for the Agincourt Health and Socio-demographic Surveillance System including community engagement; KK, ST, SN and JMP designed the parent study; PTP conceived and conceptualised this study; SN, KK, ST and JMP assisted with editing the manuscript. All authors read and approved the final manuscript.

Conflicts of Interest: The authors declare no conflict interests.

References

1. Newby, P.K.; Tucker, K.L. Empirically derived eating patterns using factor or cluster analysis: A review. *Nutr. Rev.* **2004**, *62*, 177–203. [CrossRef] [PubMed]
2. Freisling, H.; Fahey, M.T.; Moskal, A.; Ocke, M.C.; Ferrari, P.; Jenab, M.; Norat, T.; Naska, A.; Welch, A.A.; Navarro, C.; *et al.* Region-specific nutrient intake patterns exhibit a geographical gradient within and between European countries. *J. Nutr.* **2010**, *140*, 1280–1286. [CrossRef] [PubMed]
3. Moskal, A.; Pisa, P.T.; Ferrari, P.; Byrnes, G.; Freisling, H.; Boutron-Ruault, M.C.; Cadeau, C.; Nailler, L.; Wendt, A.; Kuhn, T.; *et al.* Nutrient patterns and their food sources in an International Study Setting: Report from the EPIC study. *PLoS ONE* **2014**, *9*, e98647. [CrossRef] [PubMed]
4. Hu, F.B. Dietary pattern analysis: A new direction in nutritional epidemiology. *Curr. Opin. Lipidol.* **2002**, *13*, 3–9. [CrossRef] [PubMed]
5. Freedman, L.S.; Kipnis, V.; Schatzkin, A.; Tasevska, N.; Potischman, N. Can we use biomarkers in combination with self-reports to strengthen the analysis of nutritional epidemiologic studies? *Epidemiol. Perspect. Innov.* **2010**, *7*, 2–7. [CrossRef] [PubMed]
6. O'Sullivan, A.; Gibney, M.J.; Brennan, L. Dietary intake patterns are reflected in metabolomic profiles: Potential role in dietary assessment studies. *Am. J. Clin. Nutr.* **2011**, *93*, 314–321. [CrossRef] [PubMed]
7. Van Dam, R.M. New approaches to the study of dietary patterns. *Br. J. Nutr.* **2005**, *93*, 573–574. [CrossRef] [PubMed]
8. Bertuccio, P.; Edefonti, V.; Bravi, F.; Ferraroni, M.; Pelucchi, C.; Negri, E.; Decarli, A.; La, V.C. Nutrient dietary patterns and gastric cancer risk in Italy. *Cancer Epidemiol. Biomark. Prev.* **2009**, *18*, 2882–2886. [CrossRef]
9. Bosetti, C.; Bravi, F.; Turati, F.; Edefonti, V.; Polesel, J.; Decarli, A.; Negri, E.; Talamini, R.; Franceschi, S.; La, V.C.; *et al.* Nutrient-based dietary patterns and pancreatic cancer risk. *Ann. Epidemiol.* **2013**, *23*, 124–128. [CrossRef] [PubMed]
10. Bravi, F.; Edefonti, V.; Bosetti, C.; Talamini, R.; Montella, M.; Giacosa, A.; Franceschi, S.; Negri, E.; Ferraroni, M.; La, V.C.; Decarli, A. Nutrient dietary patterns and the risk of colorectal cancer: A case-control study from Italy. *Cancer Causes Control* **2010**, *21*, 1911–1918. [CrossRef] [PubMed]
11. Bravi, F.; Edefonti, V.; Randi, G.; Garavello, W.; La, V.C.; Ferraroni, M.; Talamini, R.; Franceschi, S.; Decarli, A. Dietary patterns and the risk of esophageal cancer. *Ann. Oncol.* **2012**, *23*, 765–770. [CrossRef] [PubMed]
12. De, S.E.; Boffetta, P.; Ronco, A.L.; Deneo-Pellegrini, H.; Acosta, G.; Gutierrez, L.P.; Mendilaharsu, M. Nutrient patterns and risk of lung cancer: A factor analysis in Uruguayan men. *Lung Cancer* **2008**, *61*, 283–291. [CrossRef] [PubMed]
13. De, S.E.; Boffetta, P.; Fagundes, R.B.; Deneo-Pellegrini, H.; Ronco, A.L.; Acosta, G.; Mendilaharsu, M. Nutrient patterns and risk of squamous cell carcinoma of the esophagus: A factor analysis in uruguay. *Anticancer Res.* **2008**, *28*, 2499–2506. [PubMed]
14. De, S.E.; Ronco, A.L.; Boffetta, P.; Deneo-Pellegrini, H.; Correa, P.; Acosta, G.; Mendilaharsu, M. Nutrient-derived dietary patterns and risk of colorectal cancer: A factor analysis in Uruguay. *Asian Pac. J. Cancer Prev.* **2012**, *13*, 231–235. [CrossRef] [PubMed]
15. Deneo-Pellegrini, H.; Boffetta, P.; De, S.E.; Correa, P.; Ronco, A.L.; Acosta, G.; Mendilaharsu, M.; Silva, C.; Luaces, M.E. Nutrient-based dietary patterns of head and neck squamous cell cancer: A factor analysis in Uruguay. *Cancer Causes Control* **2013**, *24*, 1167–1174. [CrossRef] [PubMed]
16. Edefonti, V.; Bravi, F.; La, V.C.; Randi, G.; Ferraroni, M.; Garavello, W.; Franceschi, S.; Talamini, R.; Boffetta, P.; Decarli, A. Nutrient-based dietary patterns and the risk of oral and pharyngeal cancer. *Oral Oncol.* **2010**, *46*, 343–348. [CrossRef] [PubMed]
17. Edefonti, V.; Hashibe, M.; Ambrogi, F.; Parpinel, M.; Bravi, F.; Talamini, R.; Levi, F.; Yu, G.; Morgenstern, H.; Kelsey, K.; *et al.* Nutrient-based dietary patterns and the risk of head and neck cancer: A pooled analysis in the International Head and Neck Cancer Epidemiology consortium. *Ann. Oncol.* **2012**, *23*, 1869–1880. [CrossRef] [PubMed]
18. Ganganna, P.; Johnson, A.A. A new nutrient index for measuring nutritional well-being of Indian states. *Int. J. Vitam. Nutr. Res.* **1985**, *55*, 315–322. [PubMed]
19. Ishimoto, H.; Nakamura, H.; Miyoshi, T. Epidemiological study on relationship between breast cancer mortality and dietary factors. *Tokushima J. Exp. Med.* **1994**, *41*, 103–114. [PubMed]

20. Palli, D.; Russo, A.; Decarli, A. Dietary patterns, nutrient intake and gastric cancer in a high-risk area of Italy. *Cancer Causes Control* **2001**, *12*, 163–172. [CrossRef] [PubMed]

21. Ronco, A.L.; De, S.E.; Aune, D.; Boffetta, P.; Deneo-Pellegrini, H.; Acosta, G.; Mendilaharsu, M. Nutrient patterns and risk of breast cancer in Uruguay. *Asian Pac. J. Cancer Prev.* **2010**, *11*, 519–524. [PubMed]

22. Turati, F.; Edefonti, V.; Bravi, F.; Ferraroni, M.; Franceschi, S.; La, V.C.; Montella, M.; Talamini, R.; Decarli, A. Nutrient-based dietary patterns, family history, and colorectal cancer. *Eur. J. Cancer Prev.* **2011**, *20*, 456–461. [CrossRef] [PubMed]

23. Pisa, P.T.; Vorster, H.H.; Nishida, C. Cardiovascular disease and nutrition: The use of food-based dietary guidelines for prevention in Africa. *South Afr. Heart J.* **2011**, *8*, 38–47.

24. Pisa, P.T.; Behanan, R.; Vorster, H.H.; Kruger, A. Social drift of cardiovascular disease risk factors in Africans from the North West Province of South Africa: The PURE study. *Cardiovasc. J. Afr.* **2012**, *23*, 371–388. [CrossRef] [PubMed]

25. Vorster, H.H. The emergence of cardiovascular disease during urbanisation of Africans. *Public Health Nutr.* **2002**, *5*, 239–243. [PubMed]

26. Popkin, B.M. Nutrition in transition: The changing global nutrition challenge. *Asia Pac. J. Clin. Nutr.* **2001**, *10*, S13–S18. [CrossRef] [PubMed]

27. Popkin, B.M. Dynamics of the nutrition transition and its implications for the developing world. *Forum Nutr.* **2003**, *56*, 262–264. [PubMed]

28. Black, R.E.; Victora, C.G.; Walker, S.P.; Bhutta, Z.A.; Christian, P.; de Onis, M.; Ezzati, M.; Grantham-McGregor, S.; Katz, J.; Martorell, R.; *et al.* Maternal and child undernutrition and overweight in low-income and middle-income countries. *Lancet* **2013**, *382*, 427–451. [CrossRef] [PubMed]

29. Bosman, L.; Herselman, M.G.; Kruger, H.S.; Labadarios, D. Secondary analysis of anthropometric data from a South African national food consumption survey, using different growth reference standards. *Matern. Child Health J.* **2011**, *15*, 1372–1380. [CrossRef] [PubMed]

30. Jinabhai, C.C.; Reddy, P.; Taylor, M.; Monyeki, D.; Kamabaran, N.; Omardien, R.; Sullivan, K.R. Sex differences in under and over nutrition among school-going Black teenagers in South Africa: An uneven nutrition trajectory. *Trop. Med. Int. Health* **2007**, *12*, 944–952. [CrossRef] [PubMed]

31. Kimani-Murage, E.W.; Kahn, K.; Pettifor, J.M.; Tollman, S.M.; Dunger, D.B.; Gomez-Olive, X.F.; Norris, S.A. The prevalence of stunting, overweight and obesity, and metabolic disease risk in rural South African children. *BMC Public Health* **2010**, *10*, 158. [CrossRef] [PubMed]

32. Casey, B.J.; Jones, R.M.; Levita, L.; Libby, V.; Pattwell, S.S.; Ruberry, E.J.; Soliman, F.; Somerville, L.H. The storm and stress of adolescence: Insights from human imaging and mouse genetics. *Dev. Psychobiol.* **2010**, *52*, 225–235. [PubMed]

33. Huybrechts, I.; de Vriendt, T.; Breidenassel, C.; Rogiers, J.; Vanaelst, B.; Cuenca-Garcia, M.; Moreno, L.A.; Gonzalez-Gross, M.; Roccaldo, R.; Kafatos, A.; *et al.* Mechanisms of stress, energy homeostasis and insulin resistance in European adolescents—The HELENA study. *Nutr. Metab. Cardiovasc. Dis.* **2014**, *24*, 1082–1089. [CrossRef] [PubMed]

34. Kahn, K.; Tollman, S.M.; Collinson, M.A.; Clark, S.J.; Twine, R.; Clark, B.D.; Shabangu, M.; Gomez-Olive, F.X.; Mokoena, O.; Garenne, M.L. Research into health, population and social transitions in rural South Africa: Data and methods of the Agincourt Health and Demographic Surveillance System. *Scand. J. Public Health Suppl.* **2007**, *69*, 8–20. [CrossRef] [PubMed]

35. Kahn, K.; Collinson, M.A.; Gomez-Olive, F.X.; Mokoena, O.; Twine, R.; Mee, P.; Afolabi, S.A.; Clark, B.D.; Kabudula, C.W.; Khosa, A.; *et al.* Profile: Agincourt health and socio-demographic surveillance system. *Int. J. Epidemiol.* **2012**, *41*, 988–1001. [CrossRef] [PubMed]

36. Kimani-Murage, E.W.; Kahn, K.; Pettifor, J.M.; Tollman, S.M.; Klipstein-Grobusch, K.; Norris, S.A. Predictors of adolescent weight status and central obesity in rural South Africa. *Public Health Nutr.* **2011**, *14*, 1114–1122. [CrossRef] [PubMed]

37. Wrottesley, S.V.; Micklesfield, L.K.; Hamill, M.M.; Goldberg, G.R.; Prentice, A.; Pettifor, J.M.; Norris, S.A.; Feeley, A.B. Dietary intake and body composition in HIV-positive and -negative South African women. *Public Health Nutr.* **2014**, *17*, 1603–1613. [CrossRef] [PubMed]

38. Nel, J.; Steyn, J.P. *Report on South African Food Consumption Studies Undertaken among Diffirent Population Groups (1983–2000): Average Intakes of Foods Most Commonly Consumed*; Department of Health of Directorate: Pretoria, South Africa, 2002.

39. Steyn, N.; Senekal, M. *A Guide for the use of Dietary Assessment and Education Kit (DAEK)*; Medical Research Council: Cape Town, South Africa, 2005.

40. Steyn, N.P.; Senekal, M.; Norris, S.A.; Whati, L.; Mackeown, J.M.; Nel, J.H. How well do adolescents determine portion sizes of foods and beverages? *Asia Pac. J. Clin. Nutr.* **2006**, *15*, 35–42. [PubMed]

41. Langenhoven, M.L.; Kruger, M.; Gouws, E. *MRC Food Composition Tables*, 3rd ed.; Medical Research Council: Cape Town, South Africa, 1991.

42. World Health Organization. *WHO Anthro Plus for Personal Computers, Manual. Software for Assessing Growth of the World's Children and Adolescents*; WHO: Geneva, Switzerland, 2009.

43. Norris, S.; Ritcher, L. Usefulness and realibility of tanner pubertal self rating to urban black adolescents in South Africa. *J. Res. Adolesc.* **2005**, *15*, 609–624. [CrossRef]

44. McVeigh, J.A.; Norris, S.A.; Cameron, N.; Pettifor, J.M. Associations between physical activity and bone mass in black and white South African children at age 9 year. *J. Appl. Physiol.* **2004**, *97*, 1006–1012. [CrossRef] [PubMed]

45. McVeigh, J.A.; Norris, S.A. Criterion validity and test-retest realibility of a physical activity questionnaire in South African primary school-aged children. *South Afr. J. Sports Med.* **2012**, *24*, 43–48.

46. Micklesfield, L.K.; Pedro, T.M.; Kahn, K.; Kinsman, J.; Pettifor, J.M.; Tollman, S.; Norris, S.A. Physical activity and sedentary behavior among adolescents in rural South Africa: Levels, patterns and correlates. *BMC Public Health* **2014**, *14*, 40. [CrossRef] [PubMed]

47. Johnson, R.A.; Wichern, D.W. *Applied Multivariate Statistical Analysis*, 5th ed.; Prentice Hall: Upper Saddle River, NJ, USA, 2007.

48. Willet, W.C. *Nutritional Epidemiology*, 2nd ed.; Oxford University Press: New York, NY, USA, 1998.

49. Tucker, K.L. Dietary patterns, approaches, and multicultural perspective. *Appl. Physiol. Nutr. Metab.* **2010**, *35*, 211–218. [CrossRef] [PubMed]

50. Edefonti, V.; Decarli, A.; La, V.C.; Bosetti, C.; Randi, G.; Franceschi, S.; Dal, M.L.; Ferraroni, M. Nutrient dietary patterns and the risk of breast and ovarian cancers. *Int. J. Cancer* **2008**, *122*, 609–613. [CrossRef] [PubMed]

51. Edefonti, V.; Bravi, F.; Garavello, W.; La, V.C.; Parpinel, M.; Franceschi, S.; Dal, M.L.; Bosetti, C.; Boffetta, P.; Ferraroni, M.; *et al.* Nutrient-based dietary patterns and laryngeal cancer: Evidence from an exploratory factor analysis. *Cancer Epidemiol. Biomark. Prev.* **2010**, *19*, 18–27. [CrossRef]

52. Slimani, N.; Fahey, M.; Welch, A.A.; Wirfalt, E.; Stripp, C.; Bergstrom, E.; Linseisen, J.; Schulze, M.B.; Bamia, C.; Chloptsios, Y.; *et al.* Diversity of dietary patterns observed in the European Prospective Investigation into Cancer and Nutrition (EPIC) project. *Public Health Nutr.* **2002**, *5*, 1311–1328. [CrossRef] [PubMed]

53. Dugee, O.; Khor, G.L.; Lye, M.S.; Luvsannyam, L.; Janchiv, O.; Jamyan, B.; Esa, N. Association of major dietary patterns with obesity risk among Mongolian men and women. *Asia Pac. J. Clin. Nutr.* **2009**, *18*, 433–440. [PubMed]

54. Esmaillzadeh, A.; Kimiagar, M.; Mehrabi, Y.; Azadbakht, L.; Hu, F.B.; Willett, W.C. Dietary patterns, insulin resistance, and prevalence of the metabolic syndrome in women. *Am. J. Clin. Nutr.* **2007**, *85*, 910–918. [PubMed]

55. Murtaugh, M.A.; Herrick, J.S.; Sweeney, C.; Baumgartner, K.B.; Guiliano, A.R.; Byers, T.; Slattery, M.L. Diet composition and risk of overweight and obesity in women living in the southwestern United States. *J. Am. Diet. Assoc.* **2007**, *107*, 1311–1321. [CrossRef] [PubMed]

56. Paradis, A.M.; Godin, G.; Perusse, L.; Vohl, M.C. Associations between dietary patterns and obesity phenotypes. *Int. J. Obes.* **2009**, *33*, 1419–1426. [CrossRef]

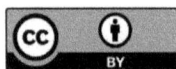

nutrients

MDPI

Article

A Dietary Pattern Derived by Reduced Rank Regression is Associated with Type 2 Diabetes in An Urban Ghanaian Population

Laura K. Frank [1,†], Franziska Jannasch [1,†], Janine Kröger [1,†], George Bedu-Addo [2,†], Frank P. Mockenhaupt [3,†], Matthias B. Schulze [1,†] and Ina Danquah [1,*]

[1]   Department of Molecular Epidemiology, German Institute of Human Nutrition Potsdam-Rehbruecke,
     Arthur-Scheunert-Allee 114-116, 14558 Nuthetal, Germany; laura.frank@dife.de (L.K.F.);
     franziska.jannasch@dife.de (F.J.); janine.kroeger@dife.de (J.K.); mschulze@dife.de (M.B.S.)
[2]   Komfo Anokye Teaching Hospital, School of Medical Sciences, Kwame Nkrumah University of Science and
     Technology, Kumasi, Ghana; gbeduaddo@gmail.com
[3]   Institute of Tropical Medicine and International Health, Charité–University Medicine Berlin,
     Campus Virchow-Klinikum, Augustenburger Platz 1, 13353 Berlin, Germany;
     frank.mockenhaupt@charite.de
*   Author to whom correspondence should be addressed; ina.danquah@dife.de;
     Tel.: +49-33200-88-2453; Fax: +49-33200-88-2437.
†   These authors contributed equally to this work.

Received: 8 May 2015; Accepted: 26 June 2015; Published: 7 July 2015

Abstract: Reduced rank regression (RRR) is an innovative technique to establish dietary patterns related to biochemical risk factors for type 2 diabetes, but has not been applied in sub-Saharan Africa. In a hospital-based case-control study for type 2 diabetes in Kumasi (diabetes cases, 538; controls, 668) dietary intake was assessed by a specific food frequency questionnaire. After random split of our study population, we derived a dietary pattern in the training set using RRR with adiponectin, HDL-cholesterol and triglycerides as responses and 35 food items as predictors. This pattern score was applied to the validation set, and its association with type 2 diabetes was examined by logistic regression. The dietary pattern was characterized by a high consumption of plantain, cassava, and garden egg, and a low intake of rice, juice, vegetable oil, eggs, chocolate drink, sweets, and red meat; the score correlated positively with serum triglycerides and negatively with adiponectin. The multivariate-adjusted odds ratio of type 2 diabetes for the highest quintile compared to the lowest was 4.43 (95% confidence interval: 1.87–10.50, *p* for trend < 0.001). The identified dietary pattern increases the odds of type 2 diabetes in urban Ghanaians, which is mainly attributed to increased serum triglycerides.

Keywords: adiponectin; biomarker; dietary pattern; HDL-cholesterol; reduced rank regression; sub-Saharan Africa; triglyceride; type 2 diabetes

---

1. Introduction

Type 2 diabetes is one of the major public health problems in sub-Saharan Africa (SSA) [1,2]. The prevalence rates are rising rapidly. Obesity, physical inactivity and urbanization substantially contribute to this development [3]. Nutritional behavior as a potentially modifiable risk factor is thought to have an important influence on the development of diabetes, but has only been insufficiently examined as a contributing factor for type 2 diabetes in SSA. The use of dietary patterns in nutritional epidemiology has increased in the past [4]. Dietary patterns reflect different combinations of food intake and allow the assessment of the overall diet instead of single nutrients or food items. Two general approaches facilitate the identification of dietary patterns: the hypothesis-oriented approach uses prior knowledge such as diet-quality scores based on diet recommendations or guidelines and the exploratory approach, such as factor and cluster analysis that are entirely empirical data-driven methods [5,6]. Reduced rank regression (RRR) has been proposed as a new dimension-reduction technique, which combines both approaches [7]. It combines the dietary information with prior scientific knowledge of the pathway from diet to disease. RRR determines linear combinations of predictor variables (e.g., food groups) by maximizing the explained variation in a set of response variables (e.g., nutrients [7–9] or biomarkers [10]) that are presumed to be related to the disease of interest. Previous studies reported strong associations between dietary patterns and type 2 diabetes by using RRR [7,11–14]. These dietary patterns were derived in Western populations but not in SSA. On the background of scarce epidemiologic data regarding nutritional behavior and type 2 diabetes in SSA, RRR appears to be a promising tool to characterize diet–disease relationships in this region. Yet, this approach remains to be attempted. Therefore, the aims of this study were, first, to identify a dietary pattern associated with serum concentrations of diabetes-related biomarkers (adiponectin, HDL-cholesterol and triglycerides) by using RRR in a training set of an urban Ghanaian study population (n = 603); second, to apply this dietary pattern score to a validation set of the same study population (n = 603); and third, to evaluate associations of the identified dietary pattern with type 2 diabetes in both sets of the urban Ghanaian study population.

2. Materials and Methods

2.1. Study Population

The Kumasi Diabetes and Hypertension (KDH) Study is an unmatched case-control study that was conducted at Komfo Anokye Teaching Hospital (KATH) in Kumasi, Ghana from August 2007 through June 2008. The primary aim was to identify risk factors for type 2 diabetes (and hypertension). The detailed description of the recruitment procedures and the characteristics of the study population are provided elsewhere [15]. Briefly, cases were recruited from the diabetes center (n = 495) and the hypertension clinic (n = 451). They encouraged their friends, neighbors and community members (n = 222) to participate in the study as potential controls. Further preliminary controls came from the outpatient department (n = 150) and hospital staff (n = 148). Every participant underwent a clinical examination and a personal interview on the socio-demographic background, the medical history, and the economic status. Fasting venous blood samples were drawn. For study purposes, type 2 diabetes was defined as having a fasting plasma glucose (FPG) $\geq$7 mmol/L and/or as being on documented anti-diabetic medication [16]. We refrained from HbA1c-based definition due to potential misclassification in individuals with hemoglobinopathies and malaria infection. Controls were defined as participants without diabetes. Of the 1466 participants included in the study, 260 were excluded from the present analysis due to missing information on nutrition (141), anthropometry (39), socio-economic status (SES, 31), genetic polymorphisms (34), and biomarkers (15). Hence, this analysis comprised 1206 individuals (668 controls, 538 diabetes cases).

All participants provided written informed consent; the study protocol was reviewed and approved by the Ethics Committee of the School of Medical Sciences, University of Science and Technology, Kumasi.

2.2. Dietary Assessment

The methods of the nutritional assessment have previously been described in detail [17]. Briefly, a locally specific food frequency questionnaire (FFQ) was applied to all participants in face-to-face interviews by trained nurses who speak the local language. This questionnaire assessed the usual weekly intake frequency of 51 food items in 10 food categories consumed during the past 12 months. Information about food groups and food categories are presented in Table S2. The food categories were starchy roots and plantain; cereals and cereal products; animal products; legumes, nuts and oilseeds; fruits; vegetables; fats and oils; salt and spices; sweets; and liquids.

No portion sizes were available. Thus, the FFQ covered intake frequencies, but not quantities of food consumption. The frequency of intake was measured using six categories: never, seldom (<time per week), 1–2 times per week, 3–4 times per week, 5–6 times per week, and daily. This FFQ has not been validated yet.

2.3. Covariate Assessment

Waist circumference (cm), hip circumference (cm), weight (kg) and height (cm) were measured (all devices Seca, Germany) by trained study personnel. BMI was calculated as weight/(height)^2 (kg/m^2), and waist-to-hip ratio (WHR) was computed as waist circumference/hip circumference. Socio-demographic data and the medical history comprised age, sex, own and family history of diabetes (yes, no), and smoking behavior (never, quit, current). SES data included information about education (none, primary, secondary, tertiary, other), literacy (able or unable to read and write), occupation (subsistence farmer, commercial farmer, casual laborer, artisan, trader, businessman/woman, public servant, unemployed, other), number of people living in the household and household assets: electricity, pipe water, fan, fridge, cupboard, radio, TV, bicycle, motor bike, car, truck and tractor and cattle (yes/no). These variables were used to construct a SES sum score. It ranges from 0 to 12 points and comprises the domains education, occupation and income. The exact procedure of the construction is depicted in Figure S1. Self-reported physical activity comprised work-related, transportation-related and leisure-time physical activity. Duration (min/week) and type (*i.e.*, intensity) of physical activity were translated into daily energy expenditure (kcal/day) as the sum of metabolic equivalents corresponding to activity intensity (mL/kg/min) × body weight (kg) × duration (min) [18].

2.4. Laboratory Procedures

Each participant provided a fasting blood sample (fluoride plasma, tubes cooled at +4 °C). FPG was measured photometrically (Glucose 201+ Analyzer, HemoCue, Ångelholm, Sweden) and is presented as plasma equivalents. Serum triglycerides and HDL-cholesterol were measured by colorimetric assays (ABX Pentra400, Horiba Medical, Reichenbach, Germany). The inter-assay CVs were 4.5% and 1.8%, respectively. The total adiponectin concentration was measured using a commercially available ELISA with intra- and inter-assay CVs of 4.9% and 6.7% (BioVendor, Heidelberg, Germany).

2.5. Statistical Analysis

2.5.1. Descriptive Analysis

For the comparison of baseline characteristics between diabetes cases and controls, the non-parametric Mann–Whitney U test was used for continuous and χ^2-test for categorical variables. Spearman correlations were used to assess the relationship between biomarkers among the control group.

2.5.2. Reduced Rank Regression

We applied RRR to derive a dietary pattern predictive of the diabetes status. This method has been described in detail by Hoffmann *et al.* [7], including SAS code and its application in nutritional epidemiology, and has been applied in recent studies of dietary patterns and chronic diseases [10]. The directed acyclic graph in Figure S2 describes the conceptual framework of the present RRR. Briefly, RRR determines linear combinations of predictor variables (e.g., food groups) that explain as much as possible variation in the response variables (e.g., biomarkers). It is based on the assumption that canonical correlations between predictor and response variables are negligibly small. In this analysis, we used 35 food items as predictor variables and serum concentrations of HDL-cholesterol, log-transformed adiponectin and log-transformed triglycerides as response variables. Thus, dietary patterns that explained a maximum of variation in these biomarkers were identified. The response variables adiponectin, HDL-cholesterol and triglycerides were chosen based on their established relationship with type 2 diabetes [19–21]. Since we are lacking an external validation population to test the robustness of our results, we randomly split our study population ($n = 1206$) into two subsamples (each $n = 603$) and performed an internal validation. We calculated the dietary pattern score in one subsample (training set) and applied this pattern score to the other (validation set). The dietary pattern score was calculated as the sum of z-standardized intakes (mean = 0, standard deviation = 1) of 35 food items multiplied by an individual weight. For the calculation of the dietary pattern score, all 35 food items were subject to analysis. However, henceforth, we will focus the description of the dietary pattern on those ten food items with the highest factor loadings. These were considered to be the main contributors to the score. Each participant received a factor score for the identified dietary pattern. These scores were used to rank participants according to the degree to which they conformed to the dietary pattern.

Based on the distribution among the control group, quintiles of the dietary pattern score were constructed. Socio-demographic and anthropometric characteristics, the SES sum score, biomarker concentrations and frequencies of food intake were calculated across the quintiles of the dietary pattern score among the control group. The differences among categorical variables (χ^2-test) and linear trends among continuous parameters (trend test) were assessed.

2.5.3. Dietary Pattern and Type 2 Diabetes

Logistic regression analysis was applied to evaluate the associations between the dietary pattern and type 2 diabetes. Odds ratios (OR) and 95% confidence intervals (CI) were calculated across the quintiles and per 1 SD of the dietary pattern score. The significance of a linear trend across the categories was tested by assigning each control the median of a category and by modeling this value as a continuous variable. For type 2 diabetes, as a rare disease with long latency, we applied the proportional odds assumption in logistic regression models and based our adjustments on previous findings. Initially we adjusted for age and sex (Model 1). Then, we further adjusted for diabetes family history (yes or no), SES sum score, smoking status (never/current or ex-smoker) and energy expenditure (kcal/day) (Model 2), and finally we adjusted for BMI and WHR (Model 3).

2.5.4. Sensitivity Analyses

We tested interactions of the association between the dietary pattern and type 2 diabetes with sex, general obesity (BMI $\geq$ 30 kg/m^2) or central adiposity (waist circumference $\geq$ 102 cm (men), $\geq$88 cm (women)) by performing stratified analyses and we evaluated the significance of cross-product terms. We also examined the sensitivity of our results and excluded participants with lipid-lowering and anti-inflammatory drug intake. We assessed the association between biomarkers of glucose metabolism (FPG and HOMA-IR) and the dietary pattern score across quintiles among the controls.

Finally, we simplified our dietary pattern score in the total study population by summing up the unweighted standardized intake of the food items with the ten highest factor loadings. To assess the importance of individual food components of the dietary pattern score for type 2 diabetes, we sequentially subtracted each component from the simplified dietary pattern score. We calculated the change in estimate (CIE) as the difference between the ORs divided by the OR from the simplified score multiplied by 100.

We defined a two-sided p-value of <0.05 as statistical significance. All statistical analyses were performed using SAS statistical software (version 9.4, SAS Institute, Cary, NC, USA).

3. Results

3.1. Study Population

The characteristics of the total study population ($n = 1206$) are presented in Table 1. Compared o the controls, the diabetes cases were on average older, had higher WHR and were of lower SES. In addition, diabetes cases had more often diabetes in their family, tended to smoke more often, and had higher intake of anti-inflammatory drugs and energy expenditure than controls. Biomarker concentrations differed significantly between diabetes cases and controls, with lower values of adiponectin and HDL-cholesterol, but higher values of serum triglycerides, FPG and HOMA-IR in the diabetes group.

Among the control group, adiponectin correlated positively with HDL-cholesterol ($r = 0.16$, $p < 0.001$) and negatively with triglycerides ($r = -0.17$, $p < 0.001$). HDL-cholesterol and triglycerides were weakly correlated with each other ($r = 0.08$, $p = 0.03$).

Table 1. Characteristics and biomarkers of 1206 urban Ghanaians of the Kumasi Diabetes and Hypertension Study.

Characteristics	Controls (n = 668)	Diabetes Cases (n = 538)
Sex (female)	516 (77.3)	396 (73.6)
Age (years)	46.8 ± 15.7	54.7 ± 13.4 *
BMI (kg/m^2)	25.8 ± 5.4	25.7 ± 4.9
Waist-to-hip ratio	0.86 ± 0.08	0.91 ± 0.07 *
Socio-economic status sum score		
Very low (0–4 points)	118 (17.7)	200 (37.2) *
Low (5–8 points)	355 (53.1)	278 (51.7)
Moderate (9–10 points)	195 (29.2)	60 (11.2)
Family history of diabetes (yes)	167 (25.0)	314 (58.4) *
Hypertension (yes)	344 (51.5)	332 (61.7) *
Smoking (ever)	27 (4.0)	40 (7.4) *
Lipid-lowering drug intake	12 (1.8)	16 (3.0)
Anti-inflammatory drug intake	6 (0.9)	18 (3.4) *
Energy expenditure (kcal/day)	1214 (848–1630)	1408 (815–1996) *
Biomarkers		
Adiponectin (mg/mL)	8.63 (6.50–11.63)	7.42 (5.36–9.98) *
HDL-cholesterol (mmol/L)	1.37 (1.13–1.62)	1.27 (1.04–1.54) *
Triglycerides (mmol/L)	1.19 (0.87–1.64)	1.36 (1.02–1.87) *
Fasting plasma glucose (mmol/L)	4.40 (4.10–4.90)	6.90 (5.30–10.30) *
HOMA-IR	1.37 (0.85–2.13)	2.00 (1.17–3.40) *

Values are expressed as mean ± standard deviation, participant number (%) or median (interquartile range); * p-value ≤ 0.05.

3.2. Dietary Pattern and Biomarkers

After a random split of our study population into two sets of equal size (each $n = 603$) and with an equal ratio of diabetes cases and controls, dietary pattern scores were derived by RRR in the training set. The intake frequencies of 35 food items were used as predictors and concentrations of adiponectin, HDL-cholesterol and triglycerides as responses; we obtained three scores. The first dietary pattern score explained 6.8% of the total variation in foods and 3.9% of the total variation in all three biomarkers and was largely driven by the explained variation in triglycerides (9.9%) and only marginally by HDL cholesterol (1.9%) and adiponectin (0.03%). The second and third RRR score explained 2.2% and 1.7% of the total biomarker variation, respectively. These were not biologically plausible. Therefore, we did not consider them for further analyses. In this training set, the identified dietary pattern was characterized by a high consumption of plantain, cassava and garden egg and a low intake of rice, juice, vegetable oil, eggs, milo (chocolate drink), sweets and red meat (Table 2).

The characteristics and biomarker concentrations across dietary pattern quintiles among the controls in the training set are shown in Table S1. Participants with higher dietary pattern score were older, heavier, of lower SES, had lower adiponectin and HDL-cholesterol, but they showed higher triglyceride concentrations.

In the next step, the identified dietary pattern score was applied to the validation set of our study population. In this set, the characteristics and distributions of biomarkers across quintiles of the pattern score among the controls were similar to those in the training set (Table 3). However, no linear trend was observed for HDL-cholesterol. The median intakes of the food items that contributed most to the dietary pattern varied across the score. For instance, participants in the highest quintile consumed plantain five-times more frequently than those in the lowest quintile. In contrast, the rice intake was five-times lower (Table 3).

Table 2. Percentage of food variation explained by first dietary pattern score and factor loadings of all 35 food items derived by reduced rank regression in the training set (*n* = 603).

Food Item	Explained Variation (%)	Factor Loading [1]
Plantain	23.6	0.31
Cassava	23.0	0.31
Garden egg	16.0	0.26
Rice	24.0	−0.32
Juice	21.7	−0.30
Vegetable oil	19.7	−0.29
Eggs	15.2	−0.25
Milo (chocolate drink)	13.3	−0.24
Sweets	11.8	−0.22
Red meat	11.2	−0.22
Groundnut	9.70	−0.20
Soft drinks	9.00	−0.19
Margarine	7.46	−0.18
Milk	6.87	−0.17
Fruits	5.37	−0.15
Carrot	3.75	−0.13
Beans	3.29	−0.12
Lettuce	2.23	−0.10
Cocoyam	2.61	0.10
Cucumber	1.70	−0.08
Millet	1.44	−0.08
Yam	1.03	−0.07
Green leaves	1.15	0.07
Coffee	0.85	−0.06
Palm oil	0.75	−0.06
Okro	0.18	0.03
Maize (banku)	0.26	0.03
Crab	0.23	0.03
Poultry	0.18	−0.03
Porridge	0.13	0.02
Alcoholic drinks	0.07	0.02
Sweet potato	0.13	−0.02
Agushie (pumpkin seeds)	0.02	0.01
Bread	0.02	−0.01
Fish	0.005	−0.004

[1] Factor loadings are correlations between food items and the dietary pattern score.

3.3. Dietary Pattern and Type 2 Diabetes

The associations with type 2 diabetes for quintiles and per 1 SD of the dietary pattern score for the training and the validation set are presented in Table 4. A higher dietary pattern score increased the odds for type 2 diabetes in both sets. In the validation set, the OR for type 2 diabetes in the highest quintile compared to the lowest was 4.43 (95% CI: 1.87–10.50), *p* for trend < 0.001 in the fully adjusted model. In the training set, this figure was 4.57 (95% CI: 2.14–9.76), *p* for trend < 0.001.

We conducted several sensitivity analyses to assess the robustness of our results. In the validation set, we examined potential modifications of the risk estimates by sex, general obesity or central adiposity. In the fully adjusted model, the associations between the dietary pattern and type 2 diabetes were consistent for men and women (men ($n = 159$): OR = 1.52 (0.99–2.34), women ($n = 444$): OR = 1.60 (1.20–2.12), *p* for interaction = 0.96), for BMI categories (<30.0 kg/m^2 ($n = 487$): OR = 1.35 (1.05–1.75), ≥30.0 kg/m^2 ($n = 116$): OR = 2.60 (1.36–4.97), *p* for interaction = 0.76) and for categories of waist circumference (<102 cm (men), <88 cm (women) ($n = 347$): OR = 1.31 (0.97–1.78), ≥102/88 cm ($n = 256$): OR = 1.83 (1.26–2.67), *p* for interaction = 0.56).

Additionally, we repeated the RRR for the identification of the dietary pattern after excluding participants with lipid-lowering (2.3%) or anti-inflammatory drug intake (2.0%). The results were virtually identical (data not shown).

We appreciated the possibility that individuals with type 2 diabetes likely present with abnormal serum concentrations of adiponectin, HDL-cholesterol and triglycerides, and that this might have distorted our findings. Hence, we investigated whether the dietary pattern score was associated with biomarkers of glucose metabolism among apparently healthy controls ($n = 343$) in the validation set. Fasting plasma glucose tended to increase across quintiles of the pattern score (mean ± sd: 4.40 ± 0.67, 4.64 ± 0.76, 4.78 ± 0.72, 4.55 ± 0.70 and 4.64 ± 0.61 mmol/L, *p* for trend = 0.13). The respective values for HOMA-IR were: median (interquartile range): 1.33 (0.96–2.15), 1.64 (0.99–2.51), 1.63 (1.03–2.51), 1.24 (0.82–1.77) and 1.38 (0.87–2.57), *p* for trend = 0.51.

Finally, we assessed the importance of individual food components for type 2 diabetes by sequential removal of each component from the simplified dietary pattern score (Table 5). This analysis was conducted in the total study population, because the associations between the dietary pattern score and type 2 diabetes were similar in the training and the validation set. The exclusion of milo (chocolate drink), juice, plantain, sweets, garden egg, red meat and rice attenuated the OR for type 2 diabetes, whereby the removal of cassava, which was positively associated with the dietary pattern score, increased the association with type 2 diabetes.

Table 3. Characteristics and biomarkers by quintiles of dietary pattern score among 343 controls in the validation set.

Characteristics	Quintile of the Dietary Pattern Score					p for trend
	1	2	3	4	5	
n	68	70	68	69	68	
Sex (female)	51 (75.0)	53 (75.7)	49 (72.1)	54 (78.3)	54 (79.4)	0.87
Age (years)	32.5 ± 13.4	40.8 ± 13.5	46.6 ± 14.0	53.0 ± 11.8	54.7 ± 14.9	<0.001
BMI (kg/m²)	24.0 ± 4.8	25.8 ± 4.7	27.1 ± 6.4	26.4 ± 6.4	27.0 ± 5.8	0.002
WHR	0.82 ± 0.08	0.85 ± 0.07	0.87 ± 0.06	0.87 ± 0.08	0.89 ± 0.08	<0.001
very low SES	3 (4.4)	8 (11.4)	5 (7.4)	21 (30.4)	16 (23.5)	<0.001
Family history of diabetes	18 (26.5)	20 (28.6)	21 (30.9)	18 (26.1)	14 (20.6)	0.73
Smoking (ever)	5 (7.4)	4 (5.7)	3 (4.4)	1 (1.5)	3 (4.4)	0.57
Energy expenditure (kcal/day)	1177 (901–1593)	1289 (949–1731)	1329 (962–1729)	1222 (1015–1687)	1245 (712–1786)	0.92
Biomarkers						
Adiponectin (mg/mL)	9.41 (6.34–11.94)	8.27 (5.86–10.57)	7.89 (5.93–11.93)	8.88 (6.79–12.53)	8.73 (6.52–12.33)	0.19
HDL-cholesterol (mmol/L)	1.37 (1.11–1.62)	1.43 (1.30–1.69)	1.35 (1.19–1.60)	1.36 (1.16–1.53)	1.38 (1.14–1.66)	0.64
Triglycerides (mmol/L)	0.97 (0.69–1.23)	1.26 (0.86–1.63)	1.10 (0.85–1.56)	1.32 (0.97–1.89)	1.48 (0.99–1.86)	<0.001
Food intake (times/week)[1]						
positive association						
Plantain	1.5 (0.5–3.5)	1.5 (1.5–3.5)	3.5 (1.5–5.5)	5.5 (3.5–7.0)	7.0 (4.5–7.0)	<0.001
Cassava	1.5 (0.5–1.5)	1.5 (1.5–3.5)	1.5 (1.5–3.5)	3.5 (1.5–3.5)	7.0 (3.5–7.0)	<0.001
Garden egg	3.5 (1.5–7.0)	3.5 (1.5–7.0)	5.5 (2.5–7.0)	7.0 (3.5–7.0)	7.0 (7.0–7.0)	<0.001
inverse association						
Rice	7.0 (5.5–7.0)	7.0 (3.5–7.0)	3.5 (3.5–7.0)	3.5 (1.5–5.5)	1.5 (0.5–3.5)	<0.001
Juice	1.5 (0.5–5.5)	1.0 (0.5–3.5)	0.5 (0–1.5)	0 (0–0.5)	0 (0–0.5)	<0.001
Vegetable oil	3.5 (1.5–7.0)	3.5 (1.5–5.5)	3.5 (1.5–3.5)	1.5 (0.5–3.5)	1.5 (0.5–3.5)	<0.001
Eggs	2.5 (1.5–3.5)	1.5 (0.5–1.5)	0.5 (0.5–1.5)	0.5 (0.5–1.5)	0.5 (0–0.5)	<0.001
Milo (chocolate drink)	3.5 (1.5–5.5)	1.5 (0.5–3.5)	1.5 (0.5–3.5)	0.5 (0–3.5)	0.5 (0–1.5)	<0.001
Sweets	0.5 (0.5–1.5)	0.5 (0.5–1.5)	0.5 (0–1.5)	0.5 (0–0.5)	0 (0–0.5)	<0.001
Red meat	3.5 (1.5–7.0)	1.5 (1.5–3.5)	1.5 (0.5–3.5)	0.5 (0.5–1.5)	0.5 (0.5–3.5)	<0.001

Values are expressed as mean ± standard deviation, participant number (%) or median (interquartile range). [1] We included 35 food items in our analysis, the ten food items that loaded highest on the dietary pattern derived by reduced rank regression are presented here.

Table 4. Odds Ratios (OR) and 95% confidence intervals for type 2 diabetes by quintiles and per 1 SD of the dietary pattern score.

	Odds Ratios (95% confidence intervals) for Quintiles					*p* for trend	OR per 1-score SD
	Quintile 1	Quintile 2	Quintile 3	Quintile 4	Quintile 5		
Training set							
No. of cases/controls	17/65	33/65	58/65	76/65	94/65		
Model 1	1.00 (ref.)	1.69 (0.85–3.37)	2.78(1.43–5.38)	3.44 (1.78–6.65)	4.05 (2.09–7.86)	<0.001	1.55 (1.27–1.88)
Model 2	1.00 (ref.)	1.98 (0.93–4.22)	3.42 (1.65–7.12)	3.84 (1.86–7.95)	5.04 (2.42–10.48)	<0.001	1.59 (1.28–1.96)
Model 3	1.00 (ref.)	1.88 (0.86–4.09)	2.95 (1.39–6.29)	3.28 (1.55–6.94)	4.57 (2.14–9.76)	<0.001	1.52 (1.22–1.89)
Validation set							
No. of cases/controls	10/69	32/70	49/70	64/68	105/70		
Model 1	1.00 (ref.)	2.50 (1.12–5.57)	3.15 (1.43–6.93)	3.76 (1.72–8.24)	6.08 (2.81–13.16)	<0.001	1.74 (1.42–2.13)
Model 2	1.00 (ref.)	2.25 (0.95–5.36)	2.86 (1.21–6.75)	3.04 (1.30–7.11)	5.04 (2.19–11.60)	<0.001	1.60 (1.28–2.00)
Model 3	1.00 (ref.)	2.26 (0.92–5.54)	2.81 (1.15–6.84)	3.20 (1.33–7.70)	4.43 (1.87–10.50)	<0.001	1.52 (1.20–1.92)

Model 1: adjusted for age (years) and sex; Model 2: adjusted for age (years), sex, diabetes family history (yes vs. no), SES sum score (metric: 0–12 points), smoking status (ever vs. never) and energy expenditure (kcal/d); Model 3: adjusted for age (years), sex, diabetes family history (yes vs. no), SES sum score (metric: 0–12 points), smoking status (ever vs. never) and energy expenditure (kcal/d), BMI (kg/m^2) and waist-to-hip ratio.

Table 5. Importance of individual components of the simplified dietary pattern score among the total study population (*n* = 1206).

Dietary Variable	OR per 1SD Score	CIE (%) [2]
Simplified dietary pattern score [1]	2.17 (1.80–2.62)	
Simplified dietary pattern score without milo (chocolate drink)	1.74 (1.47–2.07)	−19.8
Simplified dietary pattern score without juice	1.95 (1.63–2.32)	−10.1
Simplified dietary pattern score without plantain	2.02 (1.69–2.43)	−6.9
Simplified dietary pattern score without sweets	2.05 (1.71–2.46)	−5.5
Simplified dietary pattern score without garden egg	2.10 (1.74–2.52)	−5.1
Simplified dietary pattern score without red meat	2.11 (1.76–2.53)	−2.8
Simplified dietary pattern score without rice	2.12 (1.76–2.55)	−2.3
Simplified dietary pattern score without vegetable oil	2.17 (1.80–2.61)	-
Simplified dietary pattern score without eggs	2.25 (1.87–2.70)	+3.7
Simplified dietary pattern score without cassava	2.74 (2.25–3.35)	+26.3

[1] Simplified dietary pattern score: sum of unweighted standardized intake of 10 food items, which were highly loaded on the dietary pattern (plantain + cassava + garden egg − milo (chocolate drink) − red meat − juice − rice − sweets − eggs − vegetable oil); [2] CIE: Change in estimate: difference between ORs divided by OR of simplified dietary pattern score and multiplied by 100 (%); Model 3 adjustments were applied: adjusted for age, sex, diabetes family history, SES sum score, energy expenditure, BMI and waist-to-hip ratio.

4. Discussion

Due to rising prevalence rates of type 2 diabetes in SSA, it is necessary to clarify the potential importance of nutritional behavior in this region. Studies from SSA, which investigate the association between dietary patterns and type 2 diabetes are scarce. This led us to examine dietary patterns derived by RRR and their associations with type 2 diabetes in an urban Ghanaian population. In a training set, we identified a dietary pattern that was characterized by a high consumption of traditional foods and a low intake of purchased items. Participants with a higher dietary pattern score had higher concentrations of triglycerides and lower concentrations of adiponectin; the pattern score significantly increased the odds for type 2 diabetes. We verified these findings in an internal validation set of this Ghanaian study population.

The results of the present study confirm previous findings of the KDH Study. The food items that were positively associated with the dietary pattern score in the RRR (plantain and garden egg) were also included in the "traditional" dietary pattern identified by an exploratory factor analysis [17]. This "traditional" dietary pattern was characterized by high intakes of plantain, green leafy vegetables, beans, garden egg, fruits, fish, fermented maize products and palm oil and was positively associated with type 2 diabetes. Those food items that were inversely associated with the pattern score in RRR (rice, juice, eggs, milo (chocolate drink), sweets and red meat) were also included in the "purchase" pattern identified by the factor analysis. This "purchase" pattern was characterized by a high consumption of sweets, rice, red meat, poultry, eggs, milk, fruits and vegetables and a low consumption of plantain and was related to reduced odds of type 2 diabetes [17]. Moreover, previous analysis has revealed a strong association of increased triglycerides ($\geq$1.695 mmol/L) with type 2 diabetes in this study population: multivariate adjusted OR 1.83 (95% CI: 1.13–2.97) [15]. Indeed, triglycerides were the main drivers of the association between the RRR-derived dietary pattern and type 2 diabetes in the present study. Clearly, as compared to factor analysis, the RRR method is an advance for the identification of diet-disease relationships. Both approaches are dimension reduction techniques which allow the calculation of dietary pattern scores. The previous factor analysis identified dietary patterns in this population that relied only on the combined consumption of foods and drinks. Beyond this, the RRR identified a dietary pattern that affects biomarker concentrations related to diabetes risk. From the RRR, we conclude that adherence to traditional food items and low preference for purchased foods relate to increased serum triglycerides—a strong risk factor for type 2 diabetes.

To our knowledge, the present study is the first study in SSA that identified a dietary pattern by using the RRR method. Overall, few epidemiological studies investigated the association between dietary patterns derived by RRR and type 2 diabetes. Although these studies used different intermediate markers as response variables including inflammatory biomarkers [12,14], HOMA-IR [13] and HbA1c, HDL-cholesterol, C-reactive protein (CRP) and adiponectin [11]; the explained variation in biomarkers of these studies is comparable to our findings.

To investigate the generalizability of RRR-derived dietary patterns, two studies validated the association of such patterns with diabetes risk in an independent European [22] and US population [23]. The European Prospective Investigation into Cancer and Nutrition (EPIC)-InterAct study found a good generalizability for three RRR dietary pattern scores based on the American Nurses' Health Study (NHS), the German EPIC-Potsdam Study and the British Whitehall II Study [22]. The three dietary pattern scores were inversely associated with type 2 diabetes risk. In contrast, the American Framingham Offspring Study found a good generalizability for the NHS derived dietary pattern score, but the dietary pattern scores based on the European studies (EPIC-Potsdam Study and Whitehall II Study) were significantly less predictive for type 2 diabetes risk [23]. Thus the generalizability of dietary patterns associated with diabetes risk may be better in populations with comparable dietary intakes. Indeed, the transferability of previous RRR dietary patterns established in European and US populations to an urban Ghanaian population is complicated by the differences in the diet *per se*. However, all prospective studies found strong associations between dietary patterns obtained by RRR and type 2 diabetes. The strong relationships observed with the RRR method can partly be attributed to the use of disease-related biomarkers. In the Whitehall II Study, a diet high in low calories/soft drinks, onions, sugar-sweetened beverages, burgers and sausages, crisps and other snacks and white bread and low in medium-/high-fiber breakfast cereals, jam, French dressing/vinaigrette and whole meal bread was associated with a two- to threefold increase in diabetes risk by using HOMA-IR as the response variable [13]. The Insulin Resistance Atherosclerosis Study found a threefold to more than fourfold increased odds of diabetes associated with a dietary pattern high in red meat, low-fiber bread and cereal, dried beans, fried potatoes, tomato vegetables, eggs, cheese, and cottage cheese and low wine by using the inflammatory markers plasminogen activator inhibitor-1 and fibrinogen as the response variable [12]. In the NHS, Schulze *et al.* observed a pattern, which was high in sugar-sweetened soft drinks, refined grains, diet soft drinks and processed meat but low in wine, coffee, cruciferous vegetables, and yellow vegetable; this was related to a two- to threefold increase in diabetes risk by using inflammatory markers as the response variables [14]. Heidemann *et al.* found a dietary pattern among Caucasians, which was positively associated with HDL-cholesterol and adiponectin and inversely with HbA1c and CRP in the EPIC-Potsdam Study. This pattern was characterized by a high intake of fresh fruits and low intake of high-caloric soft drinks, beer, red meat, poultry, processed meat, legumes and bread (except wholegrain bread) and was inversely associated with the risk of type 2 diabetes [11].

An important difference between our observed dietary pattern and dietary patterns derived among Western populations is the inverse association of red meat with type 2 diabetes in our study population. Although not all previous meta-analyses found a positive association between red meat intake and type 2 diabetes [24], there is a large amount of epidemiologic evidence for this positive association among Western populations [25,26]. Possibly, the different types and preparation methods of red meat in urban Ghana compared to those among Western populations partially explain the inverse association with type 2 diabetes in our study. With regard to plantain—a major staple food in Ghana—we observed the highest contribution to the dietary pattern score and a positive association with type 2 diabetes. Plantain features a high glycemic index, and the content of simple sugars increases continuously during the ripening process [27]. Evidence from large epidemiologic studies showed that the glycemic index and the glycemic load are associated with a higher risk of type 2 diabetes [28]. Furthermore, frequent intake of carbohydrates has been related to an increase of fasting triglyceride concentrations and a reduction of HDL-cholesterol [29–33]. As for cassava and rice, it seemed contra-intuitive to us that its intake was positively associated with the pattern score, but inversely with type 2 diabetes. However, an inverse association between cassava flour and incident diabetes was also observed in a Brazilian study [34]. In our study population, plantain, cassava and rice were frequently consumed and the preparation methods were diverse including cooking, frying and pounding. Lacking a plausible biological explanation, we are speculating whether novel methods for the preparation of the traditional foods could explain the different associations of plantain and cassava with type 2 diabetes. Alternatively, the combined consumption of cassava and rice with other food groups [17] may represent dietary diversity, which is inversely associated with biomarkers of type 2 diabetes [35].

Notably, the biomarkers subjected to RRR in our study are similar to those in studies among Caucasian populations. However, the selection of biomarkers was limited to adiponectin, HDL-cholesterol and triglycerides based on established associations for type 2 diabetes. Inflammatory markers, such as CRP were not considered as response variables in our analysis due to the high prevalence of infectious diseases, complicating the interpretation of CRP as a risk factor for diabetes. Indeed, 13% of our study population had a *Plasmodium falciparum* infection [36]. Also, HOMA-IR was disregarded as a response variable, because of its metabolic proximity to type 2 diabetes. HOMA-IR is useful to determine pre-diabetic stages, but is not on the causal pathway for type 2 diabetes.

To the best of our knowledge, this study contributes uniquely to the literature; we are the first to identify a dietary pattern derived by RRR in an African population. We are aware that the RRR method is limited to existing studies with biomarkers or intermediate variables and knowledge of the diet–disease association. Nevertheless, this innovative method has the advantage to investigate the pathway between diet and disease as opposed to the exploratory factor analysis and cluster analysis which are entirely data driven. Given the limited data from SSA, a case-control design is useful to establish hypotheses on the relationship between dietary patterns and type 2 diabetes. However, these hypotheses require verification in prospective studies building a clear temporal relationship between dietary patterns and type 2 diabetes. Therefore, we cannot exclude that reverse causation contributes to our findings. Primarily, long-lasting type 2 diabetes might lead to changes of dietary behavior. Yet, at the time of study conduct, nutritional counseling was not part of the routine diabetes management at the hospital and thus, does not apply to our study population. Secondly, the concentrations of selected biomarkers chosen as response variables in the RRR might have changed during the course of diabetes. In this regard, we assessed whether the positive association of the dietary pattern score remained with FPG concentrations and HOMA-IR in the apparently healthy control group. Indeed, we found a nominal linear trend for FPG concentrations, while this was less clear for HOMA-IR. Also, the method of internal validation by random split technique confirmed the transferability and diabetes-association of the identified dietary pattern for urban Ghana. As for the dietary assessment, we admit that the retrospective FFQ bears the risk of under- or over-reporting of food items. The application of a locally specific FFQ by trained nurses of the same cultural background and language helped to keep these information biases to a minimum. Just since 2012, a national policy for the prevention and control of chronic non-communicable diseases exists in Ghana, including health promotions for a healthy diet [37]. Thus, public knowledge about the associations between specific food items and type 2 diabetes may not have been pronounced in the study area at the time of study conduct. Therefore, recall bias in reporting of specific foods seems unlikely in this population. Also, participants were not aware of their biomarker values at the time of dietary assessment. Even though we have adjusted for a large variety of known diabetes risk factors, we cannot rule out that unmeasured factors have influenced our observed results. Clearly, the hospital-based selection of controls helped to make the comparison groups more similar in terms of potential confounders, which are difficult to measure, such as socioeconomic background. Nevertheless, the hospital-based design leads to a study population that is not fully representative of the general one, and thus, the generalizability of our findings may be questionable.

5. Conclusions

In conclusion, we identified a dietary pattern that showed adherence to traditional food items and low preference for purchase foods in an urban Ghanaian population. This pattern was related to higher serum triglyceride concentrations and increased the risk of type 2 diabetes in this population.

Acknowledgments: The authors thank all participants at Komfo Anokye Teaching Hospital and acknowledge the study team of the KDH Study for on-site recruitment, data and sample collection as well as laboratory analyses. We thank Katrin Sprengel for performing the laboratory measurements at DIfE. This study was supported by Charité–Universitätsmedizin Berlin (grant 89539150).

Author Contributions: L.K.F. performed the statistical analysis, data interpretation and wrote the manuscript. F.J. contributed to the statistical analysis and revised the manuscript. I.D., G.B.A. and F.P.M. conceived and designed the study and were responsible for on-site recruitment and data collection. I.D., J.K. and M.B.S. supervised the study conduct, provided statistical expertise, contributed to the interpretation of data and revised the manuscript. I.D. had primary responsibility for final content. All authors read and approved the final manuscript.

Conflicts of Interest: The authors declare no conflict of interest.

References

1. Hall, V.; Thomsen, R.W.; Henriksen, O.; Lohse, N. Diabetes in sub Saharan Africa 1999–2011: Epidemiology and public health implications. A systematic review. *BMC Public Health* **2011**, *11*, 564. [CrossRef] [PubMed]

2. Mbanya, J.C.; Assah, F.K.; Saji, J.; Atanga, E.N. Obesity and type 2 diabetes in sub-Sahara Africa. *Curr. Diabetes Rep.* **2014**, *14*, 501. [CrossRef] [PubMed]

3. Mbanya, J.C.; Motala, A.A.; Sobngwi, E.; Assah, F.K.; Enoru, S.T. Diabetes in sub-Saharan Africa. *Lancet* **2010**, *375*, 2254–2266. [CrossRef]

4. Hu, F.B. Dietary pattern analysis: A new direction in nutritional epidemiology. *Curr. Opin. Lipidol.* **2002**, *13*, 3–9. [CrossRef] [PubMed]

5. Schulze, M.B.; Hoffmann, K. Methodological approaches to study dietary patterns in relation to risk of coronary heart disease and stroke. *Br. J. Nutr.* **2006**, *95*, 860–869. [CrossRef] [PubMed]

6. Tucker, K.L. Dietary patterns, approaches, and multicultural perspective. *Appl. Physiol. Nutr. Metab.* **2010**, *35*, 211–218. [CrossRef] [PubMed]

7. Hoffmann, K.; Schulze, M.B.; Schienkiewitz, A.; Nothlings, U.; Boeing, H. Application of a new statistical method to derive dietary patterns in nutritional epidemiology. *Am. J. Epidemiol.* **2004**, *159*, 935–944. [CrossRef] [PubMed]

8. Kroger, J.; Ferrari, P.; Jenab, M.; Bamia, C.; Touvier, M.; Bueno-de-Mesquita, H.B.; Fahey, M.T.; Benetou, V.; Schulz, M.; Wirfalt, E.; *et al.* Specific food group combinations explaining the variation in intakes of nutrients and other important food components in the european prospective investigation into cancer and nutrition: An application of the reduced rank regression method. *Eur. J. Clin. Nutr.* **2009**, *63* (Suppl. 4), S263–S274. [CrossRef] [PubMed]

9. DiBello, J.R.; Kraft, P.; McGarvey, S.T.; Goldberg, R.; Campos, H.; Baylin, A. Comparison of 3 methods for identifying dietary patterns associated with risk of disease. *Am. J. Epidemiol.* **2008**, *168*, 1433–1443. [CrossRef] [PubMed]

10. Hoffmann, K.; Zyriax, B.C.; Boeing, H.; Windler, E. A dietary pattern derived to explain biomarker variation is strongly associated with the risk of coronary artery disease. *Am. J. Clin. Nutr.* **2004**, *80*, 633–640. [PubMed]

11. Heidemann, C.; Hoffmann, K.; Spranger, J.; Klipstein-Grobusch, K.; Mohlig, M.; Pfeiffer, A.F.; Boeing, H. A dietary pattern protective against type 2 diabetes in the european prospective investigation into cancer and nutrition (EPIC)—Potsdam study cohort. *Diabetologia* **2005**, *48*, 1126–1134. [CrossRef] [PubMed]

12. Liese, A.D.; Weis, K.E.; Schulz, M.; Tooze, J.A. Food intake patterns associated with incident type 2 diabetes: The insulin resistance atherosclerosis study. *Diabetes Care* **2009**, *32*, 263–268. [CrossRef] [PubMed]

13. McNaughton, S.A.; Mishra, G.D.; Brunner, E.J. Dietary patterns, insulin resistance, and incidence of type 2 diabetes in the whitehall ii study. *Diabetes Care* **2008**, *31*, 1343–1348. [CrossRef] [PubMed]

14. Schulze, M.B.; Hoffmann, K.; Manson, J.E.; Willett, W.C.; Meigs, J.B.; Weikert, C.; Heidemann, C.; Colditz, G.A.; Hu, F.B. Dietary pattern, inflammation, and incidence of type 2 diabetes in women. *Am. J. Clin. Nutr.* **2005**, *82*, 675–684. [PubMed]

15. Danquah, I.; Bedu-Addo, G.; Terpe, K.J.; Micah, F.; Amoako, Y.A.; Awuku, Y.A.; Dietz, E.; van der Giet, M.; Spranger, J.; Mockenhaupt, F.P. Diabetes mellitus type 2 in urban Ghana: Characteristics and associated factors. *BMC Public Health* **2012**, *12*, 210. [CrossRef] [PubMed]

16. WHO. Definition, diagnosis and classification of diabetes mellitus and its complication: Report of a WHO consultation. Part 1: Diagnosis and classification of diabetes mellitus. World Health Organization: Geneva, 1999; Available online: http://whqlibdoc.Who.Int/hq/1999/who_ncd_ncs_99.2.Pdf (accessed on 20 March 2015).

17. Frank, L.K.; Kroger, J.; Schulze, M.B.; Bedu-Addo, G.; Mockenhaupt, F.P.; Danquah, I. Dietary patterns in urban ghana and risk of type 2 diabetes. *Br. J. Nutr.* **2014**, *112*, 89–98. [CrossRef] [PubMed]

18. Ainsworth, B.E.; Haskell, W.L.; Leon, A.S.; Jacobs, D.R., Jr.; Montoye, H.J.; Sallis, J.F.; Paffenbarger, R.S., Jr. Compendium of physical activities: Classification of energy costs of human physical activities. *Med. Sci. Sports Exerc.* **1993**, *25*, 71–80. [CrossRef] [PubMed]

19. Li, S.; Shin, H.J.; Ding, E.L.; van Dam, R.M. Adiponectin levels and risk of type 2 diabetes: A systematic review and meta-analysis. *JAMA: J. Am. Med. Assoc.* **2009**, *302*, 179–188. [CrossRef] [PubMed]

20. Drew, B.G.; Rye, K.A.; Duffy, S.J.; Barter, P.; Kingwell, B.A. The emerging role of hdl in glucose metabolism. *Nat. Rev. Endocrinol.* **2012**, *8*, 237–245. [CrossRef] [PubMed]

21. Haffner, S.M. Lipoprotein disorders associated with type 2 diabetes mellitus and insulin resistance. *Am. J. Cardiol.* **2002**, *90*, 55i–61i. [CrossRef]

22. InterAct Consortium. Adherence to predefined dietary patterns and incident type 2 diabetes in european populations: EPIC-InterAct study. *Diabetologia* **2014**, *57*, 321–333.

23. Imamura, F.; Lichtenstein, A.H.; Dallal, G.E.; Meigs, J.B.; Jacques, P.F. Generalizability of dietary patterns associated with incidence of type 2 diabetes mellitus. *Am. J. Clin. Nutr.* **2009**, *90*, 1075–1083. [CrossRef] [PubMed]

24. Micha, R.; Wallace, S.K.; Mozaffarian, D. Red and processed meat consumption and risk of incident coronary heart disease, stroke, and diabetes mellitus: A systematic review and meta-analysis. *Circulation* **2010**, *121*, 2271–2283. [CrossRef] [PubMed]

25. Pan, A.; Sun, Q.; Bernstein, A.M.; Schulze, M.B.; Manson, J.E.; Willett, W.C.; Hu, F.B. Red meat consumption and risk of type 2 diabetes: 3 cohorts of us adults and an updated meta-analysis. *Am. J. Clin. Nutr.* **2011**, *94*, 1088–1096. [CrossRef] [PubMed]

26. Feskens, E.J.M.; Sluik, D.; van Woudenbergh, G.J. Meat consumption, diabetes, and its complications. *Curr. Diabetes Rep.* **2013**, *13*, 298–306. [CrossRef] [PubMed]

27. Marriott, J.; Robinson, M.; Karikari, S.K. Starch and sugar transformation during the ripening of plantains and bananas. *J. Sci. Food Agric.* **1981**, *32*, 1021–1026. [CrossRef]

28. Bhupathiraju, S.N.; Tobias, D.K.; Malik, V.S.; Pan, A.; Hruby, A.; Manson, J.E.; Willett, W.C.; Hu, F.B. Glycemic index, glycemic load, and risk of type 2 diabetes: Results from 3 large us cohorts and an updated meta-analysis. *Am. J. Clin. Nutr.* **2014**, *100*, 218–232. [CrossRef] [PubMed]

29. Liu, S.; Manson, J.E.; Stampfer, M.J.; Holmes, M.D.; Hu, F.B.; Hankinson, S.E.; Willett, W.C. Dietary glycemic load assessed by food-frequency questionnaire in relation to plasma high-density-lipoprotein cholesterol and fasting plasma triacylglycerols in postmenopausal women. *Am. J. Clin. Nutr.* **2001**, *73*, 560–566. [PubMed]

30. Jeppesen, J.; Schaaf, P.; Jones, C.; Zhou, M.Y.; Chen, Y.D.; Reaven, G.M. Effects of low-fat, high-carbohydrate diets on risk factors for ischemic heart disease in postmenopausal women. *Am. J. Clin. Nutr.* **1997**, *65*, 1027–1033. [PubMed]

31. Mensink, R.P.; Katan, M.B. Effect of dietary fatty acids on serum lipids and lipoproteins. A meta-analysis of 27 trials. *Arterioscler. Thromb.* **1992**, *12*, 911–919. [CrossRef] [PubMed]

32. Parks, E.J. Effect of dietary carbohydrate on triglyceride metabolism in humans. *J. Nutr.* **2001**, *131*, 2772S–2774S. [PubMed]

33. Grundy, S.M.; Denke, M.A. Dietary influences on serum lipids and lipoproteins. *J. Lipid Res.* **1990**, *31*, 1149–1172. [PubMed]

34. Rosa, M.L.G.; Falcao, P.M.; Yokoo, E.M.; da Cruz, R.A.; Alcoforado, V.M.; de Souza, B.D.N.; Pinto, F.N.; Nery, A.B. Brazi's staple food and incident diabetes. *Nutrition* **2014**, *30*, 365–368. [CrossRef] [PubMed]

35. Kant, A.K.; Graubard, B.I. A comparison of three dietary pattern indexes for predicting biomarkers of diet and disease. *J. Am. Coll. Nutr.* **2005**, *24*, 294–303. [CrossRef] [PubMed]

36. Danquah, I.; Bedu-Addo, G.; Mockenhaupt, F.P. Type 2 diabetes mellitus and increased risk for malaria infection. *Emerg. Infect. Dis.* **2010**, *16*, 1601–1604. [CrossRef] [PubMed]
37. WHO. National Policy for the Prevention and Control of Chronic Non-communicable Diseases in Ghana. 2012. Available online: http://www.mindbank.info/item/1932 (accessed on 15 February 2015).

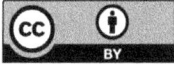

nutrients

MDPI

Article

The Relationship between Dietary Patterns and Metabolic Health in a Representative Sample of Adult Australians

Lucinda K. Bell [1], Suzanne Edwards [2] and Jessica A. Grieger [3,*]

[1] Nutrition and Dietetics, School of Health Sciences, Faculty of Medicine, Nursing and Health Sciences, Flinders University, Bedford Park 5042, Australia; E-Mail: lucy.bell@flinders.edu.au

[2] Data Management and Analysis Centre (DMAC), Faculty of Health Sciences, University of Adelaide, Adelaide 5005, Australia; E-Mail: suzanne.edwards@adelaide.edu.au

[3] Robinson Research Institute, School of Medicine, Faculty of Health Sciences, University of Adelaide, Adelaide 5005, Australia

* Author to whom correspondence should be addressed; E-Mail: jessica.grieger@adelaide.edu.au; Tel.: +61-8-8313-4086; Fax: +61-8-8313-4099.

Received: 10 June 2015 / Accepted: 31 July 2015 / Published: 5 August 2015

Abstract: Studies assessing dietary intake and its relationship to metabolic phenotype are emerging, but limited. The aims of the study are to identify dietary patterns in Australian adults, and to determine whether these dietary patterns are associated with metabolic phenotype and obesity. Cross-sectional data from the Australian Bureau of Statistics 2011 Australian Health Survey was analysed. Subjects included adults aged 45 years and over (n = 2415). Metabolic phenotype was determined according to criteria used to define metabolic syndrome (0–2 abnormalities *vs.* 3–7 abnormalities), and additionally categorized for obesity (body mass index (BMI) $\geqslant$30 kg/m^2 *vs.* BMI <30 kg/m^2). Dietary patterns were derived using factor analysis. Multivariable models were used to assess the relationship between dietary patterns and metabolic phenotype, with adjustment for age, sex, smoking status, socio-economic indexes for areas, physical activity and daily energy intake. Twenty percent of the population was metabolically unhealthy and obese. In the fully adjusted model, for every one standard deviation increase in the Healthy dietary pattern, the odds of having a more metabolically healthy profile increased by 16% (odds ratio (OR) 1.16; 95% confidence interval (CI): 1.04, 1.29). Poor metabolic profile and obesity are prevalent in Australian adults and a healthier dietary pattern plays a role in a metabolic and BMI phenotypes. Nutritional strategies addressing metabolic syndrome criteria and targeting obesity are recommended in order to improve metabolic phenotype and potential disease burden.

Keywords: dietary patterns; metabolic health; obesity; Australia, national survey; body mass index; adults

1. Introduction

Metabolic abnormalities such as insulin resistance, hypertension, dyslipidemia and abnormal glucose metabolism place individuals at increased risk of cardiovascular diseases (CVD), type 2 diabetes and mortality [1–3]. Such abnormalities are commonly associated with obesity [4], yet there are a proportion of obese individuals (approximately 10%–25%) [5] that have a normal metabolic profile [5,6]. These individuals are termed "metabolically healthy and obese". Similarly, some normal weight individuals display an abnormal metabolic profile typically seen in obese individuals and are therefore termed "metabolically unhealthy, not obese". These phenotypes may carry varying disease and mortality risk [4,7].

The dietary determinants underlying metabolic health are not fully understood. Epidemiological studies that have focused on the role of single foods and/or individual nutrients have produced inconclusive findings regarding their influence on overall (not individual markers of) metabolic health [3,8,9]. This may be due to the complex nature of diet and the synergies between dietary constituents [10,11]. Thus, dietary patterns may be a more useful means for understanding the influence of diet on metabolic health as they examine the total effect of food and nutrient combinations and are reflective of the way people eat, that is, consumption of foods or meals rather than individual dietary constituents [10,11]. One recent review highlighted the beneficial effects of foods and nutrients contained in the Mediterranean dietary pattern, the DASH (dietary approaches to stop hypertension) diet, and the Nordic diet (based on traditional foods consumed in Northern Europe), including fruits, vegetables, wholegrains, dairy, vitamin D, calcium and omega 3 fatty acids on individual markers of metabolic syndrome [12]. However, the clustering of metabolic components associated with each dietary pattern was not quantitatively assessed. Nevertheless, despite a growing body of evidence investigating and demonstrating an association between dietary patterns and metabolic abnormalities, to our knowledge, none have been conducted in Australian adults. Further, the relationship between dietary patterns and varying metabolic phenotype has rarely been investigated, with most assessing metabolic health in general, and not accounting for obesity. Whether dietary patterns are associated with varying metabolic phenotypes within the context of an obese or non-obese body mass index (BMI) in Australian adults is unknown.

Therefore, the aims of this study are: (1) to identify dietary patterns in Australian adults aged $\geqslant 45$ years; and (2) to determine whether the dietary patterns identified are associated with metabolic phenotype in those who are obese and non-obese.

2. Experimental Section

2.1. Data and Study Population

Data was from the Australian Bureau of Statistics (ABS) Confidentialised Unit Record Files (CURF) obtained in the 2011–2013 Australian Health Survey (AHS) with access to the data using the Remote Access Data Laboratory. A full description of the methods for data collection in the AHS has been reported by the ABS [13]. Within the confidentialised unit record files, survey data was collected using the *National Health Survey* (NHS), the *National Nutrition and Physical Activity Survey* (NNPAS), and the *National Health Measures Survey* (NHMS), which included a biomedical component. Both the NHS and the NNPAS were conducted using a stratified multistage area sample of private dwellings, with participants aged 2 years and over. In the NHS, 21,108 private dwellings were selected (reduced to an actual sample of 18,355 dwellings after sample loss in the field stage), in which 84.8% were fully or adequately responding households (n = 15,565). In the NNPAS, a total of 14,363 private dwellings were selected in the sample for the NNPAS (reduced to an actual sample of 12,366 dwellings after sample loss in the field stage), in which 77.0% were fully or adequately responding households to the first interview (n = 9519). Of the 30,329 respondents aged 5 years and over in the combined sample (NHS + NNPAS), 11,246 (37.1%) participated in the biomedical component (NHMS). The 2011–2012 NHS and NNPAS utilised Computer Assisted Interview instruments to collect the data [13].

Variables drawn from the datasets and included in this paper were age, sex, smoking status (categorized by the ABS as current smoker, never a smoker and previous/episodic smoker), Socio-Economic Indexes for Areas (SEIFA) derived from SEIFA deciles provided by the ABS 2011–2013 AHS, and physical activity (using the three categories provided by the ABS 2011–2013 AHS: inactive in last week, insufficiently active for health in last week, or sufficiently active for health in last week). Waist circumference and blood pressure data measured in the AHS were also used in the metabolic health definition (see below). Further details of types of data collection obtained for each survey can be found on the ABS website [13]. Adults aged 45 years and over and who had blood results recorded (at least total cholesterol) and who had the first 24-h recall completed, as this is most representative of the Australian population, were used in the current analysis (n = 2415).

2.2. Dietary Data

The 2011–2012 NNPAS collected dietary data that included: 24-h dietary recall of food, beverages, and supplements (on two separate days); usual dietary behaviours; and whether currently on a diet and for what reason. Briefly, the 24-h dietary recall questionnaire collected detailed information on all foods and beverages consumed on the day prior to interview. Where possible, at least eight days after the first interview, respondents were contacted to participate in a second 24-h dietary recall via telephone interview. The Automated Multiple-Pass Method was used to gather food intake data, where an automated questionnaire guides the interviewer through a system designed to maximise respondents' opportunities for remembering and reporting foods eaten in the previous 24 h. Interviewers also used a Food Model Booklet to assist respondents with describing the amount of food and beverages consumed. The 24-h recall data was coded using the United States Department of Agriculture Dietary Intake Data System [14]. To allow for the coding of foods and measures, and the calculation of nutrients, Food Standards Australia and New Zealand developed a food and measures database. The database contains 5644 foods and 15,847 measures in which each food within the food database has a name, associated food description, inclusions, exclusions, and an eight-digit code. The eight-digit food codes are grouped into broader food groups (2-, 3- and 5- digit levels) based on groupings used in 1995 National Nutrition Survey. For the purpose of the analysis in this study, only the first 24-h recall was used (n = 2415 (100%) of participants; n = 1883 (78%) had 2 × 24-h recalls) and the minor food group categories (*i.e.*, 5-digit level) were coded into 39 food groups (Supplementary Table S1) for use in the factor analysis (see below).

2.3. Biomedical Measures

Key biomarkers measured in the NHMS included chronic disease biomarkers, tests for diabetes, cholesterol, triglycerides, kidney disease and liver function; as well as nutrient biomarkers (iron, folate, iodine and vitamin D). For the current analysis, biomarkers for "metabolic health" were: total cholesterol, high density lipoprotein cholesterol (HDL-C), low density lipoprotein cholesterol (LDL-C), triglycerides, and glucose. All of these measurements were obtained from a blood sample in those 12 years and over, in which LDL-C, triglycerides and glucose were taken in the fasted state.

2.4. Metabolic Health

Metabolic health was defined as follows: First, the following measures were dichotomised into "normal" and "abnormal" categories, where abnormal was defined as: (i) total cholesterol ⩾ 5.5 mmol/L or having current diagnosis of high cholesterol; (ii) fasting LDL-C ⩾ 3.5 mmol/L; (iii) HDL-C (accounting for sex) < 1.0 mmol/L for males and <1.3 mmol/L for females; (iv) fasting triglycerides ⩾ 2.0 mmol/L; (v) fasting plasma glucose status > 6.0 mmol/L or having current diagnosis of type 2 diabetes or unknown type; (vi) waist circumference in males ⩾102 cm or in females ⩾88 cm; (vii) systolic blood pressure ⩾ 140 mmHg or diastolic blood pressure ⩾ 90 mmHg or having current diagnosis of hypertension. Second, based on the above "abnormal" categories, four categories relevant to metabolic health were created. That is, metabolically healthy, not obese (best outcome: 0–2 abnormal criteria and a BMI < 30 kg/m^2) [15]; metabolically unhealthy, not obese (3–7 abnormal criteria and a BMI < 30 kg/m^2); metabolically healthy and obese (0–2 abnormal criteria and a BMI ⩾ 30 kg/m^2); and metabolically unhealthy, and obese (poorest outcome: 3–7 abnormal criteria and a BMI ⩾ 30 kg/m^2). Missing values were reported for: LDL-C (n = 394, 16%), triglycerides (n = 366, 15%), fasting plasma glucose (n = 366, 15%), waist circumference (n = 97, 4%), and blood pressure (n = 87, 3.6%); variables with no missing data included total cholesterol, HDL-C, doctor-diagnosed high cholesterol, doctor-diagnosed diabetes, and doctor-diagnosed hypertension (n = 2415). Where there were missing values, the metabolic category (*i.e.*, normal/abnormal) for that measurement (e.g., LDL-C) was coded as "normal".

2.5. Factor Analysis

Dietary patterns were derived using factor analysis with factor loadings extracted using the principal component method and varimax/orthogonal rotation. The number of dietary patterns identified was based on eigenvalues > 1.5, on identification of a break point in the scree plot, and on interpretability [16]. Using these criteria, a three-factor solution was chosen and rerun with the resulting factor scores saved and converted to *z*-scores for analysis. Items with factor loadings > 0.25 were considered as items of relevance for the identified factor. These items represent the foods most highly related to the identified factor [17]. Foods that cross-loaded on several factors were retained. Inter-item reliability for each factor was assessed using Cronbach's α coefficients.

2.6. Statistical Analyses

Frequencies and descriptive data were assessed as *n* (%) or mean (standard deviation, SD). Ordinal logistic regression analysis (*i.e.*, 1. metabolically healthy, not obese (best outcome); 2. metabolically unhealthy, not obese; 3. metabolically healthy, and obese; and 4. metabolically unhealthy and obese (poorest outcome)) was used to determine the association between the dietary patterns and metabolic health, after adjusting for dietary energy intake (Model 1) and further adjusting for age, sex, smoking status, Socio-Economic Indexes for Areas (SEIFA) quintile, and physical activity (Model 2). The proportional odds assumption was tested and appeared reasonable. Multivariable linear regression was performed to investigate the association between number of metabolic abnormalities and the dietary patterns, also with adjustments for age, sex, smoking status, SEIFA quintile, physical activity, and daily energy intake. Population weights were applied (supplied by the ABS) to produce estimates at the population level using the "surveyreg" and "surveylogistic" procedures in SAS. The statistical software used within the Remote Access Data Laboratory was SAS 9.1 (SAS Institute Inc., Cary, NC, USA).

3. Results

Characteristics of the 2415 adults included in the analysis are reported in Table 1. The mean number of metabolic abnormalities was 2.2 and the median was 2.0. In the sample, 12% were metabolically healthy and obese; 48% were metabolically healthy, not obese; 20% were metabolically unhealthy, and obese; and 20% were metabolically unhealthy, not obese. In males and females combined, the most prevalent metabolic abnormality was high waist circumference (48%), followed by high LDL-C (43%), high total cholesterol (42%), high blood pressure (38%), low HDL-C (22%), high triglycerides (17%), and high plasma glucose (7%).

3.1. Dietary Patterns

Three dietary patterns were identified (Table 2). The variance explained by each factor was 9.8%, 7.5%, and 4.6%, respectively. Factor 1 was labelled Red meat and vegetable as red meat and several types of vegetables loaded on this pattern. Factor 2 was labelled Refined and processed as added sugar, full fat dairy, unsaturated spreads, cakes, pastries, and processed meat loaded on this pattern, while fresh fruit and vegetables were inversely correlated. Factor 3 was labelled Healthy as wholegrains, fresh fruit, dried fruit, legumes and low fat dairy loaded on this pattern, while take-away foods, soft drinks, alcoholic drinks, and fried potato were inversely correlated.

Table 1. Descriptive characteristics of the Australian sample aged 45 years and over, participating in the 2011–2013 Australian Health Survey.

	All (n = 2415)	Red Meat and Vegetable			Refined and Processed			Healthy		
		Tertile 1	Tertile 2	Tertile 3	Tertile 1	Tertile 2	Tertile 3	Tertile 1	Tertile 2	Tertile 3
Males/females (%)	48/52	49/51	43/57	53/47	37/63	43/57	66/34	53/47	43/57	50/50
Age group (%)										
45–60 years	54	60	50	52	53	55	53	57	54	50
61–70 years	25	20	27	27	27	22	24	26	23	25
>70 years	21	20	23	21	20	22	22	17	23	25
BMI (%)										
Obese (≥30 kg/m^2)	31	40	32	32	27	34	33	33	33	28
Overweight (25–29.99 kg/m^2)	40	30	39	39	43	38	38	44	35	40
Normal/underweight (<25 kg/m^2)	29	30	29	29	31	28	29	23	32	32
Metabolic abnormalities (%)										
0	10	13	12	11	14	10	12	10	14	12
1–2	49	50	49	48	48	52	48	49	49	51
3–5	40	36	38	39	37	37	39	40	36	36
6–7	1	2	1	1	1	1	1	1	2	1
Physical activity (%)										
Inactive	22	25	17	24	17	24	25	22	26	17
Insufficiently active	26	23	31	25	24	24	32	27	24	29
Sufficiently active for health	52	52	51	51	59	52	43	51	50	54
SEIFA quintile (%)										
Quintile 1 (lowest)	19	17	20	18	17	18	21	19	18	20
Quintile 2	19	21	18	19	16	21	20	21	19	17
Quintile 3	21	22	19	22	19	20	23	19	22	20
Quintile 4	19	19	19	18	22	17	17	19	17	20
Quintile 5 (highest)	23	21	24	23	26	24	19	22	23	22
Smoking status (%)										
Current smoker	10	11	11	9	9	9	12	14	11	5
Never a smoker	47	46	47	48	50	47	43	39	47	54
Previous/episodic smoker	43	44	42	44	41	44	45	47	42	41

BMI: body mass index; SEIFA: Socio-Economic indexes for areas.

Table 2. Dietary patterns of the adults aged 45 years and over participating in the 2011–2013 Australian Health Survey.

Red Meat and Vegetable		Refined and Processed		Healthy	
Food Group	Factor Loading	Food Group	Factor Loading	Food Group	Factor Loading
Yellow or red vegetables	0.59	Added sugar	0.56	Whole grains	0.36
Potatoes	0.57	Full-fat dairy products	0.41	Fresh fruit	0.35
Red meats	0.50	Unsaturated spreads	0.36	Low-fat dairy products	0.33
Other vegetables	0.33	Cakes, biscuits, sweet pastries	0.32	Dried fruit	0.32
Cruciferous vegetables	0.29	Processed meat	0.25	Legumes	0.29
		Canned fruit	0.25	Unsaturated spreads	0.25
		Soft drinks	0.25		
Meat-based mixed dishes	−0.40	Other vegetables	−0.26	Take-away foods	−0.28
		Fresh fruit	−0.32	Soft drinks	−0.33
				Alcoholic drinks	−0.40
				Fried potatoes	−0.42

3.2. Dietary Patterns and Metabolic Health

In the ordinal logistic regression analysis, after adjustment for energy intake, there was a significant association between the four metabolic profile categories and the Refined and processed dietary pattern, such that for every one standard deviation increase in the Refined and processed pattern, the odds of having a more metabolically healthy profile decreased by 14% (odds ratio (OR) 0.86, 95% confidence interval (CI): 0.76, 0.98), while for every one standard deviation increase in the Healthy dietary pattern, the odds of having a more metabolically healthy profile increased by 18% (OR 1.18, 95% CI: 1.06, 1.31). In the fully adjusted models, only the association between the Healthy dietary pattern and a healthier metabolic profile remained significant (Table 3).

Table 3. Odds ratios (95% confidence interval (CI)) for metabolic profile [1], according to dietary pattern.

Metabolic Profile	Model 1 [2]	95% CI	Model 2 [3]	95% CI
Red meat and vegetable	0.97	0.88, 1.08	0.99	0.89, 1.10
Refined and processed	0.86	0.76, 0.98 *	0.92	0.81, 1.04
Healthy	1.18	1.06, 1.31 †	1.16	1.04, 1.29 †

[1] Metabolic profile (ordinal logistic regression analysis with outcomes: 1. metabolically healthy, not obese (best outcome); 2. metabolically unhealthy, not obese; 3. metabolically healthy, and obese; and 4. metabolically unhealthy and obese (poorest outcome). Probabilities modelled are cumulated over the lower ordered values and metabolically healthy, not obese, is the lowest of the lower ordered values). [2] Adjusted for energy intake (energy $p = 0.0728$). [3] Adjusted for age (45–60; 61–70; > 70), sex, smoking status (Current smoker Never a smoker Previous/episodic smoker), socio-economic indexes for areas quintile, physical activity level. * $p < 0.05$; † $p < 0.01$.

3.3. Dietary Patterns and Metabolic Abnormalities

In linear regression, a significant association was found between number of metabolic abnormalities and the Refined and processed dietary pattern (Model 1, $p = 0.0089$), such that for every one standard deviation increase in the Refined and processed pattern, the average number of metabolic abnormalities increases by 0.104 (Table 4). In the adjusted model however, the association did not reach statistical significance. In the unadjusted and adjusted analyses, there was no association for any of the dietary patterns and being metabolically healthy (0–2 abnormalities) or metabolically unhealthy (3–7 abnormalities) (Table 5).

Table 4. Linear regression estimates for number of metabolic abnormalities, according to dietary pattern.

Metabolic Number	Model 1 Estimate [1]	95% CI	Model 2 Adjusted Estimate [2]	95% CI
Red meat and vegetable	0.0007	−0.07, 0.07	−0.004	−0.07, 0.07
Refined and processed	0.10	0.03, 0.18	0.07	−0.01, 0.15
Healthy	−0.06	−0.13, 0.01	−0.04	−0.11, 0.03

[1] Adjusted for energy intake ($p = 0.0109$); [2] Adjusted for energy intake, age (45–60; 61–70; > 70), sex, smoking status (current smoker, never a smoker, previous/episodic smoker), socio-economic indexes for areas quintile, physical activity level (inactive, insufficiently active, sufficiently active); CI, confidence interval.

Table 5. Odds ratios for metabolic health [1], according to dietary pattern.

Metabolic Health	Model 1 [2]	95% CI	Model 2 [3]	95% CI
Red meat and vegetable	1.00	0.90, 1.11	1.01	0.91, 1.12
Refined and processed	0.89	0.78, 1.02	0.94	0.82, 1.07
Healthy	1.10	0.98, 1.23	1.08	0.96, 1.21

[1] Metabolically healthy (0–2 abnormalities) *vs.* those who are metabolically unhealthy (3–7 abnormalities); [2] Adjusted for energy intake (not significant); [3] Adjusted for energy intake, age (45–60; 61–70; >70), sex, smoking status (current smoker, never a smoker, previous/episodic smoker), socio-economic indexes for areas quintile, physical activity level (inactive, insufficiently active, sufficiently active); CI, confidence interval.

4. Discussion

To our knowledge, this is the first study reporting on the prevalence of metabolic health in a sample of adult Australians, and identifying associations between metabolic phenotype and current dietary patterns. We report that nearly half of the sample had a metabolically healthy profile (*i.e.*, metabolically healthy and not obese), while 40% of the remaining sample was metabolically unhealthy (regardless of BMI), and 12% were metabolically healthy and obese. The prevalence of the latter phenotype identified in this population is intermediate compared to 19% of adults (*n* = 4541) from the Atherosclerosis Risk in Communities study [18]; 8.2% reported in Thai men and women aged 18–59 years [19]; while in a sample of 780 women, 28% of women with normal BMI were metabolically unhealthy [20]. Further, in a population-based sample of 2803 women and 2557 men from Switzerland, six different criteria were used to define metabolically healthy obesity, with prevalence rates varying between 3.3% and 32.1% in men and between 11.4% and 43.3% in women [21]. Although differences in metabolic health criteria exist between studies, the fact that nearly half of our population was metabolically unhealthy is of concern as the biomarkers used to define metabolic health can be modified, particularly through diet and lifestyle changes. Irrespective of metabolic health, 71% of our population was either overweight or obese, which, in addition to poor metabolic health, has been consistently shown to play a key role in several chronic diseases [4,22].

Three dietary patterns were identified in the dietary pattern analysis. The dietary patterns resemble other dietary patterns, common in previous studies such as a prudent diet, similar to our red meat and vegetable pattern, a western diet, similar to our refined and processed pattern, and a healthy diet, comparable to our healthy pattern. After adjusting for energy intake only, we found that the odds for having a more metabolically healthy profile decreased by 14% following higher consumption of the refined and processed pattern, while the odds of having a more metabolically healthy profile increased by 16% with increasing consumption of the healthy dietary pattern (adjusted analysis). Only two other studies, to our knowledge, were found that assessed diet and metabolic health with or without obesity [3,23]. In a sample of 45–85 year old men and women participating in National Health and Nutrition Examination Survey, 2007–2008 and 2009–2010, there were no significant differences in the Healthy Eating Index (2005) between those who were metabolically healthy and obese compared to those metabolically unhealthy and obese [23]. In a cross-sectional study of 6964 women in the US, food intake, as measured by a food frequency questionnaire, was not significantly different between obese women who were metabolically healthy or metabolically unhealthy [3]. That is, consumption of for example, fruits, vegetables, refined grains, sugar sweetened beverages, low/high fat dairy or take-away foods, were not different between those with or without metabolic syndrome (defined using both the American Heart Association/National Heart, Lung, and Blood Institute guidelines [24] and the homeostatic model assessment for insulin resistance [25,26]). That study however assessed single food group intakes rather than a complete dietary pattern, and the criteria for metabolic health between our study and that study was different. For example, our study used fasting plasma glucose status > 6.0 mmol/L or having current diagnosis of type 2 diabetes or unknown type, and systolic blood pressure ⩾ 140 mmHg or diastolic blood pressure ⩾ 90 mmHg, compared to that study using elevated blood pressure (⩾ 130/⩾ 85 mmHg) or drug therapy for hypertension, elevated glucose (⩾ 5.6 mmol/L) or drug therapy for hyperglycemia. Given the limited results, drawing conclusions on the impact of metabolic health and obesity requires further investigation. However our results indicate that a healthier dietary pattern, consisting of wholegrains, fruit, legumes and low fat dairy is associated with a more metabolically healthy profile and these foods should be promoted to assist metabolic parameters.

We found no associations between metabolic health, as a continuous number of abnormalities, or between those considered metabolically healthy or metabolically unhealthy, and any of the dietary patterns. This contrasts with previous studies that have shown a Western dietary pattern was associated with incidence of metabolic syndrome over 9 years [27], metabolic abnormalities in 20,827 Chinese adults [28], as well as individual components of the metabolic syndrome [29,30]. A vegetarian dietary pattern was associated with a lower risk of metabolic syndrome in older adults in the US [31]; lower adherence to a Mediterranean dietary pattern was associated with greater number of metabolic syndrome parameters [32]; and men and women in the highest quartile of carbohydrate pattern (containing high intake of glutinous rice, fermented fish, chili paste, and bamboo shoots) had an 82% and 60% greater odds of having metabolic syndrome, respectively, than those in the lower quartiles of the carbohydrate pattern [33]. Similarly, a recent review by Calton *et al.*, highlighted the beneficial effects of the Mediterranean dietary pattern, the DASH diet, and the Nordic diet on metabolic syndrome components [12]. Additional large population studies are required to assist in drawing conclusions on the relationship between dietary patterns and metabolic health.

The pathophysiology of metabolically healthy obesity is likely the result of a number of underlying mechanisms and the interaction between genetic, environmental, and behavioral factors [34]. All of these factors have been shown to be related to fat distribution and accumulation, in addition to insulin resistance. Thus, the phenotype of those who are metabolically unhealthy and obese compared to those who are metabolically healthy and obese is different [35]. In particular, those who are metabolically unhealthy and obese have a greater proportion of subcutaneous fat [36] as well as increased markers of inflammation [37] compared to those who are metabolically unhealthy and obese. However, a recent meta-analysis of 20 studies (n = 359,137) reported a general non-significant relationship between metabolically healthy obesity and cardiovascular disease risk [15], indicating the metabolically healthy obese phenotype does not appear to confer greater risk for cardiovascular disease. These outcomes may lend support to our results in which we found no significant associations between number of metabolic abnormalities and dietary patterns, albeit an increased odds of having a more metabolically healthy profile with a healthier dietary pattern rather than a refined pattern.

Strengths of our study include the large population assessed and the rigorous data collection methods employed within the Australian Health Survey. Limitations to the study include the heterogeneous nature of the metabolic phenotype definition. However, we limited our criteria of metabolic phenotype to <3 abnormalities which several previous studies have also used [15], and our definition of metabolic health included waist circumference, rather than BMI as a marker of adiposity, as although BMI is useful in estimating body fatness, waist circumference provides an estimate of visceral adiposity and has been associated with insulin resistance, type 2 diabetes, and cardiovascular events [38]. Fasting glucose was also used to determine metabolic health, which has limitations in that in only provides a snap-shot of glucose regulation [39]; however the survey did not measure insulin resistance, thus we used the best marker available. Limitations of our study include its cross-sectional nature which does not assess change in diet and participants may have improved their diet if they had diagnosis of poor metabolic profile. That is, if participants were aware they had high blood pressure they may have reduced their sodium intake or increased their dairy intake; or if they had high cholesterol, they may have reduced their saturated fat and increased the unsaturated fat intake, hence improving diet quality. As such, capturing a single day of intake would have not have picked up these changes in diet. Further, using a 24-h recall, usual intake of an individual cannot be assessed, thus repeated 24-h recalls are needed to get population distributions of habitual intake. However, as the multiple pass system was used rather than a self-administered 24-h recall, this provides greater precision and provides the respondent with a number of occasions in which to reflect and accurately report on their intake by a trained researcher. Additionally, the survey was conducted over a year, thereby capturing seasonal intakes of different foods. Longitudinal studies would be ideal to capture any changes in diet and/or risk for developing adverse metabolic outcomes. The variance explained by our factors was lower than other previous studies [40–43], however the low variance could be partially explained by the fact that a number of participants were not eating some of the food groups thereby skewing the data and potentially indicating lower communality amongst the measured variables. Nevertheless, the Kaiser-Meyer-Olkin measure of sampling adequacy was greater than 0.5 indicating that factor analysis was appropriate for this data set and the food groups loading on the factors were varied and many were greater than the 0.25 cut-off value, suggesting our population had a varied diet that was, nevertheless, still specific to the identified factors. Finally, although we had some missing values for some of the metabolic markers, given the large sample size in this dataset, the number of missing values is unlikely to have influenced the results.

5. Conclusions

In summary, we identified that 20% of Australian adults aged $\geqslant$ 45 years were metabolically unhealthy and obese. Higher consumption of an unhealthier dietary pattern, characterised by refined and processed foods was associated with decreased likelihood of having a healthy metabolic and BMI profile, while the reverse was apparent for the healthy dietary pattern. Nutritional strategies addressing metabolic syndrome criteria and targeting obesity are recommended in order to improve metabolic phenotype and potential disease burden.

Acknowledgments: The authors declare that there were no other personal or financial conflicts of interest. Findings based on use of ABS confidentialised unit record files data.

Author Contributions: Jessica A. Grieger devised the aims and wrote the manuscript; Suzanne Edwards performed the statistical analyses; Lucinda K. Bell assisted with interpretation of the results and writing of the manuscript.

Conflicts of Interest: The authors declare no conflict of interest.

References

1. Grundy, S.M.; Brewer, H.B., Jr.; Cleeman, J.I.; Smith, S.C., Jr.; Lenfant, C. Definition of metabolic syndrome: Report of the National Heart, Lung, and Blood Institute/American Heart Association conference on scientific issues related to definition. *Circulation* **2004**, *109*, 433–438. [CrossRef] [PubMed]
2. Grundy, S.M.; Cleeman, J.I.; Daniels, S.R.; Donato, K.A.; Eckel, R.H.; Franklin, B.A.; Gordon, D.J.; Krauss, R.M.; Savage, P.J.; Smith, S.C., Jr.; *et al.* Diagnosis and management of the metabolic syndrome: An American Heart Association/National Heart, Lung, and Blood Institute Scientific Statement. *Circulation* **2005**, *112*, 2735–2752. [CrossRef] [PubMed]
3. Kimokoti, R.W.; Judd, S.E.; Shikany, J.M.; Newby, P.K. Food intake does not differ between obese women who are metabolically healthy or abnormal. *J. Nutr.* **2014**, *144*, 2018–2026. [CrossRef] [PubMed]
4. Pajunen, P.; Kotronen, A.; Korpi-Hyovalti, E.; Keinanen-Kiukaanniemi, S.; Oksa, H.; Niskanen, L.; Saaristo, T.; Saltevo, J.T.; Sundvall, J.; Vanhala, M.; *et al.* Metabolically healthy and unhealthy obesity phenotypes in the general population: The FIN-D2D Survey. *BMC Public Health* **2011**, *11*. [CrossRef] [PubMed]
5. Bluher, M. The distinction of metabolically "healthy" from "unhealthy" obese individuals. *Curr. Opin. Lipidol.* **2010**, *21*, 38–43. [CrossRef] [PubMed]
6. Sims, E.A. Are there persons who are obese, but metabolically healthy? *Metabolism* **2001**, *50*, 1499–1504. [CrossRef] [PubMed]
7. Hinnouho, G.M.; Czernichow, S.; Dugravot, A.; Batty, G.D.; Kivimaki, M.; Singh-Manoux, A. Metabolically healthy obesity and risk of mortality: Does the definition of metabolic health matter? *Diabetes Care* **2013**, *36*, 2294–2300. [CrossRef] [PubMed]
8. Lee, K. Metabolically obese but normal weight (MONW) and metabolically healthy but obese (MHO) phenotypes in Koreans: Characteristics and health behaviors. *Asia Pac. J. Clin. Nutr.* **2009**, *18*, 280–284. [PubMed]
9. Shin, J.Y.; Kim, J.Y.; Kang, H.T.; Han, K.H.; Shim, J.Y. Effect of fruits and vegetables on metabolic syndrome: A systematic review and meta-analysis of randomized controlled trials. *Int. J. Food Sci. Nutr.* **2015**, *66*, 416–425. [CrossRef] [PubMed]
10. Hu, F.B. Dietary pattern analysis: A new direction in nutritional epidemiology. *Curr. Opin. Lipidol.* **2002**, *13*, 3–9. [CrossRef] [PubMed]
11. Moeller, S.M.; Reedy, J.; Millen, A.E.; Dixon, L.B.; Newby, P.K.; Tucker, K.L.; Krebs-Smith, S.M.; Guenther, P.M. Dietary patterns: Challenges and opportunities in dietary patterns research an Experimental Biology workshop, 1 April 2006. *J. Am. Diet. Assoc.* **2007**, *107*, 1233–1239. [CrossRef] [PubMed]

12. Australian Bureau of Statistics. Australian Health Survey 2011–13, Expanded CURF, RADL. Findings based on use of ABS CURF data. Available online: http://www.abs.gov.au/ausstats/abs@.nsf/Lookup/D9707300945AE90FCA257B8D00229E78?opendocument (accessed on 13 January 2015).

13. Calton, E.; James, A.; Pannu, P.; Soares, M. Certain dietary patterns are beneficial for the metabolic syndrome: Reviewing the evidence. *Nutr. Res.* **2014**, *34*, 559–568. [CrossRef] [PubMed]

14. Raper, N.; Perloff, B.; Ingwersen, L.; Steinfeldt, L.; Anand, J. An overview of USDA's dietary intake data system. *J. Food Compos. Anal.* **2004**, *17*, 545–555. [CrossRef]

15. Roberson, L.L.; Aneni, E.C.; Maziak, W.; Agatston, A.; Feldman, T.; Rouseff, M.; Tran, T.; Blaha, M.J.; Santos, R.D.; Sposito, A.; *et al.* Beyond BMI: The "metabolically healthy obese" phenotype & its association with clinical/subclinical cardiovascular disease and all-cause mortality—A systematic review. *BMC Public Health* **2014**, *14*, 14. [PubMed]

16. Schulze, M.B.; Hoffmann, K.; Kroke, A.; Boeing, H. An approach to construct simplified measures of dietary patterns from exploratory factor analysis. *Br. J. Nutr.* **2003**, *89*, 409–419. [CrossRef] [PubMed]

17. Kline, P.K. *An Easy Guide to Factor Analysis*; Routledge: London, UK; New York, NY, USA, 1994.

18. Cui, Z.; Truesdale, K.P.; Bradshaw, P.T.; Cai, J.; Stevens, J. Three-year weight change and cardiometabolic risk factors in obese and normal weight adults who are metabolically healthy: The atherosclerosis risk in communities study. *Int. J. Obes. (Lond.)* **2015**. [CrossRef] [PubMed]

19. Hwang, L.C.; Bai, C.H.; Sun, C.A.; Chen, C.J. Prevalence of metabolically healthy obesity and its impacts on incidences of hypertension, diabetes and the metabolic syndrome in Taiwan. *Asia Pac. J. Clin. Nutr.* **2012**, *21*, 227–233. [PubMed]

20. Kip, K.E.; Marroquin, O.C.; Kelley, D.E.; Johnson, B.D.; Kelsey, S.F.; Shaw, L.J.; Rogers, W.J.; Reis, S.E. Clinical importance of obesity *versus* the metabolic syndrome in cardiovascular risk in women: A report from the Women's Ischemia Syndrome Evaluation (WISE) study. *Circulation* **2004**, *109*, 706–713. [CrossRef] [PubMed]

21. Velho, S.; Paccaud, F.; Waeber, G.; Vollenweider, P.; Marques-Vidal, P. Metabolically healthy obesity: Different prevalences using different criteria. *Eur. J. Clin. Nutr.* **2010**, *64*, 1043–1051. [CrossRef] [PubMed]

22. Manabe, I. Chronic inflammation links cardiovascular, metabolic and renal diseases. *Circ. J.* **2011**, *75*, 2739–2748. [CrossRef] [PubMed]

23. Camhi, S.M.; Whitney Evans, E.; Hayman, L.L.; Lichtenstein, A.H.; Must, A. Healthy eating index and metabolically healthy obesity in U.S. adolescents and adults. *Prev. Med.* **2015**, *77*, 23–27. [CrossRef] [PubMed]

24. Alberti, K.G.; Eckel, R.H.; Grundy, S.M.; Zimmet, P.Z.; Cleeman, J.I.; Donato, K.A.; Fruchart, J.C.; James, W.P.; Loria, C.M.; Smith, S.C., Jr.; *et al.* Harmonizing the metabolic syndrome: A joint interim statement of the International Diabetes Federation Task Force on Epidemiology and Prevention; National Heart, Lung, and Blood Institute; American Heart Association; World Heart Federation; International Atherosclerosis Society; and International Association for the Study of Obesity. *Circulation* **2009**, *120*, 1640–1645. [PubMed]

25. Balkau, B.; Charles, M.A. Comment on the provisional report from the WHO consultation. European Group for the Study of Insulin Resistance (EGIR). *Diabet. Med.* **1999**, *16*, 442–443. [PubMed]

26. Matthews, D.R.; Hosker, J.P.; Rudenski, A.S.; Naylor, B.A.; Treacher, D.F.; Turner, R.C. Homeostasis model assessment: Insulin resistance and β-cell function from fasting plasma glucose and insulin concentrations in man. *Diabetologia* **1985**, *28*, 412–419. [CrossRef] [PubMed]

27. Lutsey, P.L.; Steffen, L.M.; Stevens, J. Dietary intake and the development of the metabolic syndrome: The Atherosclerosis Risk in Communities study. *Circulation* **2008**, *117*, 754–761. [CrossRef] [PubMed]

28. He, Y.; Li, Y.; Lai, J.; Wang, D.; Zhang, J.; Fu, P.; Yang, X.; Qi, L. Dietary patterns as compared with physical activity in relation to metabolic syndrome among Chinese adults. *Nutr. Metab. Cardiovasc. Dis.* **2013**, *23*, 920–928. [CrossRef] [PubMed]

29. Arisawa, K.; Uemura, H.; Yamaguchi, M.; Nakamoto, M.; Hiyoshi, M.; Sawachika, F.; Katsuura-Kamano, S. Associations of dietary patterns with metabolic syndrome and insulin resistance: A cross-sectional study in a Japanese population. *J. Med. Investig.* **2014**, *61*, 333–344. [CrossRef]

30. Panagiotakos, D.B.; Pitsavos, C.; Skoumas, Y.; Stefanadis, C. The association between food patterns and the metabolic syndrome using principal components analysis: The ATTICA Study. *J. Am. Diet. Assoc.* **2007**, *107*, 979–987. [CrossRef] [PubMed]

31. Rizzo, N.S.; Sabate, J.; Jaceldo-Siegl, K.; Fraser, G.E. Vegetarian dietary patterns are associated with a lower risk of metabolic syndrome: The adventist health study 2. *Diabetes Care* **2011**, *34*, 1225–1227. [CrossRef] [PubMed]

32. Viscogliosi, G.; Cipriani, E.; Liguori, M.L.; Marigliano, B.; Saliola, M.; Ettorre, E.; Andreozzi, P. Mediterranean dietary pattern adherence: Associations with prediabetes, metabolic syndrome, and related microinflammation. *Metab. Syndr. Relat. Disord.* **2013**, *11*, 210–216. [CrossRef] [PubMed]

33. Aekplakorn, W.; Satheannoppakao, W.; Putwatana, P.; Taneepanichskul, S.; Kessomboon, P.; Chongsuvivatwong, V.; Chariyalertsak, S. Dietary pattern and metabolic syndrome in Thai adults. *J. Nutr. Metab.* **2015**, *2015*. [CrossRef] [PubMed]

34. Rice, T.; Perusse, L.; Bouchard, C.; Rao, D.C. Familial clustering of abdominal visceral fat and total fat mass: The Quebec Family Study. *Obes. Res.* **1996**, *4*, 253–261. [CrossRef] [PubMed]

35. Naukkarinen, J.; Heinonen, S.; Hakkarainen, A.; Lundbom, J.; Vuolteenaho, K.; Saarinen, L.; Hautaniemi, S.; Rodriguez, A.; Fruhbeck, G.; Pajunen, P.; *et al.* Characterising metabolically healthy obesity in weight-discordant monozygotic twins. *Diabetologia* **2014**, *57*, 167–176. [CrossRef] [PubMed]

36. Koster, A.; Stenholm, S.; Alley, D.E.; Kim, L.J.; Simonsick, E.M.; Kanaya, A.M.; Visser, M.; Houston, D.K.; Nicklas, B.J.; Tylavsky, F.A.; *et al.* Body fat distribution and inflammation among obese older adults with and without metabolic syndrome. *Obesity (Silver Spring)* **2010**, *18*, 2354–2361. [CrossRef] [PubMed]

37. Esser, N.; L'Homme, L.; de Roover, A.; Kohnen, L.; Scheen, A.J.; Moutschen, M.; Piette, J.; Legrand-Poels, S.; Paquot, N. Obesity phenotype is related to NLRP3 inflammasome activity and immunological profile of visceral adipose tissue. *Diabetologia* **2013**, *56*, 2487–2497. [CrossRef] [PubMed]

38. Lebovitz, H.E.; Banerji, M.A. Point: Visceral adiposity is causally related to insulin resistance. *Diabetes Care* **2005**, *28*, 2322–2325. [CrossRef] [PubMed]

39. Bonora, E.; Tuomilehto, J. The pros and cons of diagnosing diabetes with A1C. *Diabetes Care* **2011**, *34*, S184–S190. [CrossRef] [PubMed]

40. Sculze, M.; Hoffmann, K.; Kroke, A.; Boeing, H. Dietary patterns and their association with food and nutrient intake in the European Prospective Investigation into Cancer and Nutrition (EPIC)-Potsdam study. *Br. J. Nutr.* **2001**, *85*, 363–373. [CrossRef]

41. Petersen, S.B.; Rasmussen, M.A.; Olsen, S.F.; Vestergaard, P.; Molgaard, C.; Halldorsson, T.I.; Strom, M. Maternal dietary patterns during pregnancy in relation to offspring forearm fractures: Prospective study from the Danish National Birth Cohort. *Nutrients* **2015**, *7*, 2382–2400. [CrossRef] [PubMed]

42. Sun, J.; Buys, N.J.; Hills, A.P. Dietary pattern and its association with the prevalence of obesity, hypertension and other cardiovascular risk factors among Chinese older adults. *Int. J. Environ. Res. Public Health* **2014**, *11*, 3956–3971. [CrossRef] [PubMed]

43. Grieger, J.A.; Grzeskowiak, L.E.; Clifton, V.L. Preconception dietary patterns in human pregnancies are associated with preterm delivery. *J. Nutr.* **2014**, *144*, 1075–1080. [CrossRef] [PubMed]

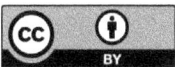

nutrients

MDPI

Article

Associations between Dietary Patterns and Impaired Fasting Glucose in Chinese Men: A Cross-Sectional Study

Meilin Zhang [1], Yufeng Zhu [1], Ping Li [1], Hong Chang [1,2], Xuan Wang [1], Weiqiao Liu [3], Yuwen Zhang [3] and Guowei Huang [1,*]

[1] Department of Nutrition and Food Science, School of Public Health, Tianjin Medical University, 22 Qixiangtai Road, Heping District, Tianjin 300070, China; E-Mails: defjmmm@163.com (M.Z.); zhuyufeng5580@163.com (Y.Z.); lp900221@gmail.com (P.L.); changhong@tmu.edu.cn (H.C.); wangxuan@tmu.edu.cn (X.W.)

[2] Department of Rehabilitation and Sports Medicine, Tianjin Medical University, 22 Qixiangtai Road, Heping District, Tianjin 300070, China

[3] Health Education and Guidance Center of Heping District, 97 Hualong Road, Heping District, Tianjin 300040, China; E-Mails: hptjjs@126.com (W.L.); zyw19830910@gmail.com (Y.Z.)

* Author to whom correspondence should be addressed; E-Mail: huangguowei@tmu.edu.cn; Tel.: +86-22-8333-6606; Fax: +86-22-8333-6603.

Received: 16 July 2015 / Accepted: 15 September 2015 / Published: 21 September 2015

Abstract: Few studies have examined the association between Asian dietary pattern and prediabetes, in particular, the Chinese diet. We conducted a cross-sectional study to identify dietary patterns associated with impaired fasting glucose (IFG) which considered a state of prediabetes in Chinese men. The study included 1495 Chinese men aged 20 to 75 years. Information about diet was obtained using an 81-item food frequency questionnaire (FFQ), and 21 predefined food groups were considered in a factor analysis. Three dietary patterns were generated by factor analysis: (1) a vegetables-fruits pattern; (2) an animal offal-dessert pattern; and (3) a white rice-red meat pattern. The multivariate-adjusted odds ratio (OR) of IFG for the highest tertile of the animal offal-dessert pattern in comparison with the lowest tertile was 3.15 (95% confidence intervals (CI): 1.87–5.30). The vegetables-fruits dietary pattern was negatively associated with the risk of IFG, but a significant association was observed only in the third tertile. There was no significant association between IFG and the white rice-red meat pattern. Our findings indicated that the vegetables-fruits dietary pattern was inversely associated with IFG, whereas the animal offal-dessert pattern was associated with an increased risk of IFG in Chinese men. Further prospective studies are needed to elucidate the diet-prediabetes relationships.

Keywords: dietary pattern; factor analysis; prediabetes; impaired fasting glucose; men; China

1. Introduction

Impaired fasting glucose (IFG) is a common glucose disorder, and considered a state of prediabetes associated with increased risk of diabetes [1] and complications or cardiovascular disease [2–4]. Currently, the prevalence of prediabetes in Chinese adults was 15.5%, accounting for 148.2 million adults with prediabetes [5]. More importantly, 5%–10% of people per year with prediabetes will progress to diabetes [6]. Contrary to the relative irreversibility of diabetes, IFG does not typically present with clinical symptoms and can be treated using appropriate dietary intervention measures, thereby delaying or preventing diabetes [7,8]. Currently, many epidemiological studies focus on the dietary pattern and diabetes. Assessing dietary patterns enables the analysis of potentially interactive and antagonistic effects of different nutrients. The healthy balanced dietary pattern, characterized by a diet with a frequent intake of raw and salad vegetables, fruits in both summer and winter, fish, pasta and rice, and low intake of fried foods, sausages, fried fish, and tubers, may be negatively associated with the risk of having undiagnosed diabetes [9]. From the Framingham Offspring Study, it was suggested that consumption of a diet rich in fruits, vegetables, whole grains, and reduced fat dairy protects against insulin resistance phenotypes (impaired glucose tolerance and IFG) and displacing these healthy choices with refined grains, high fat dairy, sweet baked foods, candy, and sugar sweetened soda promotes impaired glucose tolerance and IFG [10]. Few studies have examined the association between Asian dietary pattern and prediabetes, in particular, the Chinese diet. Among Japanese men, a dietary pattern characterized by frequent consumption of dairy products and fruits and vegetables but low alcohol intake may be associated with a decreased risk of developing prediabetes [11]. From the 2002 China National Nutrition and Health Survey, the New Affluence pattern (mainly well-to-do individuals) characterized by living in urban areas, being less physical active, having more smokers, alcohol users, and overweight individuals, and having a higher intake of animal foods and soybean productswas associated with a substantially higher risk of prediabetes in Chinese adults [12].

Due to the rapid economic and social changes, Chinese dietary patterns and lifestyle have changed substantially, we sought to determine the influence of specific dietary patterns on prediabetes in the Chinese population. The objective of this study was to determine the association between various dietary patterns and IFG among Chinese men.

2. Materials and Methods

2.1. Population

A total of 1615 subjects aged 20–75 years were performed routine health check-up in Health Education and Guidance Center of Heping District, Tianjin, China in 2014. Participants with fasting plasma glucose (FPG) concentration of 110–126 mg/dL (6.1–7.0 mmol/L) were classified as IFG [1], those with a fasting glucose concentration <110 mg/dL (<6.1 mmol/L) were classified as normoglycemic, those with a fasting glucose concentration of ⩾126 mg/dL (7.0 mmol/L) or self-reported current diabetes treatments were excluded. The final cross-sectional study population comprised 1459 participants. The study protocol was approved by the Ethics Committee of Tianjin Medical University. Written informed consent was obtained from all participates.

2.2. Data Collection

Height was measured without shoes to the nearest 1 cm and weight measured in light clothing to the nearest 0.1 kg on a beam balance scale. Body mass index (BMI) was calculated as weight in kilograms divided by the square of the height in meters (kg/m^2). Venous blood samples were taken from all participants after an overnight fast (12 h at least) and the samples were stored at $-80\ °C$ until assessment assays were performed. Serum total cholesterol (TC) and triglyceride (TG) were measured by routine enzymatic methods. Serum high-density lipoprotein cholesterol (HDL-C) and low-density lipoprotein cholesterol (LDL-C) were measured using colorimetric method. Plasma glucose and lipid levels were determined by automatic biochemical analyzer (TBA-40, Tokyo, Japan).

Information about demographic characteristics and lifestyle habits, including smoking, drinking, and physical activity, were collected by trained interviewers. Current smokers were defined as those who smoked at least one cigarette per day and non-smokers were defined as those who were either former smokers or never smoked a cigarette in their lives. Those who stopped smoking for less than a year were classified as smokers. A participant was classified as "drinker" in case of having drunk beer or any other alcoholic beverage once a week on average during the last year, excluding those who drank beer or any other alcoholic beverage once during festivals.

Physical activity was recorded as a three level variable (light, moderate, and heavy), as recommended by the China Nutrition Society.

2.3. Dietary Assessment

Dietary data were collected by trained dietitians during a structured interview. A validated semi-quantitative food frequency questionnaire (FFQ) was used to assess the dietary intake [13]. Participants were asked to report their frequency of consumption of each food item during the past month. The food frequency questionnaire consisted of 81 items, including seven frequency categories as follows: (1) almost never eat or drink; (2) less than once per week; (3) once a week; (4) 2–3 times per week; (5) 4–6 times per week; (6) once a day; (7) twice or more per day. According to the similarity of nutrient profiles and culinary usage among the foods and the grouping scheme used in other studies, we collapsed the 81 food items into 21 predefined food groups. Information on frequency of intake and portion size was used to calculate the amount of each food item consumed on average, using China Food Composition Table (2009) as the database. Four three-day 24-h recalls (24h) in three consecutive days (including two weekdays and one weekend day) were completed to determine the validity of FFQ. Nutrients intake assessed by the FFQ and the average of 24h correlated well, with the correlation coefficients being 0.52–0.64 for macronutrients and 0.29–0.76 for micronutrients.

2.4. Statistical Analysis

Descriptive data for study populations are presented as the median (range) for continuous variables and as percentages for categorical variables. To compare the general characteristics according to IFG status, continuous variables were examined using Wilcoxon rank sum test and chi-square test for categorical variables. p trend was calculated using generalized linear models for continuous variables. Factor analysis (principal component) was used to extract the participants' dietary patterns among the 21 predefined food groups. To simplify the interpretation, the factors were rotated by orthogonal transformation (varimax rotation) to maintain uncorrelated factor variables called principal factor or patterns. After evaluating the eigenvalues ($\geqslant 1.5$), screen plot test, and factor interpretability, three factors were retained. Items were retained in a factor if they had an absolute correlation $\geqslant 0.20$ with that factor. Tertiles were categorized across the scores of each dietary pattern based on the distribution of the scores for all the participants and used for further analysis. Relationships between tertile categories of dietary pattern scores and IFG status were examined using logistic regression by three different models. Odds ratios (OR) and corresponding 95% confidence intervals (CI) were calculated. Model 1 was used to calculate the crude OR, and model 2 was adjusted for age, BMI, total energy intake, drinking, smoking, and physical activity. A linear trend across increasing quartiles was tested using the median value of each quartile as a continuous variable based on linear regression. All statistical operations were performed using SPSS Version 19.0 (IBM, Chicago, IL, USA). All reported p values were two-sided and a $p < 0.05$ was considered significant.

3. Results

The general characteristics of the study population according to IFG status are presented in Table 1. Compared with participants without IFG, participants with IFG tended to be older, have higher BMI, TC, LDL-C, FPG, and TG levels ($p < 0.05$).

Table 1. General characteristics of study population.

Characteristics	IFG Status		p [1]
	No (1327)	Yes (132)	
Age (year)	41.0 (32.0–50.0)	50.0 (41.0–58.0)	0.000
BMI (kg/m²)	25.1 (23.0–27.1)	26.3 (24.4–28.5)	0.000
TC (mmol/L)	4.8 (4.3–5.3)	5.1 (4.6–5.8)	0.000
TG (mmol/L)	1.4 (0.9–2.0)	1.7 (1.2–2.7)	0.000
HDL-C (mmol/L)	1.1 (1.0–1.3)	1.1 (1.0–1.3)	0.546
LDL-C(mmol/L)	3.0 (2.5–3.5)	3.2 (2.8–3.8)	0.000
FPG(mmol/L)	5.4 (5.2–5.7)	6.4 (6.2–6.6)	0.000
Total energy intake (kcal)	2086.9 (1646.1–2603.7)	2049.1 (1595.1–2481.7)	0.827
Smoking (%)			0.067
Current	41.5	48.5	
Past	12.4	15.9	
Never	46.1	35.6	
Drinking (%)			0.015
Everyday	8.7	16.7	
Sometimes	71.4	66.7	
Past	8.0	9.1	
Never	11.9	7.6	
Physical activity (%)			
Light	80.8	81.0	0.970
Middle	51.5	60.3	0.136
Heavy	35.2	38.8	0.525

IFG, impaired fasting glucose; BMI: Body mass index; TC: total cholesterol; TG: triglycerides; HDL-C: high-density lipoprotein cholesterol; LDL-C: low-density lipoprotein cholesterol; FPG: fasting plasma glucose; [1] Analysis of Wilcoxon rank sum test or chi-squared test.

Factor analysis identified three major dietary patterns among the 21 food groups, and the associated factor loading scores with absolute values ≥ 0.20 are shown in Table 2. The "vegetables-fruits" dietary pattern was characterized by high intakes of vegetables, fruits, tubers, seaweeds and mushrooms, coarse cereals, and low intakes of alcohol. The "animal offal-dessert pattern" included high intakes of animal offal, dessert, fast food and beverages. The "white rice-red meat pattern" included high intakes of white rice, red meat, poultry, and eggs. Each dietary pattern explained 16.8%, 8.7%, and 7.8% of the variation in food intake, respectively.

Table 2. Factor loadings for the three major dietary patterns derived from principal components analysis with orthogonal rotation.

Foods/Food Groups	Vegetables-Fruits Pattern	Animal Offal-Dessert Pattern	White Rice-Red Meat Pattern
White rice	−0.132	−0.077	0.628
Vegetables	0.698	0.091	0.220
Coarse cereals	0.533	−0.244	0.152
Refined wheat	0.419	−0.116	0.006
Tubers	0.618	0.036	−0.114
Fruits	0.582	0.311	0.086
Seaweeds and mushrooms	0.575	0.250	0.198
Soybean products	0.474	−0.064	0.341
Red meat	−0.050	0.123	0.750
Poultry	0.108	0.161	0.610
Peanuts	0.408	0.230	−0.014
Seafood	0.354	0.454	0.039
Dairy products	0.272	0.115	−0.018
Eggs	0.206	−0.038	0.576

Table 2. *Cont.*

Foods/Food Groups	Vegetables-Fruits Pattern	Animal Offal-Dessert Pattern	White Rice-Red Meat Pattern
Tea	0.203	0.288	−0.063
Dessert	0.167	0.636	−0.007
Condiments	0.133	0.348	0.236
Animal offal	0.090	0.648	0.115
Alcohol beverages	0.015	0.347	−0.022
Fast food	0.004	0.603	0.021
Beverages	−0.094	0.595	0.053
Variance of explained (%)	16.8	8.7	7.8

Factor loadings with absolute values ⩾ 0.20 were listed in the table among 21 food groups.

The distribution of characteristics by dietary pattern score tertiles is presented in Table 3. Increasing scores in the vegetables-fruits patterns were correlated with a decreased percent energy from fat (*p* for trend <0.001), whereas the percent energy from carbohydrate increased as the score of the vegetables-fruits pattern increased. Animal offal-dessert pattern and white rice-red meat pattern, however, has an inverse relationship with the percent energy from fat and carbohydrate. The vegetables-fruits pattern score was associated with a high intake of fiber and low intake of cholesterol, whereas the dessert pattern and white rice-red meat pattern score were associated with a low intake of fiber and high intake of cholesterol. The fatty acids were significantly associated with dietary pattern scores. The vegetables-fruits pattern score was associated with a lower intake of total fatty acids, saturated fatty acid and monounsaturated fatty acids, whereas the animal offal-dessert pattern and white rice-red meat pattern score was positively associated with the intakes of total fatty acids, saturated fatty acid, monounsaturated fatty acids, and polyunsaturated fatty acids. Regarding mineral intake, iron intake was positively associated with the scores of the vegetables-fruits pattern and animal offal-dessert pattern. Magnesium intake was positively associated with the scores of the vegetables-fruits pattern and negatively associated with scores of animal offal-dessert pattern and white rice-red meat pattern. Zinc was positively associated with the scores of the white rice-red meat pattern. Selenium was positively associated with animal offal-dessert pattern.

Table 3. Distribution of characteristics by the tertiles of dietary pattern scores.

Characteristics	Vegetables-Fruits Pattern			*p* Trend [2]
	T1 (*n* = 486) [1]	T2 (*n* = 486)	T3 (*n* = 487)	
Age (year)	38.5 (32.0–44.0)	41.0 (32.0–51.0)	45.0 (37.0–54.0)	0.000
BMI (kg/m^2)	25.2 (23.1–27.3)	25.0 (22.9–27.1)	25.2 (23.5–27.2)	0.743
Energy (kcal)	1555.4 (1296.3–1889.5)	2052.6 (1752.7–2363.4)	2687.6 (2321.8–3207.0)	0.000
Fat (g)	50.0 (45.5–54.7)	48.1 (42.4–54.2)	46.8 (38.8–52.7)	0.000
Fat (% energy)	21.0 (18.5–23.9)	19.8 (17.2–22.4)	19.3 (16.3–21.3)	0.000
Protein (g)	89.4 (84.2–94.7)	89.8 (84.8–95.9)	89.0 (82.2–97.8)	0.962

Table 3. *Cont.*

Characteristics	Vegetables-Fruits Pattern			p Trend [2]
	T1 (n = 486) [1]	T2 (n = 486)	T3 (n = 487)	
Protein (% energy)	16.9 (15.5–18.3)	16.6 (15.6–17.7)	16.1 (15.1–17.4)	0.000
Carbohydrate (g)	335.0 (312.0–350.5)	340.6 (317.1–358.8)	343.3 (315.6–369.1)	0.000
Carbohydrate (% energy)	59.8 (54.5–64.1)	62.0 (57.4–65.7)	63.1 (59.1–66.8)	0.000
Fiber (g)	19.1 (17.2–20.9)	20.6 (18.3–22.7)	22.9 (20.1–26.5)	0.000
Cholesterol (g)	564.2 (458.3–662.5)	537.5 (446.6–627.1)	498.2 (392.4–610.2)	0.000
Total fatty acids (g)	39.1 (35.1–44.7)	38.8 (32.7–46.2)	38.2 (30.8–46.1)	0.010
SFA (g)	11.7 (10.4–13.9)	11.4 (9.7–13.9)	10.9 (8.8–13.1)	0.000
MUFAs (g)	13.8 (12.3–16.1)	13.4 (11.3–16.0)	12.7 (10.2–15.3)	0.000
PUFAs (g)	10.0 (8.7–11.5)	9.9 (8.0–12.4)	10.1 (7.7–13.6)	0.096
Magnesium, Mg (mg)	444.9 (420.2–465.8)	466.3 (438.1–490.0)	497.3 (461.6–531.0)	0.000
Iron, Fe (mg)	37.8 (35.0–39.8)	37.0 (33.9–39.2)	36.8 (33.6–39.6)	0.001
Mg/Fe ratio	11.6 (11.1–12.4)	12.4 (11.6–13.3)	13.2 (12.4–14.7)	0.000
Zinc, Zn (mg)	14.4 (13.7–15.3)	14.3 (13.5–15.4)	14.4 (13.2–15.6)	0.053
Selenium, Se (mg)	65.4 (58.7–71.0)	63.9 (57.30–70.2)	60.8 (53.6–71.4)	0.088
Animal giblets-dessert pattern				
Age (year)	46.0 (38.0–55.0)	41.0 (33.0–50.0)	37.5 (31.0–44.0)	0.000
BMI (kg/m^2)	25.0 (23.1–27.1)	25.3 (23.1–27.2)	25.1 (23.1–27.2)	0.733
Energy (kcal)	1966.7 (1561.7–2397.1)	1951.0 (1564.9–2434.7)	2324.1 (1913.5–3033.2)	0.000
Fat (g)	44.7 (39.1–50.5)	48.5 (43.9–53.8)	51.4 (46.9–58.3)	0.000
Fat (% energy)	18.2 (15.5–20.9)	20.0 (17.9–22.5)	21.2 (19.3–23.7)	0.000
Protein (g)	89.9 (84.2–95.9)	90.0 (85.2–95.5)	88.5 (82.4–96.4)	0.274
Protein (% energy)	16.7 (15.4–17.9)	16.7 (15.6–17.9)	16.1 (15.0–17.5)	0.000
Carbohydrate (g)	348.0 (324.4–367.2)	336.3 (314.4–353.3)	333.9 (308.5–352.0)	0.000
Carbohydrate (% energy)	63.5 (58.5–67.9)	60.8 (55.9–64.9)	61.2 (56.7–64.5)	0.000
Fiber (g)	21.3 (18.9–23.9)	20.6 (18.4–23.1)	20.0 (17.2–22.5)	0.000
Cholesterol (g)	512.0 (408.8–592.0)	535.9 (444.9–646.8)	550.8 (450.1–668.9)	0.000
Total fatty acids (g)	36.7 (30.9–43.5)	39.3 (34.6–44.7)	40.6 (34.2–49.4)	0.000
SFA (g)	10.8 (9.1–12.8)	11.6 (9.9–13.4)	11.8 (9.8–14.5)	0.000
MUFAs (g)	12.6 (10.5–14.8)	13.6 (11.6–15.5)	14.2 (11.8–16.7)	0.000
PUFAs (g)	9.6 (7.7–12.1)	10.0 (8.5–11.9)	10.5 (8.5–12.7)	0.000
Magnesium, Mg (mg)	481.5 (455.9–508.3)	462.6 (437.1–495.4)	451.0 (413.3–478.6)	0.000
Iron, Fe (mg)	37.3 (34.8–39.5)	37.5 (34.5–39.9)	36.7 (33.1–39.3)	0.002
Mg/Fe ratio	12.7 (11.9–13.7)	12.2 (11.4–13.2)	11.8 (10.9–13.0)	0.000
Zinc, Zn (mg)	14.4 (13.4–15.3)	14.4 (13.6–15.3)	14.4 (13.4–15.7)	0.224
Selenium, Se (mg)	58.7 (53.0–64.9)	63.8 (58.2–69.0)	70.1 (61.9–78.7)	0.000
White rice-red meat pattern				
Age (year)	45.0 (36.8–52.0)	41.0 (33.0–51.0)	38.0 (32.0–46.0)	0.000
BMI (kg/m^2)	25.0 (23.1–27.1)	25.1 (23.2–27.0)	25.3 (23.0–27.5)	0.337
Energy (kcal)	1739.0 (1379.5–2209.7)	1999.7 (1662.4–2485.3)	2440.6 (2052.9–2958.4)	0.000
Fat (g)	44.6 (39.5–49.1)	48.6 (43.3–53.7)	52.4 (47.0–59.9)	0.000
Fat (% energy)	18.1 (15.3–20.6)	20.1 (17.8–22.6)	21.4 (19.4–24.0)	0.000
Protein (g)	84.7 (79.9–88.9)	90.4 (85.1–95.2)	95.3 (88.6–102.9)	0.000
Protein (% energy)	15.6 (14.6–16.7)	16.7 (15.6–17.8)	17.2 (16.1–18.6)	0.000
Carbohydrate (g)	350.7 (335.3–370.6)	337.9 (318.6–358.8)	321.0 (293.8–345.4)	0.000
Carbohydrate (% energy)	64.2 (60.3–68.8)	61.6 (57.6–65.5)	59.1 (54.5–63.4)	0.000
Fiber (g)	21.4 (19.3–23.4)	20.8 (18.5–23.3)	19.3 (16.7–22.5)	0.000
Cholesterol (g)	468.0 (373.0–553.4)	540.6 (453.0–634.3)	603.2 (502.7–752.3)	0.000
Total fatty acids (g)	35.3 (30.3–39.8)	38.9 (33.2–45.1)	43.3 (37.3–51.3)	0.000
SFA (g)	9.8 (8.7–11.2)	11.5(9.9–13.3)	13.5(11.6–15.9)	0.000
MUFAs (g)	11.7 (10.0–13.1)	13.5 (11.6–15.5)	15.6 (13.6–18.3)	0.000
PUFAs (g)	9.6 (7.6–11.3)	10.2 (8.6–12.4)	10.5 (8.5–13.2)	0.000
Magnesium, Mg (mg)	475.9 (451.4–505.0)	466.9 (439.8–495.6)	450.9 (415.0–482.3)	0.000
Iron, Fe (mg)	37.2 (34.5–39.4)	37.4 (34.4–39.7)	37.0 (34.2–39.5)	0.871
Mg/Fe ratio	12.7 (11.8–13.7)	12.4 (11.4–13.4)	11.9 (11.1–13.0)	0.000
Zinc, Zn (mg)	13.5 (12.7–14.1)	14.4 (13.7–15.1)	15.6 (14.7–16.6)	0.000
Selenium, Se (mg)	64.3 (57.4–70.9)	64.5 (57.2–70.8)	62.0 (54.9–70.5)	0.835

[1] Tertiles of dietary pattern scores; [2] p trend was calculated using generalized linear models for continuous variables; p trend of nutrient consumption was adjusted for total energy intake. Abbreviation: SFA: saturated fatty acids; PUFAs: polyunsaturated fatty acids; MUFAs: monounsaturated fatty acids; BMI: Body mass index.

The ORs and 95% CIs of IFG were analyzed across the tertiles of dietary pattern scores (Table 4). The OR (95% CI) in the highest tertiles of the vegetables-fruits dietary pattern compared to those in the lowest tertiles in crude model was 1.15 (0.75–1.75), but a significant association was observed in multivariate model 2 (OR: 0.57, 95% CI: 0.34–0.95). Population in the highest tertile of the animal offal-dessert pattern score had an increased risk of IFG in the multivariate-adjusted models when compared with those in the lowest tertile (OR: 2.89, 95% CI: 1.76–4.75) in the multivariate model and this association was stronger (OR: 3.15, 95% CI: 1.87–5.30) in multivariate model 2. The white rice-red meat pattern was not significantly associated with IFG in any of the models.

Table 4. Distribution of characteristics by the tertiles of dietary pattern scores.

Dietary Pattern		No. of IFG	Crude Model	Multivatiate Model 1 [1]	Multivatiate Model 2 [2]
Vegetables-fruits pattern	T1 [3]	45	1.00	1.00	1.00
	T2	36	0.78 (0.50–1.24)	0.63 (0.39–1.02)	0.57 (0.31–1.09)
	T3	51	1.15 (0.75–1.75)	0.73 (0.46–1.15)	0.57 (0.34–0.95)
	p trend [4]		0.151	0.700	0.013
Animal offal-dessert pattern	T1	37	1.00	1.00	1.00
	T2	45	1.24 (0.78–1.95)	1.84 (1.13–2.99)	1.86 (1.14–3.02)
	T3	50	1.39 (0.89–2.17)	2.89 (1.76–4.75)	3.15 (1.87–5.30)
	p trend		0.370	0.001	0.035
White rice-red meat pattern	T1	49	1.00	1.00	1.00
	T2	48	0.98 (0.64–1.49)	1.14 (0.74–1.76)	1.13 (0.73–1.76)
	T3	35	0.69 (0.44–1.10)	0.91 (0.59–1.53)	0.92 (0.55–1.52)
	p trend		0.095	0.942	0.557

[1] Adjusted for age and body mass index; [2] Model 1 + additional adjustment for total energy intake, drinking status, smoking status, physical activity status; [3] Tertiles of dietary pattern scores; [4] Tests for trend were conducted by assigning the median value to each tertile of food intake as a continuous variable. Abbreviation: IFG, impaired fasting glucose.

4. Discussion

We examined associations between dietary patterns and IFG. We identified three major dietary patterns: a vegetables-fruits food pattern (rich in vegetables, fruits, tubers, seaweeds and mushrooms, coarse cereals, and low intake of alcohol), an animal offal-dessert pattern (rich in animal offal, dessert, fast food, and beverages) and a white rice-red meat pattern(rich in white rice, red meat, poultry, and eggs). A vegetables-fruits food pattern and an animal offal-dessert food pattern were associated with IFG; however, a white rice-red meat food pattern was not associated with IFG.

To the best of our knowledge, there have been few studies published that have examined the relationship between dietary patterns, derived by factor analysis, and IFG [9–12]. The prudent dietary pattern, which was rich in fruits and vegetables [9,14], particularly the high green leafy vegetables intake [15], was associated with a reduced risk of type 2 diabetes. In the Da Qing study for diabetes prevention conducted in China, a diet high in vegetables and fruits was associated with a lower incidence of diabetes [16]. The preventive effects of fruits and vegetables have been hypothesized to be mediated by antioxidants [17], and results of some follow-up studies have supported this hypothesis [18–20]. Our findings on the relation between the dietary pattern reflecting vegetable and fruit intake and prediabetes risk is in line with results of previous studies, which have shown an inverse association between consumption of fruits and vegetables and the risk of type 2 diabetes. Our results also showed that the vegetables-fruits pattern score was associated with high intakes of magnesium and iron. Magnesium is an essential cofactor for multiple enzymes involved in glucose metabolism and has been discovered to play a role in the development of diabetes [21]. Animal studies have shown that low magnesium diet can lead to impaired insulin secretion and action [22] and magnesium supplementation decrease the incidence of diabetes [23]. The green leafy vegetables have a high content of magnesium [24], which could reduce the risk of prediabetes and diabetes. In the Chinese population, the main source of iron is from plant foods, which contain mainly non-heme iron. Iron status is associated with diabetes in China [25]. Iron overload may stimulate oxidative stress and inflammation, thus promoting the development of diabetes [26,27]. The intake of iron was positively related to the risk of diabetes, whilst magnesium intake was inversely related. Although our results showed that the vegetables-fruits pattern score was associated with high intakes of iron, a strong inverse association between magnesium: iron intake ratio and diabetes could explain this pattern was negatively associated with IFG [28]. In our study, it was shown that the magnesium: iron intake ratio was increased across the tertile in this pattern. Moreover, vegetables and fruits are rich in dietary fiber, which is a known protective factor for diabetes. Recently, Frank *et al.* found a dietary pattern among urban Ghanaian population, which was characterized by a high consumption of plantain, cassava, and garden egg, and a low intake of rice, juice, vegetable oil, eggs, chocolate drink, sweets, and red meat was related to higher serum triglyceride concentrations and increased the risk of type 2 diabetes [29]. However, an inverse association between cassava flour and incident diabetes was also observed in a Brazilian study [30]. As for cassava, a major carbohydrate source in Africa, contains potentially diabetogenic chemicals, however, its consumption could be considered in diets for the prevention and control of diabetes. The preparation methods were diverse including cooking, frying, and pounding. The different associations of cassava with diabetes could be explained by novel methods for the preparation of the cassava. Alternatively, the combined consumption of cassava and rice with other food groups [31] may represent dietary diversity, which is inversely associated with biomarkers of type 2 diabetes [32]. In the present study, however, the tubers in this dietary pattern were not apparently associated with IFG. The lack of an association may reflect low consumption of tubers in the Chinese men; mean daily intake is 52.9 g for tubers (Appendix).

This study also found that an animal offal-dessert pattern characterized by high intake of animal offal, dessert, fast food and beverages was positively associated with IFG. The animal offal are generally high in saturated fatty acid, cholesterol, iron, and selenium, and desserts contribute importantly to glycemic load (GL), which appear to be associated with increased IFG risk. In the Nurses' Health Study (NHS), Schulze et al. observed a pattern, which was high in sugar-sweetened soft drinks, refined grains, diet soft drinks, and processed meat but low in wine, coffee, cruciferous vegetables, and yellow vegetables, was associated with an increased risk of diabetes [33]. Desserts and sweets have been found to be part of the Western dietary pattern associated with higher diabetes risk [34, 35]. In addition, our study showed that the animal offal-dessert pattern score was associated with a low intake of magnesium and a higher intake of selenium and iron. A cross-sectional study in Chinese population explored a significant positive correlation between dietary selenium intake and the prevalence of diabetes [36]. The findings of our study suggest a significant positive association between dietary selenium intake and animal offal-dessert pattern, consistent with the conclusions of studies on associations between dietary selenium and diabetes [37], supplementary selenium and diabetes [38], and serum selenium and diabetes [39,40]. An increased level of dietary selenium intake may increase the release of glucagon, which can lead to hyperglycemia [41]. Moreover, a high level of dietary selenium intake may stimulate the release of glucagon or may induce overexpression of glutathione peroxidase 1 (GPx1), which is a type of antioxidant selenoprotein. The high activity of GPx1 can interfere with insulin signaling, which is critical to the regulation of glucose levels and the prevention of diabetes [42]. Thus, the animal offal-dessert pattern was associated with an increased risk of IFG in our study.

Our findings demonstrated that the white rice-red meat pattern characterized by white rice, red meat, poultry, and eggs was not associated with IFG. In China, white rice is a staple food and major source of calories contributing to a high dietary GL. The cooked rice, congee (rice porridge) and rice noodle are the three most common white rice-based foods. The Shanghai Women's Health Study has linked higher dietary GL, primarily from white rice, to an increased risk of diabetes [43]. However, the association between rice intake and diabetes has been inconsistent in China [44,45]. Study in a single province (Jiangsu China) observed a significantly positive association between white rice intake and hyperglycemia risk, whereas no association was observed in a Hong Kong population [45]. Compared with the refined grains (such as white rice), the coarse cereals were low in glycemic index (GI) and rich in fiber may lower the risk of diabetes [46]. It was suggested that high intakes of refined grains intake and usual diets with high GL diet were associated with reduced β-cell function in pre-diabetic Japanese-Brazilians [47]. The updated analyses from three large US cohorts and meta analyses provide evidence that higher dietary GI and GL are associated with increased risk of diabetes, participants who consumed diets with high GI or high GL and low cereal fiber had a nearly 40% higher risk of compared with those whose diets were high in cereal fiber and low in GI or GL [48]. A systematic review and meta-analysis of cohort studies of meat consumption and diabetes risks suggested that meat consumption increased the risk of diabetes [49], particularly processed red meat was associated with an increased risk of diabetes [50]. Eggs, generally regarded as an important dietary source of protein, are commonly consumed in China. Findings from some studies suggest that dietary cholesterol from eggs leads to a modest increase in blood concentrations of total and LDL-C [51–53], which have been found to be positively related to diabetes risk [52,54]. On the other hand, eggs contain many other potentially beneficial nutrients, such as monounsaturated fats, minerals, essential amino acids, folate, and other B vitamins. Moreover, consumption of eggs instead of carbohydrate-rich foods may raise HDL-C levels and decrease blood glycemic and insulinemic responses [55]. The data from a representative sample in Jiangsu Province, China indicate that consumption of more than 1 egg/day is associated with significantly elevated risk for diabetes [56]. It was reported that the traditional south pattern of rice as the major staple food in conjunction with pork and vegetable dishes was associated with lower risk of general and abdominal obesity [57]. The rice rich "traditional" pattern was associated with reduced weight gain in Jiangsu province of China [58]. Moreover, the "Green Water" dietary pattern, characterized by high intakes of rice and vegetables and moderate intakes in animal foods was related to the lowest prevalence of metabolic syndrome (MS) (15.9%) in a large-scale, nationally-representative sample of Chinese adults [59]. However, our study showed that there was no relationship between white rice-red meat pattern and IFG. On one hand, the factor loading of white rice in this pattern derived from principal components analysis was 0.628, which was higher than the factor loading of coarse cereals (0.152). Although the white rice contains higher dietary GI and GL, the consumption of white rice in our study was 131.7 g/day (Appendix), which was lower than the southern city. The prospective study conducted in Shanghai, China, reported a diabetes relative risk of 1.78 (95% CI: 1.48–2.15) comparing middle-aged women who consumed ⩾300 g/day (versus <200 g/day) of white rice [43]. On the other hand, although the higher contribution to this dietary pattern score was red meat, poultry, and egg, the lack of an association may reflect moderate consumption of red meat in the Chinese men; the mean daily intake was 49.3 g for red meat, 25.1 g for poultry and 62.5 g for egg (Appendix). Additionally, we found the white rice-red meat pattern score was associated with a low intake of magnesium and high intake of zinc. Zinc content is highest in animal-source foods, relatively high in whole-grain cereals, and low in refined cereals and vegetables [60]. Zinc has been postulated that zinc deficiency may aggravate the insulin resistance in noninsulin dependent diabetes mellitus over a six year follow-up study [61]. From above we did not conclude the white rice-red meat pattern score was associated with IFG. Further study will be performed to determine the casual role of white rice-red meat pattern and IFG.

Several potential limitations of this study need to be highlighted. First, because of the cross-sectional design of our study, we cannot assess the causal relationships between dietary patterns and the risk of IFG. Second, because of the nature of the self-reporting questionnaire, recall bias exists and the food intake may be not exact. Third, oral glucose tolerance tests were not performed, possibly leading to an underestimate of the diagnosis of prediabetes. Finally, even though we have adjusted for confounders that related prediabetes risk, we cannot rule out that unmeasured factors have influenced our observed results. The health checkup center-based design leads to a study population that is not fully representative of the general one, and thus, the generalizability of our findings may be questionable. In addition, the lack of racial diversity limits our ability to generalize our results to other populations. Despite these limitations, this study could reveal the relationships between dietary patterns and IFG in Chinese men.

5. Conclusions

The vegetables-fruits dietary pattern, which was characterized by high intakes of fruits and vegetables, and low consumption of alcohol, appears to be negatively associated with IFG in Chinese

Nutrients **2015**, *7*, 8072–8089

men. Whereas, the animal offal-dessert pattern, which was characterized by frequent consumption of animal offal and dessert might be associated with an increased risk of developing IFG in Chinese men. Further large prospective epidemiologic studies to investigate the effect of those dietary patterns on IFG in Chinese populations are needed in the future.

Acknowledgments: This research was supported by a grant from the National Science and Technology Support Program (No. 2012BAI02B02).

Author Contributions: Meilin Zhang and Yufeng Zhu participated in planning and designing of the study, data acquisition, analysis of the data and drafted the manuscript. Guowei Huang participated in planning and designing of the study, and drafting the manuscript. Hong Chang and Xuan Wang performed the statistical analyses. Weiqiao Liu and Yuwen Zhang conceived of the study and participated in its design. Ping Li participated in interpreting and presenting the results. All the authors have read and approved the final manuscript.

Conflicts of Interest: The authors declare no conflict of interest.

Appendix

Table A1. Intakes of selected dietary items according to tertiles of dietary pattern score among Chinese men.

Dietary Items	All subjects	Vegetables-Fruits Pattern			Animal offal-Dessert Pattern			White Rice-Red Meat Pattern		
		T1 [1]	T2	T3	T1	T2	T3	T1	T2	T3
White rice (g)	131.7 (128.7–184.4)	131.7 (128.7–360.4)	141.8 (128.7–184.4)	131.7 (65.9–184.4)	180.2 (128.7–198.5)	131.7 (128.7–184.4)	131.7 (65.9–184.4)	70.9 (64.4–131.7)	131.7 (128.7–184.4)	198.5 (180.2–368.8)
Vegetables (g)	309.7 (217.6–436.5)	209.4 (155.6–282.4)	304.5 (236.4–382.6)	458.0 (361.3–612.6)	308.6 (216.5–441.7)	291.9 (210.8–410.8)	337.8 (230.6–457.5)	278.9 (195.8–384.3)	304.2 (215.4–420.3)	358.7 (262.2–488.9)
Coarse cereals (g)	82.4 (47.3–130.6)	46.7 (18.7–82.4)	82.4 (54.7–129.0)	129.0 (82.4–188.7)	116.7 (60.9–166.4)	76.8 (46.7–129.0)	74.6 (32.9–116.7)	76.8 (32.9–116.7)	82.4 (53.8–129.0)	107.6 (53.8–164.7)
Refined wheat (g)	140.8 (94.5–196.4)	95.4 (67.9–135.8)	147.8 (107.0–194.4)	185.0 (135.5–272.6)	147.0 (96.3–194.6)	137.5 (93.0–188.2)	140.2 (94.5–206.3)	147.0 (95.5–204.8)	143.1 (95.5–191.2)	136.3 (92.2–194.4)
Tubers (g)	52.9 (28.3–94.0)	28.3 (17.9–45.1)	52.9 (35.6–64.9)	100.5 (52.9–141.6)	52.0 (28.2–93.8)	45.1 (27.3–82.8)	52.9 (28.3–100.5)	45.1 (27.8–100.5)	52.9 (28.3–82.8)	51.1 (28.3–82.8)
Fruits (g)	228.2 (134.5–344.2)	136.5 (89.8–210.7)	230.6 (164.5–311.1)	341.1 (241.3–473.2)	198.3 (110.8–296.0)	203.7 (120.3–308.8)	281.9 (182.2–418.2)	201.0 (121.6–336.5)	236.1 (126.7–339.2)	242.9 (147.5–355.2)
Seaweeds and mushrooms (g)	15.7 (8.6–27.3)	8.6 (6.1–13.2)	15.7 (8.6–25.0)	28.6 (15.7–39.3)	12.1 (7.9–25.0)	13.2 (7.9–25.0)	21.4 (12.1–30.3)	12.1 (7.9–25.0)	13.2 (8.6–28.6)	17.5 (10.3–28.6)
Soybean products (g)	78.8 (46.1–127.7)	46.4 (27.1–77.6)	78.8 (52.4–120.3)	103.1 (78.8–152.2)	81.2 (46.4–139.3)	78.8 (46.4–126.0)	77.5 (45.1–104.0)	64.5 (36.1–82.3)	78.8 (46.4–116.5)	93.7 (68.8–150.7)
Red meat (g)	49.3 (31.9–81.6)	41.0 (33.4–74.8)	41.0 (33.4–85.3)	51.7 (31.9–81.6)	37.4 (19.9–71.3)	41.0 (33.8–74.8)	67.4 (37.4–85.6)	31.9 (13.9–37.4)	51.7 (34.0–71.3)	85.6 (67.7–107.2)
Poultry (g)	25.1 (10.1–50.3)	25.1 (10.1–30.2)	25.1 (10.1–30.2)	25.1 (12.1–50.3)	25.1 (10.1–30.2)	25.1 (10.1–30.2)	25.1 (12.1–50.3)	12.1 (6.0–25.1)	25.1 (11.4–30.2)	50.3 (25.1–70.4)
Peanuts (g)	11.1 (6.9–23.6)	6.9 (0.0–11.1)	11.1 (6.9–23.6)	23.6 (8.3–38.7)	6.9 (0.0–20.9)	8.3 (6.9–23.6)	13.9 (6.9–34.7)	11.1 (6.6–23.6)	11.1 (6.9–26.4)	8.3 (4.2–23.6)
Seafood (g)	25.7 (17.6–43.0)	22.2 (11.8–32.5)	25.1 (19.7–43.0)	38.2 (22.2–69.3)	21.5 (10.9–34.2)	23.7 (18.6–40.8)	38.9 (22.2–69.3)	25.7 (17.1–43.0)	24.2 (18.6–44.3)	27.0 (18.6–44.3)
Dairy products (g)	78.3 (17.9–178.6)	48.7 (10.5–95.5)	90.7 (21.0–178.6)	114.7 (46.2–199.6)	46.2 (17.9–146.9)	70.3 (19.1–148.0)	95.5 (48.7–191.1)	77.2 (17.9–178.6)	86.6 (19.1–178.6)	78.3 (17.9–147.0)
Eggs (g)	62.5 (36.6–77.1)	56.3 (28.4–73.7)	66.4 (49.3–77.1)	69.0 (50.3–78.0)	69.0 (49.3–73.7)	66.4 (49.3–77.1)	57.2 (31.2–78.0)	47.4 (25.9–61.2)	61.5 (49.3–74.3)	77.1 (69.0–94.2)
Tea (mL)	192.9 (21.4–364.3)	107.1 (0.0–300.0)	171.4 (37.5–342.9)	300.0 (42.9–600.0)	96.4 (0.0–321.4)	171.4 (42.9–342.9)	257.1 (85.7–600.0)	182.1 (42.9–428.6)	214.3 (42.9–385.7)	150.0 (0.0–342.9)
Dessert (g)	14.4 (3.1–29.4)	13.2 (3.1–23.2)	13.9 (3.1–25.4)	17.5 (3.1–43.2)	3.1 (0.0–11.0)	14.4 (4.3–22.8)	32.3 (17.5–57.0)	13.2 (0.0–27.7)	15.2 (3.1–26.5)	15.3 (3.1–30.6)
Condiments (g)	14.3 (3.5–29.6)	12.9 (2.5–29.4)	14.5 (2.9–29.3)	16.4 (5.1–31.9)	6.8 (1.4–17.8)	14.3 (3.9–29.3)	25.1 (13.2–32.5)	8.4 (2.5–17.8)	15.7 (4.2–29.6)	20.0 (5.1–32.5)
Animal offal (g)	6.4 (0.0–15.3)	6.4 (0.0–15.3)	6.4 (0.0–15.3)	6.4 (0.0–21.6)	0.0 (0.0–6.4)	6.4 (0.0–13.5)	20.6 (7.9–40.7)	6.4 (0.0–15.3)	6.4 (0.0–15.3)	8.1 (0.0–19.9)
Alcohol beverages (mL)	71.4 (0.0–233.9)	65.9 (0.0–205.4)	61.8 (0.0–222.6)	83.2 (0.0–273.6)	29.6 (0.0–107.7)	79.6 (14.3–250.0)	148.2 (29.6–367.9)	79.1 (0.0–250.0)	65.4 (0.0–219.7)	65.4 (0.0–219.6)
Fast food (g)	18.6 (5.3–42.6)	17.5 (5.3–37.3)	18.6 (5.3–38.4)	19.4 (5.3–47.9)	5.3 (0.0–14.9)	18.6 (8.9–32.3)	45.7 (24.6–74.6)	17.0 (0.0–37.6)	19.3 (5.3–42.2)	19.3 (5.3–45.7)
Beverages (mL)	27.7 (0.0–84.0)	41.1 (0.0–84.0)	26.8 (0.0–83.1)	26.8 (0.0–82.1)	0.0 (0.0–26.8)	27.7 (0.0–68.8)	84.0 (29.5–206.3)	26.8 (0.0–82.1)	26.8 (0.0–81.2)	31.4 (0.0–133.9)

[1] Tertiles of dietary pattern scores.

Nutrients **2015**, 7, 8072–8089

References

1. American Diabetes Association. Standards of medical care in diabetes-2012. *Diabetes Care* **2012**, *35*, S11–S63.
2. Schmidt, M.I.; Duncan, B.B.; Bang, H.; Pankow, J.S.; Ballantyne, C.M.; Golden, S.H.; Folsom, A.R.; Chambless, L.E. Identifying individuals at high risk for diabetes—The Atherosclerosis Risk in Communities study. *Diabetes Care* **2005**, *28*, 2013–2018. [CrossRef] [PubMed]
3. Levitzky, Y.S.; Pencina, M.J.; D'Agostino, R.B.; Meigs, J.B.; Murabito, J.M.; Vasan, R.S.; Fox, C.S. Impact of impaired fasting glucose on cardiovascular disease. *J. Am. Coll. Cardiol.* **2008**, *51*, 264–270. [CrossRef] [PubMed]
4. Ford, E.S.; Zhao, G.X.; Li, C.Y. Pre-Diabetes and the risk for cardiovascular disease asystematic review of the evidence. *J. Am. Coll. Cardiol.* **2010**, *55*, 1310–1317. [CrossRef] [PubMed]
5. Xu, Y.; Wang, L.M.; He, J.; Bi, Y.F.; Li, M.; Wang, T.G.; Wang, L.H.; Jiang, Y.; Dai, M.; Lu, J.L.; *et al.* Prevalence and Control of Diabetes in Chinese Adults. *J. Am. Med. Assoc.* **2013**, *310*, 948–958. [CrossRef] [PubMed]
6. Tabak, A.G.; Herder, C.; Rathmann, W.; Brunner, E.J.; Kivimaki, M. Prediabetes: A high-risk state for diabetes development. *Lancet* **2012**, *379*, 2279–2290. [CrossRef]
7. Diabetes Prevention Program Research Group. Reduction in the incidence of type 2 diabetes with lifestyle intervention or metformin. *N. Engl. J. Med.* **2002**, *346*, 393–403.
8. Perreault, L.; Pan, Q.; Mather, K.J.; Watson, K.E.; Hamman, R.F.; Kahn, S.E.; Diabetes Prevention Program Research Group. Effect of regression from prediabetes to normal glucose regulation on long-term reduction in diabetes risk: Results from the Diabetes Prevention Program Outcomes Study. *Lancet* **2012**, *379*, 2243–2251. [CrossRef]
9. Williams, D.E.; Prevost, A.T.; Whichelow, M.J.; Cox, B.D.; Day, N.E.; Wareham, N.J. A cross-sectional study of dietary patterns with glucose intolerance and other features of the metabolic syndrome. *Br. J. Nutr.* **2000**, *83*, 257–266. [CrossRef] [PubMed]
10. Liu, E.; McKeown, N.M.; Newby, P.K.; Meigs, J.B.; Vasan, R.S.; Quatromoni, P.A.; D'Agostino, R.B.; Jacques, P.F. Cross-sectional association of dietary patterns with insulin-resistant phenotype among adults without diabetes in the Framinham Offspring study. *Br. J. Nutr.* **2009**, *102*, 576–583. [CrossRef] [PubMed]
11. Mizoue, T.; Yamaji, T.; Tabata, S.; Yamaguchi, K.; Ogawa, S.; Mineshita, M.; Kono, S. Dietary patterns and glucose tolerance abnormalities in Japanese men. *J. Nutr.* **2006**, *136*, 1352–1358. [PubMed]
12. He, Y.N.; Hu, Y.; Ma, G.; Feskens, E.J.; Zhai, F.; Yang, X.; Li, Y. Dietary Patterns and Glucose Tolerance Abnormalities in Chinese Adults. *Diabetes Care* **2009**, *32*, 1972–1976. [PubMed]
13. Jia, Q.; Xia, Y.; Zhang, Q.; Wu, H.; Du, H.; Liu, L.; Wang, C.; Shi, H.; Guo, X.; Liu, X.; *et al.* Dietary patterns are associated with prevalence of fatty liver disease in adults. *Eur. J. Clin. Nutr.* **2015**, *69*, 914–921. [CrossRef] [PubMed]
14. Montonen, J.; Knekt, P.; Harkanen, T.; Jarvinen, R.; Heliovaara, M.; Aromaa, A.; Reunanen, A. Dietary patterns and the incidence of type 2 diabetes. *Am. J. Epidemiol.* **2005**, *161*, 219–227. [CrossRef] [PubMed]
15. Li, M.; Fan, Y.; Zhang, X.; Hou, W.; Tang, Z. Fruit and vegetable intake and risk of type 2 diabetes mellitus: Meta-analysis of prospective cohort studies. *BMJ Open* **2014**, *4*, e005497. [CrossRef] [PubMed]
16. Pan, X.R.; Li, G.W.; Hu, Y.H.; Wang, J.X.; Yang, W.Y.; An, Z.X.; Hu, Z.X.; Lin, J.; Xiao, J.Z.; Cao, H.B.; *et al.* Effects of diet and exercise in preventing NIDDM in people with impaired glucose tolerance: The Da Qing IGT and diabetes study. *Diabetes Care* **1997**, *20*, 537–544. [CrossRef] [PubMed]
17. Hamer, M.; Chida, Y. Intake of fruit, vegetables, and antioxidants and risk of type 2 diabetes: Systematic review and meta-analysis. *J. Hypertens.* **2007**, *25*, 2361–2369. [CrossRef] [PubMed]
18. Feskens, E.J.; Virtanen, S.M.; Räsänen, L.; Tuomilehto, J.; Stengård, J.; Pekkanen, J.; Nissinen, A.; Kromhout, D. Dietary factors determining diabetes and impaired glucose tolerance: A 20-year follow-up of the Finnish and Dutch cohorts of the Seven Countries Study. *Diabetes Care* **1995**, *18*, 1104–1112. [CrossRef] [PubMed]
19. Salonen, J.T.; Nyyssönen, K.; Tuomainen, T.P.; Mäenpää, P.H.; Korpela, H.; Kaplan, G.A.; Lynch, J.; Helmrich, S.P.; Salonen, R. Increased risk of non-insulin dependent diabetes mellitus at low plasma vitamin E concentrations: A four year follow up study in men. *BMJ* **1995**, *311*, 1124–1127. [CrossRef] [PubMed]
20. Reunanen, A.; Knekt, P.; Aaran, R.K.; Aromaa, A. Serum antioxidants and risk of non-insulin dependent diabetes mellitus. *Eur. J. Clin. Nutr.* **1998**, *52*, 89–93. [CrossRef] [PubMed]

21. Barbagallo, M.; Dominguez, L.J.; Galioto, A.; Ferlisi, A.; Cani, C.; Malfa, L.; Pineo, A.; Busardo, A.; Paolisso, G. Role of magnesium in insulin action, diabetes and cardio-metabolic syndrome X. *Mol. Aspects. Med.* **2003**, *24*, 39–52. [CrossRef]

22. Suarez, A.; Pulido, N.; Casla, A.; Casanova, B.; Arrieta, F.J.; Rovira, A. Impaired tyrosine-kinase activity of muscle insulin receptors from hypomagnesaemic rats. *Diabetologia* **1995**, *38*, 1262–1270. [PubMed]

23. Balon, T.W.; Gu, J.L.; Tokuyama, Y.; Jasman, A.P.; Nadler, J.L. Magnesium supplementation reduces development of diabetes in a rat model of spontaneous NIDDM. *Am. J. Physiol.* **1995**, *269*, E745–E752. [PubMed]

24. Lopez-Ridaura, R.; Willett, W.C.; Rimm, E.B.; Liu, S.; Stampfer, M.J.; Manson, J.E.; Hu, F.B. Magnesium intake and risk of type 2 diabetes in men and women. *Diabetes Care* **2004**, *27*, 134–140. [CrossRef] [PubMed]

25. Shi, Z.; Hu, X.; Yuan, B.; Pan, X.; Meyer, H.E.; Holmboe-Ottesen, G. Association between serum ferritin, hemoglobin, iron intake, and diabetes in adults in Jiangsu, China. *Diabetes Care* **2006**, *29*, 1878–1883. [CrossRef] [PubMed]

26. Fernandez-Real, J.M.; Lopez-Bermejo, A.; Ricart, W. Cross-talk between iron metabolism and diabetes. *Diabetes* **2002**, *51*, 2348–2354. [CrossRef] [PubMed]

27. Swaminathan, S.; Fonseca, V.A.; Alam, M.G.; Shah, S.V. The role of iron in diabetes and its complications. *Diabetes Care* **2007**, *30*, 1926–1933. [CrossRef] [PubMed]

28. Shi, Z.M.; Hu, X.S.; Yuan, B.J.; Gibson, R.; Dai, Y.; Garg, M. Association between magnesium: Iron intake ratio and diabetes in Chinese adults in Jiangsu Province. *Diabet. Med.* **2008**, *25*, 1164–1170. [CrossRef] [PubMed]

29. Frank, L.K.; Jannasch, F.; Kröger, J.; Bedu-Addo, G.; Mockenhaupt, F.P.; Schulze, M.B.; Danquah, I. A dietary pattern derived by reduced rank regression is associated with type 2 diabetes in an urban Ghanaian population. *Nutrients* **2015**, *7*, 5497–5514. [CrossRef] [PubMed]

30. Rosa, M.L.; Falcão, P.M.; Yokoo, E.M.; da Cruz Filho, R.A.; Alcoforado, V.M.; de Souza Bda, S.; Pinto, F.N.; Nery, A.B. Brazil's staple food and incidents diabetes. *Nutrition* **2014**, *30*, 365–368. [CrossRef] [PubMed]

31. Frank, L.K.; Kroger, J.; Schulze, M.B.; Bedu-Addo, G.; Mockenhaupt, F.P.; Danquah, I. Dietary patterns in urban Ghana and risk of type 2 diabetes. *Br. J. Nutr.* **2014**, *112*, 89–98. [CrossRef] [PubMed]

32. Kant, A.K.; Graubard, B.I. A comparison of three dietary pattern indexes for predicting biomarkers of diet and disease. *J. Am. Coll. Nutr.* **2005**, *24*, 294–303. [CrossRef] [PubMed]

33. Schulze, M.B.; Hoffmann, K.; Manson, J.E.; Willett, W.C.; Meigs, J.B.; Weikert, C.; Heidemann, C.; Colditz, G.A.; Hu, F.B. Dietary pattern, inflammation, and incidence of type 2 diabetes in women. *Am. J. Clin. Nutr.* **2005**, *82*, 675–684. [PubMed]

34. Fung, T.T.; Schulze, M.; Manson, J.E.; Willett, W.C.; Hu, F.B. Dietary patterns, meat intake, and the risk of type 2 diabetes in women. *Arch. Intern. Med.* **2004**, *164*, 2235–2240. [CrossRef] [PubMed]

35. Van Dam, R.M.; Rimm, E.B.; Willett, W.C.; Stampfer, M.J.; Hu, F.B. Dietary patterns and risk for type 2 diabetes mellitus in U.S. men. *Ann. Intern. Med.* **2002**, *136*, 201–209. [CrossRef] [PubMed]

36. Wei, J.; Zeng, C.; Gong, Q.Y.; Yang, H.B.; Li, X.X.; Lei, G.H.; Yang, T.B. The association between dietary selenium intake and diabetes: A cross-sectional study among middle-aged and older adults. *Nutr. J.* **2015**, *14*, 18. [CrossRef] [PubMed]

37. Stranges, S.; Sieri, S.; Vinceti, M.; Grioni, S.; Guallar, E.; Laclaustra, M.; Muti, P.; Berrino, F.; Krogh, V. A prospective study of dietary selenium intake and risk of type 2 diabetes. *BMC Public Health.* **2010**, *10*, 564. [CrossRef] [PubMed]

38. Stranges, S.; Marshall, J.R.; Natarajan, R.; Donahue, R.P.; Trevisan, M.; Combs, G.F.; Cappuccio, F.P.; Ceriello, A.; Reid, M.E. Effects of long-term selenium supplementation on the incidence of type 2 diabetes: A randomized trial. *Ann. Intern. Med.* **2007**, *147*, 217–223. [CrossRef] [PubMed]

39. Bleys, J.; Navas-Acien, A.; Guallar, E. Serum selenium and diabetes in U.S. adults. *Diabetes Care* **2007**, *30*, 829–834. [CrossRef] [PubMed]

40. Laclaustra, M.; Navas-Acien, A.; Stranges, S.; Ordovas, J.M.; Guallar, E. Serum selenium concentrations and diabetes in U.S. adults: National Health and Nutrition Examination Survey (NHANES) 2003–2004. *Environ. Health. Perspect.* **2009**, *117*, 1409–1413. [CrossRef] [PubMed]

41. Satyanarayana, S.; Sekhar, J.R.; Kumar, K.E.; Shannika, L.B.; Rajanna, B.; Rajanna, S. Influence of selenium (antioxidant) on gliclazide induced hypoglycaemia/anti hyperglycaemia in normal/alloxan-induced diabetic rats. *Mol. Cell. Biochem.* **2006**, *283*, 123–127. [CrossRef] [PubMed]

42. Goldstein, B.J.; Mahadev, K.; Wu, X. Redox paradox: Insulin action is facilitated by insulin-stimulated reactive oxygen species with multiple potential signaling targets. *Diabetes* **2005**, *54*, 311–321. [CrossRef] [PubMed]

43. Villegas, R.; Liu, S.; Gao, Y.T.; Yang, G.; Li, H.; Zheng, W.; Shu, X.O. Prospective study of dietary carbohydrates, glycemic index, glycemic load, and incidence of type 2 diabetes mellitus in middle-aged Chinese women. *Arch. Intern. Med.* **2007**, *167*, 2310–2316. [CrossRef] [PubMed]

44. Shi, Z.; Taylor, A.W.; Hu, G.; Gill, T.; Wittert, G.A. Rice intake, weight change and risk of the metabolic syndrome development among Chinese adults: The Jiangsu Nutrition Study (JIN). *Asia Pac. J. Clin. Nutr.* **2012**, *21*, 35–43. [PubMed]

45. Yu, R.; Woo, J.; Chan, R.; Sham, A.; Ho, S.; Tso, A.; Cheung, B.; Lam, T.H.; Lam, K. Relationship between dietary intake and the development of type 2 diabetes in a Chinese population: The Hong Kong Dietary Survey. *Public Health Nutr.* **2011**, *14*, 1133–1141. [CrossRef] [PubMed]

46. Kaur, K.D.; Jha, A.; Sabikhi, L.; Singh, A.K. Significance of coarse cereals in health and nutrition: A review. *J. Food Sci. Technol.* **2014**, *51*, 1429–1441. [CrossRef] [PubMed]

47. Sartorelli, D.S.; Franco, L.J.; Damião, R.; Gimeno, S.; Cardoso, M.A.; Ferreira, S.R. Dietary glycemic load, glycemic index, and refined grains intake are associated with reduced beta-cell function in prediabetic Japanese migrants. *Arq. Bras. Endocrinol. Metabol.* **2009**, *53*, 429–434. [CrossRef] [PubMed]

48. Bhupathiraju, S.N.; Tobias, D.K.; Malik, V.S.; Pan, A.; Hruby, A.; Manson, J.E.; Willett, W.C.; Hu, F.B. Glycemic index, glycemic load, and risk of type 2 diabetes: Results from 3 large US cohorts and an updated meta-analysis. *Am. J. Clin. Nutr.* **2014**, *100*, 218–232. [CrossRef] [PubMed]

49. Aune, D.; Ursin, G.; Veierod, M.B. Meat consumption and the risk of type 2 diabetes: A systematic review and meta-analysis of cohort studies. *Diabetologia* **2009**, *52*, 2277–2287. [CrossRef] [PubMed]

50. Pan, A.; Sun, Q.; Bernstein, A.M.; Schulze, M.B.; Manson, J.E.; Willett, W.C.; Hu, F.B. Red meat consumption and risk of type 2 diabetes: 3 cohorts of US adults and an updated meta-analysis. *Am. J. Clin. Nutr.* **2011**, *94*, 1088–1096. [CrossRef] [PubMed]

51. Nakamura, Y.; Iso, H.; Kita, Y.; Ueshima, H.; Okada, K.; Konishi, M.; Inoue, M.; Tsugane, S. Egg consumption, serum total cholesterol concentrations and coronary heart disease incidence: Japan Public Health Center-based prospective study. *Br. J. Nutr.* **2006**, *96*, 921–928. [CrossRef] [PubMed]

52. Howell, W.H.; McNamara, D.J.; Tosca, M.A.; Smith, B.T.; Gaines, J.A. Plasma lipid and lipoprotein responses to dietary fat and cholesterol: A meta-analysis. *Am. J. Clin. Nutr.* **1997**, *65*, 1747–1764. [PubMed]

53. McNamara, D.J. Eggs and heart disease risk: Perpetuating the misperception. *Am. J. Clin. Nutr.* **2002**, *5*, 333–335.

54. Howard, B.V.; Knowler, W.C.; Vasquez, B.; Kennedy, A.L.; Pettitt, D.J.; Bennett, P.H. Plasma and lipoprotein cholesterol and triglyceride in the Pima Indian population: Comparison of diabetics and nondiabetics. *Arteriosclerosis* **1984**, *4*, 462–471. [CrossRef] [PubMed]

55. Pelletier, X.; Thouvenot, P.; Belbraouet, S.; Chayvialle, J.A.; Hanesse, B.; Mayeux, D.; Debry, G. Effect of egg consumption in healthy volunteers: Influence of yolk, white or whole-egg on gastric emptying and on glycemic and hormonal responses. *Ann. Nutr. Metab.* **1996**, *40*, 109–115. [CrossRef]

56. Shi, Z.; Yuan, B.; Zhang, C.; Zhou, M.; Holmboe-Ottesen, G. Egg consumption and the risk of diabetes in adults, Jiangsu, China. *Nutrition* **2011**, *27*, 194–198. [CrossRef] [PubMed]

57. Zhang, J.G.; Wang, Z.H.; Wang, H.J.; Du, W.W.; Su, C.; Zhang, J.; Jiang, H.R.; Zhai, F.Y.; Zhang, B. Dietary patterns and their associations with general obesity and abdominal obesity among young Chinese women. *Eur. J. Clin. Nutr.* **2015**, *69*, 1009–1014. [CrossRef] [PubMed]

58. Shi, Z.; Yuan, B.; Hu, G.; Dai, Y.; Zuo, H.; Holmboe-Ottesen, G. Dietary pattern and weight change in a 5 year follow up among Chinese adults: Results from Jiangsu nutrition and health study. *Br. J. Nutr.* **2011**, *105*, 1047–1054. [CrossRef] [PubMed]

59. He, Y.; Li, Y.; Lai, J.; Wang, D.; Zhang, J.; Fu, P.; Yang, X.; Qi, L. Dietary patterns as compared with physical activity in relation to metabolic syndrome among Chinese adults. *Nutr. Metab. Cardiovasc. Dis.* **2013**, *23*, 920–928. [CrossRef] [PubMed]

60. Brown, K.H.; Rivera, J.A.; Bhutta, Z.; Gibson, R.S.; King, J.C.; Lonnerdal, B.; Ruel, M.T.; Sandtrom, B.; Wasantwisut, E.; *et al.* International Zinc Nutrition Consultative Group (IZiNCG) technical document #1. Assessment of the risk of zinc deficiency in populations and options for its control. *Food Nutr. Bull.* **2004**, *25*, S99–S203. [PubMed]

61. Vashum, K.P.; McEvoy, M.; Shi, Z.; Milton, A.H.; Islam, M.R.; Sibbritt, D.; Patterson, A.; Byles, J.; Loxton, D.; Attia, J. Is dietary zinc protective for type 2 diabetes? Results from the Australian longitudinal study on women's health. *BMC Endocr. Disord.* **2013**, *13*, 40. [CrossRef] [PubMed]

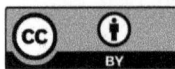

nutrients

MDPI

Article

Dietary Patterns during Pregnancy Are Associated with Risk of Gestational Diabetes Mellitus

Dayeon Shin, Kyung Won Lee and Won O. Song *

Department of Food Science and Human Nutrition, Michigan State University, 469 Wilson Road,
Trout FSHN Building, East Lansing, MI 48824, USA; shinda@msu.edu (D.S.); kyungwon@msu.edu (K.W.L.)
*   Correspondence: song@msu.edu; Tel.: +1-517-353-3332; Fax: +1-517-353-8963

Received: 11 August 2015 ; Accepted: 4 November 2015 ; Published: 12 November 2015

Abstract: Maternal dietary patterns before and during pregnancy play important roles in the development of gestational diabetes mellitus (GDM). We aimed to identify dietary patterns during pregnancy that are associated with GDM risk in pregnant U.S. women. From a 24 h dietary recall of 253 pregnant women (16–41 years) included in the National Health and Nutrition Examination Survey (NHANES) 2003–2012, food items were aggregated into 28 food groups based on Food Patterns Equivalents Database. Three dietary patterns were identified by reduced rank regression with responses including prepregnancy body mass index (BMI), dietary fiber, and ratio of poly- and monounsaturated fatty acids to saturated fatty acid: "high refined grains, fats, oils and fruit juice", "high nuts, seeds, fat and soybean; low milk and cheese", and "high added sugar and organ meats; low fruits, vegetables and seafood". GDM was diagnosed using fasting plasma glucose levels $\geqslant 5.1$ mmol/L for gestation <24 weeks. Multivariable logistic regression models were used to estimate adjusted odds ratio (AOR) and 95% confidence intervals (CIs) for GDM, after controlling for maternal age, race/ethnicity, education, family poverty income ratio, marital status, prepregnancy BMI, gestational weight gain, energy intake, physical activity, and log-transformed C-reactive protein (CRP). All statistical analyses accounted for the appropriate survey design and sample weights of the NHANES. Of 249 pregnant women, 34 pregnant women (14%) had GDM. Multivariable AOR (95% CIs) of GDM for comparisons between the highest *vs.* lowest tertiles were 4.9 (1.4–17.0) for "high refined grains, fats, oils and fruit juice" pattern, 7.5 (1.8–32.3) for "high nuts, seeds, fat and soybean; low milk and cheese" pattern, and 22.3 (3.9–127.4) for "high added sugar and organ meats; low fruits, vegetables and seafood" pattern after controlling for maternal sociodemographic variables, prepregnancy BMI, gestational weight gain, energy intake and log-transformed CRP. These findings suggest that dietary patterns during pregnancy are associated with risk of GDM after controlling for potential confounders. The observed connection between a high consumption of refined grains, fat, added sugars and low intake of fruits and vegetables during pregnancy with higher odds for GDM, are consistent with general health benefits of healthy diets, but warrants further research to understand underlying pathophysiology of GDM associated with dietary behaviors during pregnancy.

Keywords: dietary patterns; reduced rank regression; gestational diabetes mellitus; National Health and Nutrition Examination Survey

1. Introduction

Gestational diabetes mellitus (GDM) is indicated when any degree of glucose intolerance is recognized for the first time during pregnancy, regardless of whether the condition may have predated the pregnancy or persisted after the pregnancy [1]. In the U.S., approximately 1%–14% of all pregnancies have been reported to be complicated by GDM, which accounts for more than 200,000 cases annually [2].

Several studies reported how macro- or micro-nutrient intakes during pregnancy are related to GDM risk [3–6]. In 171 nulliparous Chinese pregnant women, macronutrient intake estimated from a 24 h recall at 24–28 weeks of gestation were associated with glucose tolerance in pregnancy [3]. Chinese women with GDM had a significantly lower polyunsaturated fat intake (% total fat) compared to women without GDM (28.2% *vs.* 31.6% of total fat). Women with GDM had significantly higher saturated fat intake compared to those without GDM (46.1% *vs.* 42.1% of total fat) [3]. In a study of 504 Italian pregnant women, Bo *et al.* [4] found that every 10% increase in saturated fat (% total fat) at 24 to 28 weeks of gestation was associated with an increased risk for GDM, whereas every 10% increase of polyunsaturated fat (% total fat) was associated with 15% reduction of GDM risk. In a prospective cohort study entitled, Pregnancy, Infection, and Nutrition (PIN) of 1698 U.S. pregnant women, women with GDM consumed a lower percentage of energy from carbohydrates and a higher percentage of energy from fat in the second trimester than women with normal glucose tolerance did [5]. In another prospective cohort study of 3158 U.S. pregnant women, Qiu *et al.* [6] reported that the dietary heme iron intake in the first trimester was associated with an increased risk for GDM. The current body of literature indicates that high intake of saturated fat, *n*-3 fatty acids, and dietary heme iron is associated with increased risk for GDM, whereas polyunsaturated fat intake may be protective against GDM risk. However, the studies reviewed vary widely for time point of pregnancy and diet assessment, dietary assessment tools (24 h recalls *vs.* food frequency questionnaires (FFQs), and diagnostic criteria for GDM (75 g or 100 g oral glucose).

Analyses of overall food patterns account for any interactions or synergistic effects among individual foods or nutrients [7]. In literature on dietary patterns in pregnant populations, factors analysis or principal component analysis ("foods group-driven") [8–12] were used to derive dietary patterns and related to pregnancy complications or birth outcomes. Reduced rank regression methods ("biomarker or nutrient-driven") have been introduced to better assess the diet-disease relations compared to using factor analysis and principal component analysis [13], but the method has been underutilized among pregnant women. The reduced rank regression method has only been reported in the studies that assessed dietary patterns during pregnancy in relation to spina bifida [14] and congenital heart defect [15] in Netherlands. Dietary patterns derived using the reduced rank regression method is expected to explain the maximum variation of GDM-related maternal nutrients and biomarkers as response variables in women with GDM.

A few studies have examined the association between dietary patterns during pregnancy and the risk of GDM in U.S. representative pregnant women. The role of dietary patterns during pregnancy in relation to GDM risk is still uncertain. We hypothesized that dietary patterns during pregnancy derived from reduced rank regression are differentially associated with the risk of GDM.

2. Methods

2.1. Study Population

We used public domain data from the continuous National Health and Nutrition Examination (NHANES) 2003–2004, 2005–2006, 2007–2008, 2009–2010, and 2011–2012 for this study. Data from the NHANES 2003–2012 were combined for this study with greater statistical reliability. The NHANES is a program of studies cross-sectionally designed to assess the health and nutritional status of civilian, non-institutionalized population in the U.S. conducted by the National Center for Health Statistics (NCHS), Centers for Disease Control and Prevention (CDC). The NHANES used a stratified multistage probability sample that was based on the selection of counties, blocks, households, and finally persons within households. The NHANES survey is unique in that it combines interviews and physical examinations. The participants were interviewed for the information of age, race/ethnicity, education level, marital status, family poverty income ratio, and physical activity. Reproductive health interviews obtained information on month of gestation at the time of the survey. Pregnancy status was based on a positive urine pregnancy test. Prepregnancy weight was self-reported during the weight history questionnaire interview. A complete description of data-collection procedures and analytic guidelines has been provided elsewhere [16,17].

The 2003–2012 NHANES dataset included 761 pregnant women. Subjects were excluded if they reported unreliable dietary data, as defined by the NCHS ($n = 24$) and had missing data of gestational weeks ($n = 105$), measured height, weight and self-reported prepregnancy weight ($n = 35$), glucose and insulin levels ($n = 310$), and CRP levels ($n = 1$). Pregnant women who did not participate in the fasting subsample for glucose and insulin were excluded from the analysis ($n = 33$). Lastly, pregnant women who were already diagnosed with GDM were excluded ($n = 4$). The final analytic sample size was 249 pregnant women. NHANES protocol was reviewed and approved by the NCHS Research Ethics Review Board [18].

2.2. Dietary Assessment

What We Eat in America, component of the NHANES 2003–2012 collected dietary information by using an interviewer-administered 24 h recall that used automated multiple pass methodology developed by the U.S. Department of Agriculture (USDA) [19]. A second dietary recall, 3–10 days after the first dietary recall, was obtained by using phone calls [20]. Although two 24 h dietary recalls were collected in the 2007–2010 NHANES, only the first recall data are recommended to be used by the NCHS as different methods were used to collect dietary data, *i.e.*, day 1 by in-person and day 2 by phone calls [20]. A single 24 h recall has also been reported to be adequate to estimate mean group dietary intake [21].

Dietary pattern analysis was performed in two steps to identify dietary patterns as predictors of the responses to GDM. In the first step, food items were aggregated into 28 food groups, which are comparable with the grouping schemes reported in the Food Patterns Equivalents Database (FPED) 2011–2012 [22] (as shown in Table 1). The USDA's food code from an individual's day 1 dietary recall of NHANES was matched to the USDA food code of FPED 2011–2012. Since the components of FPED 2011–2012 are presented per 100 g of food and beverages, an individual's food intake in grams was divided by 100 g and multiplied by the number of FPED equivalents in FPED 2011–2012 [23]. To derive optimal dietary patterns, total fruit, total vegetables, total red and orange vegetables, total starch vegetables, total grains, total protein foods, total meat, poultry, and seafood, and total dairy from the original FPED 2011–2012's subgroups were removed because a total subgroup is the summation of its subgroup components. For example, total dairy is the summation of milk, yogurt, and cheese. In the second step, dietary pattern analysis was performed with the reduced rank regression method. The reduced rank regression method extracts linear combinations from predicting variables while maximizing the variance explained within a set of response variables [13]. We used PROC PLS with the reduced rank regression method option to drive dietary patterns using SAS software (version 9.3; SAS Institute, Cary, NC, U.S.). The analysis began with the selection of the 28 food groups on the basis of the number of cup equivalents of fruit, vegetables, and dairy; ounce equivalents of grains and protein foods; teaspoon equivalents of added sugars; gram equivalents of solid fats and oils; and number of alcoholic drinks as independent or exposure variables. This was followed by the choice of the prepregnancy BMI, nutrient intake, and maternal biomarkers related to GDM as response measures following log transformation. The predicting variables are the food groups from a 24 h recall, and the final set of response measures are prepregnancy BMI, dietary fiber, and poly- and monounsaturated fatty acids to saturated fatty acid. The final number of response variables indicating the greatest explanation of the total variation in foods groups and in biomarkers was obtained by sensitivity analysis (Table S1).

Table 1. Food patterns equivalents database (FPED) 2011–2012 food groups and modified groups used in the present study.

FPED [1] 2011–2012 Food Groups	Original FPED 2011–2012 Subgroups	Modified FPED 2011–2012 Subgroups
Fruit	1. Total fruit 2. Citrus, melons, and berries 3. Other fruits 4. Fruit juice	*Removed* 1. Citrus, melons, and berries 2. Other fruits 3. Fruit juice
Vegetables	5. Total vegetables 6. Dark green vegetables 7. Total red and orange vegetables 8. Tomatoes 9. Other red and orange vegetables (excludes, tomatoes) 10. Total starchy vegetables 11. Potatoes (white potatoes) 12. Other starchy vegetables (excludes white potatoes) 13. Other vegetables 14. Beans and peas computed as vegetables	*Removed* 4. Dark green vegetables *Removed* 5. Tomatoes 6. Other red and orange vegetables (excludes, tomatoes) *Removed* 7. Potatoes (white potatoes) 8. Other starchy vegetables (excludes white potatoes) 9. Other vegetables 10. Beans and peas computed as vegetables
Grains	15. Total grains 16. Whole grains 17. Refined grains	*Removed* 11. Whole grains 12. Refined grains
Protein Foods	18. Total protein foods 19. Total meat, poultry, and seafood 20. Meat (beef, veal, pork, lamb, game) 21. Cured meat (frankfurters, sausage, corned beef, cured ham and luncheon meat made from beef, pork, poultry) 22. Organ meat (from beef, veal, pork, lamb, game, poultry) 23. Poultry (chicken, turkey, other fowl) 24. Seafood high in *n*-3 fatty acids 25. Seafood low in *n*-3 fatty acids 26. Eggs 27. Soybean products (excludes calcium fortified soy milk and mature soybeans) 28. Nuts and seeds 29. Beans and peas computed as protein foods	*Removed* *Removed* 13. Meat (beef, veal, pork, lamb, game) 14. Cured meat (frankfurters, sausage, corned beef, cured ham and luncheon meat made from beef, pork, poultry) 15. Organ meat (from beef, veal, pork, lamb, game, poultry) 16. Poultry (chicken, turkey, other fowl) 17. Seafood high in *n*-3 fatty acids 18. Seafood low in *n*-3 fatty acids 19. Eggs 20. Soybean products (excludes calcium fortified soy milk and mature soybeans) 21. Nuts and seeds *Removed*
Dairy	30. Total dairy (milk, yogurt, cheese, whey) 31. Milk (includes calcium fortified soy milk) 32. Yogurt 33. Cheese	*Removed* 22. Milk (includes calcium fortified soy milk) 23. Yogurt 24. Cheese
Oils	34. Oils	25. Oils
Solid Fats	35. Solid fats	26. Solid fats
Added Sugars	36. Added sugars	27. Added sugars
Alcoholic Drinks	37. Alcoholic drinks	28. Alcoholic drinks

USDA's Food Patterns Equivalents Database 2011–2012 (FPED 2011–2012) converts foods and beverages in the Food and Nutrient Database for Dietary Studies (FNDDS) 2011–2012 to 37 Food Patterns (FP) components [23].
[1] The FPED provides an unique research tool to evaluate food and beverage intakes of Americans compared to recommendations of the 2010 Dietary Guidelines for Americans.

The relationship between the 28 food groups and the identified dietary patterns was indicated by factor loadings, which represent the correlation coefficients between the food groups and the dietary patterns. The dietary patterns were labeled on the basis of food groups that loaded highest and/or lowest in the respective dietary pattern. Each pregnant woman was assigned a score of the derived dietary patterns, calculated as the product of the food group value and its factor loading and summed across the food groups.

2.3. Maternal Biomarkers

All the blood measurements used in this study were drawn, analyzed, and reported as part of the NHANES 2003–2012 surveys dataset. A fasting blood glucose test was performed on eligible participants who were examined in the morning session after a nine-hour fast [24]. Plasma glucose was measured using an enzyme hexokinase method [24]. For NHANES 2003–2004, glucose and insulin measurements were performed by Diabetes Diagnostic Laboratory at University of Missouri (Columbia, MO, USA) [25], and for NHANES 2005–2012, glucose and insulin measurements were performed by the Fairview Medical Center Laboratory at the University of Minnesota (Minneapolis, MN, USA) [24]. Insulin was measured using Tosoh AIA-PACK IRI immunoenzymometric assay in NHANES 2003–2004 [25], and the Merocodia Insulin ELISA Immunoassay in NHANES 2005–2012 [24]. Insulin resistance was estimated using the homeostatic model assessment for insulin resistance (HOMA-IR) by the following formula: fasting insulin (μU/mL) × fasting glucose (mmol/L)/22.5 [26]. Glycohemoglobin (HbA1C) was measured using a Tosoh A1C 2.2 Plus Glycohemoglobin Analyzer (Tosoh Medics Inc., San Francisco, CA, USA) or a Tosoh G7 Automated HPLC Analyzer (Tosoh Medics Inc., San Francisco, CA, USA) [27]. CRP (nmol/L) was measured by latex-enhanced nephelometry [28]. Vitamin C (μmol/L) level in serum was measured using isocratic high performance liquid chromatography (HPLC) with electrochemical detection at 650 mV1 [29]. Lastly, vitamin D (nmol/L) concentration was measured by using the Diasorin 25-OH-Vitamin D assay (DiaSorin Inc., Stillwater, MN, USA) [30].

2.4. Outcome Variables

In this cross-sectional study, the average gestational age of study participants was 20 weeks. GDM was diagnosed according to the 2010 International Association of Diabetes and Pregnancy Study Groups (IADPSG) Consensus Panel [31] if the following criteria were met: fasting plasma glucose level ⩾ 5.1 mmol/L before 24 weeks of gestation.

2.5. Covariates

Analyses were adjusted for maternal age, race/ethnicity, family poverty income ratio, education, marital status, and physical activity level. Maternal age was controlled in continuous variables. The study group consisted of Mexican-American or other Hispanic, non-Hispanic White, non-Hispanic Black and other race. Family poverty income ratio was divided into three categories: ⩽1.85, 1.85–4 and >4. Maternal education was grouped by the number of completed years of school: less than high school, high school diploma and more than high school. Marital status was divided into three groups: married/living with a partner, widowed/divorced/separated and single. Physical activity level was divided into four groups: no activity, 0–500 MET-minutes/week, 500–1000 MET-minutes/week and ⩾1000 MET minutes/week.

2.6. Statistical Analyses

Maternal characteristics were expressed as numbers (weighted percentages) by the status of GDM. The Chi-square test was performed to test the association between maternal characteristic and the status of GDM. The risk for GDM was categorized as yes or no, and multivariable logistic regression models were applied to estimate odds ratios (ORs) (95% CI) of the risk for GDM across tertiles of dietary pattern scores. The *p* for trend across tertiles was computed by treating dietary pattern scores as continuous variables. We first ran models testing crude associations, then models were adjusted in three ways: (1) maternal age, race/ethnicity, education, family poverty income ratio and marital status; (2) model 1 + prepregnancy BMI + gestational weight gain + energy intake; (3) model 2 + log-transformed CRP concentrations.

To analyze the magnitude of collinearity, the variance inflation factor (VIF) was used to test with VIF <5 set as the acceptable level [32]. NHANES uses a complex sample survey design including a multistage cluster sample and weighting methodology that oversamples certain groups of individuals to ensure adequate statistical power. All analyses were carried out using SAS software, which incorporates appropriate sampling weights to adjust for the complex sampling weights. Sampling weights associated with the smallest subsample (fasting subsample) were used as recommended by the NHANES [33].

3. Results

Pregnant women's characteristics according to the status of GDM are shown in Table 2. Pregnant women with GDM generally had a family poverty income ratio ≤1.85 and were less likely to be involved in physical activity compared to women without GDM. Multi-collinearity between age, race/ethnicity, family poverty income ratio, education, marital status, and physical activity did not exist. The VIF for the all confounding variables were less than 2.

Table 2. Maternal characteristics in relation to gestational diabetes mellitus (GDM).

	GDM		No GDM		*p* Value [2]
	n	Wt'd% [1]	*n*	Wt'd% [1]	
Age					
≤25	17	57.4	94	37.2	0.22
26–35	14	38.7	110	56.0	
≥35	3	3.9	11	6.8	
Race					
Mexican American or other Hispanic	10	20.9	74	21.3	0.60
Non-Hispanic white	18	62.9	96	54.7	
Non-Hispanic black	4	14.3	32	14.3	
Other including multi-racial	2	1.9	13	9.6	
Family poverty income ratio					
≤1.85	20	62.6	108	38.1	0.02
1.85–4	5	5.9	60	35.8	
>4	9	31.5	47	26.1	
Education level					
≤11th Grade	12	37.7	75	21.2	0.23
High School Grade	5	8.2	38	19.7	
Above College	17	54.1	102	59.1	
Marital status					
Married or living with a partner	29	86.8	171	85.9	0.76
Widowed/divorced/separated	1	4.1	7	2.2	
Single	4	9.2	37	11.9	
Parity (*n* = 179)					
None	1	12.7	12	6.7	0.46
1	14	51.7	79	47.2	
2	10	34.6	38	33.0	
≥3	1	1.1	24	13.0	
Trimester of pregnancy					
1st trimester	12	50.9	39	29.3	0.15
2nd trimester	12	26.9	86	34.2	
3rd trimester	10	22.3	90	36.5	
Prepregnancy weight status					
BMI < 25 kg/m^2	8	29.4	133	61.7	0.06
BMI ≥ 25 kg/m^2	26	70.6	82	38.2	
Gestational weight gain					
Inadequate	8	14.9	59	29.9	0.07
Adequate	3	12.0	49	23.4	
Excessive	23	73.0	107	46.7	

Table 2. *Cont.*

	GDM		No GDM		*p* Value [2]
	n	Wt'd% [1]	*n*	Wt'd% [1]	
Physical activity (*n* = 154)					
None	6	29.1	8	10.1	0.02
0 to <500 MET-min/week	10	44.7	66	48.8	
500 to <1,000 MET-min/week	5	21.8	23	14.9	
≥1000 MET-min/week	3	4.4	33	26.3	
C-reactive protein					
>28.6 nmol/L	29	82.0	164	73.5	0.41
≤28.6 nmol/L	5	18.0	51	26.5	

[1] Wt'd%: Weighted %. Sample weights are created in the National Health and Nutrition Examination Survey (NHANES) to account for the complex survey design (including oversampling of some subgroups), survey non-responses, and post-stratification. When a sample is weighted in NHANES, it is representative of the U.S. civilian non-institutionalized Census population. Weighted percentages may not sum up to 100 due to rounding. [2] *p* Value obtained from Chi-square tests.

Dietary patterns were derived using the reduced rank regression method. The reduced rank regression method derives dietary patterns from predictors to maximize the explained variation of pre-defined set of responses chosen [34]. Responses chosen for reduced rank regression were prepregnancy BMI and nutrients that have bene consistently associated with GDM in the literature such as dietary fiber and ratio of poly- and monounsaturated fatty acids to saturated fatty acids [4,5,35]. Sensitivity analysis using different numbers of response variables (different sets for prepregnancy BMI and GDM-related nutrients including or excluding GDM-related biomarkers) indicated that the greatest explanation of the total variation in foods and in responses was obtained using prepregnancy BMI, dietary fiber, and ratio of poly- and monounsaturated fatty acids to saturated fatty acids (Table S1). Three factors were extracted with reduced rank regression, explaining the 45.9% of the total variation in the response variables and the 15.0% variation in food groups (Table S2). Three dietary patterns were derived using reduced rank regression. Loading values for each of the 28 food groups for the reduced rank regression obtained dietary patterns are presented in Table S3. The "high refined grains, fats, oils and fruit juice" pattern was characterized by high loadings of refined grains, solid fats, oils, and fruit juice. The "high nuts, seeds, fat and soybean; low milk and cheese" pattern was characterized by high loadings of nuts and seeds, solid fats, soybean products and low loadings of milk and cheese. The "high added sugar and organ meats; low fruits, vegetables and seafood" pattern was represented by high loadings of added sugars and organ meats and low loadings of fruits and vegetables and seafood (Table S3).

Maternal characteristics according to the tertiles of three dietary patterns' scores are presented in Table 3. Total energy intake and dietary fiber intake were differed significantly by the tertiles of "high refined grains, fats, oils and fruit juice" dietary pattern score. Total energy intake, total fat and saturated fat intake as percentages of energy, dietary fiber, ratio of poly- and monounsaturated fatty acids to saturated fatty acid, and serum vitamin D significantly differed by the tertiles of "high nuts, seeds, fat and soybean; low milk and cheese" dietary pattern score. Prepregnancy BMI, carbohydrate, protein and monounsaturated fatty acids intake as percentages of energy, dietary fiber, and HOMA-IR significantly differed by the tertiles of "high added sugar and organ meats; low fruits, vegetables and seafood" dietary pattern score (Table 3).

Table 3. Maternal characteristics by the tertiles of dietary pattern scores.

	"High Refined Grains, Fats, Oils and Fruit Juice" Pattern				"High Nuts, Seeds, Fat and Soybean; Low Milk and Cheese" Pattern				"High Added Sugar and Organ Meats; Low Fruits, Vegetables and Seafood" Pattern			
	Tertile 1 (n = 83)	Tertile 2 (n = 83)	Tertile 3 (n = 83)	p trend	Tertile 1 (n = 83)	Tertile 2 (n = 83)	Tertile 3 (n = 83)	p trend	Tertile 1 (n = 83)	Tertile 2 (n = 83)	Tertile 3 (n = 83)	p trend
Age (year)	25.7 ± 0.6 [1]	28 ± 0.9	27.5 ± 0.7	0.06	28.6 ± 0.8	26.8 ± 0.79	26.0 ± 0.6	0.05	28.8 ± 0.9	26.6 ± 0.6	26.6 ± 0.8	0.09
Prepregnancy BMI (kg/m²)	25.4 ± 1.2	27.6 ± 0.9	25.4 ± 0.7	0.07	26.0 ± 1.3	25.8 ± 0.9	26.8 ± 1.1	0.76	24.9 ± 1.2	24.6 ± 0.8	28.3 ± 1.1	0.008
Total energy (kcal/day)	1985.0 ± 125.1	2539.2 ± 137.7	2811.3 ± 153.7	0.0007	2866.5 ± 113.0	2116.6 ± 118.0	2320.3 ± 105.5	<0.0001	2658.1 ± 127.1	2230.0 ± 187.5	2463.5 ± 96.1	0.12
Carbohydrate (% of energy/day)	53.1 ± 2.3	52.7 ± 1.1	54.1 ± 1.7	0.82	52.7 ± 1.9	55.7 ± 1.5	50.9 ± 1.4	0.83	48.9 ± 1.4	51.6 ± 1.2	57.3 ± 1.7	0.008
Protein (% of energy/day)	15.9 ± 0.8	14.0 ± 0.4	14.1 ± 0.5	0.09	14.7 ± 0.6	14.9 ± 0.7	14.4 ± 0.5	0.05	16.6 ± 1.0	15.5 ± 0.9	12.8 ± 0.5	<0.0001
Total fat (% of energy/day)	31.7 ± 1.9	34.5 ± 1.2	33.9 ± 1.3	0.46	33.7 ± 1.6	30.8 ± 1.3	36.1 ± 1.1	0.02	35.6 ± 1.1	33.8 ± 1.6	31.6 ± 1.3	0.05
MUFA (% of energy/day)	11.9 ± 0.8	12.6 ± 0.5	12.2 ± 0.5	0.73	12.2 ± 0.7	11.6 ± 0.5	13.1 ± 0.5	0.12	13.0 ± 0.4	12.7 ± 0.6	11.4 ± 0.5	0.02
SFA (% of energy/day)	10.8 ± 0.7	11.5 ± 0.6	11.0 ± 0.6	0.69	12.4 ± 0.6	10.5 ± 0.7	10.5 ± 0.5	0.04	12.2 ± 0.6	10.9 ± 0.8	10.6 ± 0.5	0.15
Dietary fiber (g/day)	10.9 ± 1.0	16.6 ± 0.6	26.1 ± 1.2	<0.0001	20.7 ± 1.2	15.8 ± 1.5	15.7 ± 0.8	0.004	19.9 ± 1.3	14.8 ± 1.3	18.3 ± 1.3	0.03
Fatty acids ratio [2]	1.6 ± 0.1	1.6 ± 0.1	1.8 ± 0.1	0.54	1.3 ± 0.1	1.6 ± 0.1	2.1 ± 0.1	<0.0001	1.6 ± 0.1	1.8 ± 0.1	1.6 ± 0.1	0.59
Glycohemoglobin (%)	4.9 ± 0.1	4.9 ± 0.1	5.0 ± 0.1	0.34	4.9 ± 0.1	5.0 ± 0.1	5.0 ± 0.1	0.54	5.0 ± 0.1	4.9 ± 0.1	5.0 ± 0.1	0.50
HOMA-IR	2.2 ± 0.2	2.5 ± 0.3	2.4 ± 0.3	0.67	2.2 ± 0.2	2.1 ± 0.2	2.9 ± 0.4	0.25	2.2 ± 0.2	1.8 ± 0.2	3.0 ± 0.3	0.02
Fasting glucose (mmol/L)	4.7 ± 0.1	4.6 ± 0.1	4.8 ± 0.1	0.20	4.6 ± 0.1	4.8 ± 0.1	4.7 ± 0.1	0.36	4.6 ± 0.1	4.6 ± 0.1	4.8 ± 0.1	0.08
Serum Vitamin C (μmol/L)	62.5 ± 4.5	56.8 ± 3.4	68.1 ± 3.4	0.15	62.5 ± 2.8	68.1 ± 4.0	62.5 ± 5.1	0.78	62.5 ± 2.3	73.8 ± 3.4	56.8 ± 5.1	0.12
Serum Vitamin D (nmol/L)	65.4 ± 4.7	77.6 ± 8.0	70.6 ± 6.0	0.36	72.6 ± 4.0	78.1 ± 8.2	61.2 ± 4.2	0.04	70.1 ± 3.7	77.1 ± 8.7	67.4 ± 5.5	0.59
C-reactive protein (nmol/L)	57.1 ± 6.7	66.7 ± 8.6	57.1 ± 7.6	0.91	47.6 ± 4.8	57.1 ± 5.7	76.2 ± 9.5	0.07	66.7 ± 8.6	57.1 ± 5.7	66.7 ± 6.7	0.24

[1] Mean ± SE (all such values); [2] Ratio of poly- and monounsaturated fatty acids to saturated fatty acid. BMI: body mass index. HOMA-IR: the homeostatic model assessment for insulin resistance. MUFA: monounsaturated fatty acids. SFA: saturated fatty acids.

Covariate-adjusted multivariable logistic regression analyses showed that all three dietary patterns were significantly and positively associated with a higher GDM risk (Table 4). In the fully adjusted multivariable model 4, comparing pregnant women in the highest tertile with those in the lowest reference tertile of "high refined grains, fats, oils and fruit juice" pattern, pregnant women had a higher odds of developing GDM (OR 4.9; 95% CI 1.4–17.0). Pregnant women in the highest tertile of the "high nuts, seeds, fat and soybean; low milk and cheese" pattern had higher odds of GDM (OR 7.5; 95% CI 1.8–32.3) than those in the lowest tertile (model 4). Pregnant women in the highest tertile of "high added sugar and organ meats; low fruits, vegetables and seafood" pattern had higher odds of GDM (OR 21.1; 95% CI 4.0–109.8) than those in the lowest tertile (model 3). The significant relationship between the "added sugar, low fruits and vegetables" diet and GDM persisted after controlling for log-transformed CRP (OR 22.3; 95% CI 3.9–127.4) (model 4).

Table 4. Odds ratios (and 95% CIs) for risk of gestational diabetes mellitus (GDM) according to the tertiles of dietary pattern score derived from reduced rank regression (n = 249).

	Tertile 1	Tertile 2	Tertile 3	p Trend
"High Refined Grains, Fats, Oils and Fruit Juice" Pattern				
GDM/pregnancies	8/83	11/83	15/83	
Model 1	1.0	1.1 (0.3–3.9)	3.7 (0.9–15.7)	0.09
Model 2	1.0	1.7 (0.5–5.8)	5.1 (1.1–24.0) *	0.04
Model 3	1.0	1.3 (0.5–3.7)	4.9 (1.4–17.3) *	0.009
Model 4	1.0	1.4 (0.4–4.5)	4.9 (1.4–17.0) *	0.007
"High Nuts, Seeds, Fat and Soybean; Low Milk and Cheese" Pattern				
GDM/pregnancies	9/83	11/83	14/83	
Model 1	1.0	4.7 (1.9–11.5) *	5.2 (2.2–12.2) *	0.004
Model 2	1.0	4.2 (1.6–11.1) *	5.7 (2.1–15.2) *	0.001
Model 3	1.0	5.5 (2.5–12.1) *	8.2 (1.8–37.4) *	0.01
Model 4	1.0	5.3 (2.3–12.2) *	7.5 (1.8–32.3) *	0.009
"High Added Sugar and Organ Meats; Low Fruits, Vegetables and Seafood" Pattern				
GDM/pregnancies	5/83	8/83	21/83	
Model 1	1.0	1.7 (0.4–7.0)	15.4 (4.5–52.0) *	0.0004
Model 2	1.0	2.2 (0.3–14.1)	20.0 (4.2–95.9) *	0.0004
Model 3	1.0	2.9 (0.6–13.1)	21.1 (4.0–109.8) *	<0.0001
Model 4	1.0	3.2 (0.7–15.7)	22.3 (3.9–127.4) *	<0.0001

Model 1: Crude association between dietary patterns and gestational diabetes mellitus; Model 2: Adjusted for age, race/ethnicity, family poverty income ratio, education level, and marital status. Model 3: Adjusted for model 2 + energy intake, prepregnancy body mass index (BMI), and gestational weight gain. Model 4: Adjusted for model 3 + log-transformed C-reactive protein (CRP); * p < 0.05.

4. Discussion

In this cross-sectional study, three dietary patterns during pregnancy were identified with the choice of response variables including prepregnancy BMI, ratio of poly- and monounsaturated fatty acids to saturated fatty acids and dietary fiber: "high refined grains, fats, oils and fruit juice" pattern, "high nuts, seeds, fat and soybean; low milk and cheese" pattern, and "high added sugar and organ meats; low fruits, vegetables and seafood" pattern. Despite small differences, all three dietary patterns were associated with increased risks for GDM. Among three dietary patterns, the strongest relationship to the GDM risk was found for "high added sugar and organ meats; low fruits, vegetables and seafood" pattern. The positive association of the "high added sugar and organ meats; low fruits, vegetables and seafood" pattern with GDM, was largely explained by the high consumption of added sugars and low consumption of fruits and vegetables. Sugar-sweetened beverages are one of the leading sources of added sugars in the American diet [36]. In the Nurses' Health Study II, intake of sugar-sweetened coke before pregnancy was positively associated with the risk of GDM [37]. Compared to women who consumed one serving/month, those women who consumed ⩾5 servings/week of sugar sweetened coke had a 22% greater risk for GDM (relative risk (RR) 1.22; 95% CI 1.01–1.47). Epidemiologic studies demonstrate that high consumption of sugar-sweetened beverages was associated with increased risk for type 2 diabetes among general adult populations [38–40]. High sugar intake is also associated with high energy intake and hence obesity which is associated with risk of GDM. The high levels of rapidly absorbable carbohydrates in the form of added sugars of sugar sweetened beverages [40] may increase the levels of fasting blood glucose levels and insulin resistance. In our study, low intake of fruits and vegetables pattern was associated with an increased risk for GDM. Although the biological mechanisms for the inverse associations of fruits and vegetable intake and GDM risk are not clear, Bazzano *et al.* [41] explained that fruit and green leafy vegetables may contribute to a decreased incidence of type 2 diabetes through their low energy density, low glycemic load and high fiber. This mechanism may partially explain the association of low intake of fruits and vegetables in relation to decreased risk for GDM. Our findings are further supported by the findings from the Nurses' Health Study II [8]. Women in the lowest quintile of the prudent pattern characterized by a high intake of fruit, vegetables, and green leafy vegetables (lowest adherence) were associated with increased risks for GDM compared to those women in the highest quintile (highest adherence) (RR 1.39; 95% CI 1.08–1.80). In the same prospective cohort of Nurses' Health Study II, intake of whole fruits and green leafy green vegetables was inversely associated with incidence of type 2 diabetes in the middle-aged U.S. women [42].

The association with "high refined grains, fats, oils and fruit juice" pattern was largely explained by high intakes of refined grains and solid fats. Our findings are in accordance with the evidence of positive associations of the "Western" dietary pattern, characterized by high intakes of refined grains and solid fats with GDM in pregnant women [8]. In the Nurses' Health Study II [8], the "Western" dietary pattern before pregnancy characterized by high intake of red meat, processed meat, refined grain products, and sweets were associated with the risk of GDM. In contrast, the "Western" dietary pattern in the first month of pregnancy, which included red and processed meats, sugar-sweetened beverages, and refined grains, was not associated with the risk of GDM in the prospective cohort study of Project Viva [43]. The authors explained that once insulin resistance has been established from years of dietary patterns characterized by the "Western" dietary pattern, what women eat in the first few months of pregnancy may not have additional effect on the risk of GDM.

The positive association of "high nuts, seeds, fat and soybean; low milk and cheese" pattern with GDM was partly explained by low intakes of fruits, tomatoes, and beans and peas although high nuts and seeds would be expected to be protective on GDM risk. Low intake of fruits may partially explain the positive association between "high nuts, seeds, fat and soybean; low milk and cheese" pattern and the risk for GDM. Low consumption of fruits, lack of phytonutrients, including carotenoids and vitamins such as vitamin C [44], found to have preventive effect on GDM [45] may explain the association.

There are inconsistent findings regarding the relationship between elevated CRP and the risk for GDM. Elevated maternal CRP concentration in the first trimester of pregnancy has been reported to be positively associated with the risk for GDM in the third trimester [46,47]. In contrast, maternal serum levels of CRP were not associated with the risk for GDM but significantly correlated with prepregnancy obesity in a cross-sectional study [48]. In our study, CRP levels (⩽28.6 nmol/L *vs.* >28.6 nmol/L) were not significantly differed by the status for GDM. For this reason, after adjustment for CRP levels, the significant relationship between dietary patterns and the risk for GDM persisted.

The strengths of this study are that first, the reduced rank regression method allowed for a hypothesis regarding pathways (by the response variables) between diet and disease (GDM) to be evaluated [34]. Although traditional principal component analysis seems beneficial in the past, the pattern solely focused on inter-correlations among food groups, which may not represent diet qualities relevant to specific disease etiology [34]. Reduced rank regression is useful for etiological investigation explaining how a certain dietary pattern is associated with the health outcome of

Nutrients **2015**, *7*, 9369–9382

interest [49]. In our study, a great number of potential confounders such as physical activity, prepregnancy BMI and gestational weight gain were controlled in the analysis. Lastly, we also demonstrated that multi-collinearity among covariates did not exist.

The study has several limitations. Due to the use of cross-sectional study design of NHANES, we cannot provide evidence of a causal relationship between dietary patterns during pregnancy and the risk for GDM. Particularly, this could be the result of reverse causality in which subjects may change or adapt to different styles of diet after the diagnosis for GDM. Another limitation is that a history of family type 2 diabetes was not controlled for in our analysis. Due to the relatively small sample size of pregnant women included in this study, low statistical power may cause the wide confidence intervals in our analysis. It is possible that women with GDM are consuming foods high in added sugars and solid fats without recognizing that they are diagnosed with GDM. Lastly, FFQ would have been better to capture dietary patterns than 24 h recalls.

5. Conclusions

In conclusion, dietary patterns during pregnancy were associated with increased risks for GDM. Women in the third tertile of "high refined grains, fats, oils and fruit juice", "high nuts, seeds, fat and soybean; low milk and cheese" and "high added sugar and organ meats; low fruits, vegetables and seafood" dietary patterns were all significantly associated with increased risk for GDM. Prospective and cohort studies are needed to further evaluate and monitor changes in dietary patterns before to during pregnancy and its effect on the risk for GDM in consideration of GDM-related lifestyle factors such as physical activity levels.

Supplementary Materials: The following are available online at www.mdpi.com/2072-6643/7/11/5472/s1, Table S1: Response variables to derive dietary patterns using reduced rank regression, Table S2: Variations explained by food groups and response variables by extracted dietary patterns, Table S3: Loadings of food groups in dietary pattern scores in pregnant women.

Acknowledgments: The manuscript was prepared using NHANES 2003–2012 data obtained from the Centers for Disease Control and Prevention. The first author (Dayeon Shin) would like to appreciate the College of Agriculture and Natural Resources at Michigan State University for providing a dissertation completion fellowship to conduct this research. The study was based on the first author (Dayeon Shin)'s doctoral dissertation by Michigan State University.

Author Contributions: Dayeon Shin designed the study, analyzed the data, and prepared the first draft of manuscript under the guidance of Won O. Song. Kyung Won Lee provided inputs for the data analysis and helped to prepare the manuscript. Won O. Song guided the manuscript development and substantially revised the paper. All authors critically reviewed the manuscript and approved the final version submitted for publication.

Conflicts of Interest: Conflicts of Interest: The authors declare no conflict of interest.

References

1. The Expert Committee on the Diagnosis and Classification of Diabetes Mellitus. Report of the expert committee on the diagnosis and classification of diabetes mellitus. *Diabetes Care* **2003**, *26* (Suppl. S1), S5–S20.
2. American Diabetes Association. Diagnosis and classification of diabetes mellitus. *Diabetes Care* **2014**, *37*, S81–S90.
3. Wang, Y.; Storlien, L.H.; Jenkins, A.B.; Tapsell, L.C.; Jin, Y.; Pan, J.F.; Shao, Y.F.; Calvert, G.D.; Moses, R.G.; Shi, H.L.; *et al.* Dietary variables and glucose tolerance in pregnancy. *Diabetes Care* **2000**, *23*, 460–464. [CrossRef] [PubMed]
4. Bo, S.; Menato, G.; Lezo, A.; Signorile, A.; Bardelli, C.; de Michieli, F.; Massobrio, M.; Pagano, G. Dietary fat and gestational hyperglycaemia. *Diabetologia* **2001**, *44*, 972–978. [CrossRef] [PubMed]
5. Saldana, T.M.; Siega-Riz, A.M.; Adair, L.S. Effect of macronutrient intake on the development of glucose intolerance during pregnancy. *Am. J. Clin. Nutr.* **2004**, *79*, 479–486. [PubMed]
6. Qiu, C.; Zhang, C.; Gelaye, B.; Enquobahrie, D.A.; Frederick, I.O.; Williams, M.A. Gestational diabetes mellitus in relation to maternal dietary heme iron and nonheme iron intake. *Diabetes Care* **2011**, *34*, 1564–1569. [CrossRef] [PubMed]

7. Hu, F.B. Dietary pattern analysis: A new direction in nutritional epidemiology. *Curr. Opin. Lipidol.* **2002**, *13*, 3–9. [CrossRef] [PubMed]
8. Zhang, C.; Schulze, M.B.; Solomon, C.G.; Hu, F.B. A prospective study of dietary patterns, meat intake and the risk of gestational diabetes mellitus. *Diabetologia* **2006**, *49*, 2604–2613. [CrossRef] [PubMed]
9. Brantsaeter, A.L.; Haugen, M.; Samuelsen, S.O.; Torjusen, H.; Trogstad, L.; Alexander, J.; Magnus, P.; Meltzer, H.M. A dietary pattern characterized by high intake of vegetables, fruits, and vegetable oils is associated with reduced risk of preeclampsia in nulliparous pregnant Norwegian women. *J. Nutr.* **2009**, *139*, 1162–1168. [CrossRef] [PubMed]
10. Englund-Ogge, L.; Brantsaeter, A.L.; Sengpiel, V.; Haugen, M.; Birgisdottir, B.E.; Myhre, R.; Meltzer, H.M.; Jacobsson, B. Maternal dietary patterns and preterm delivery: Results from large prospective cohort study. *BMJ* **2014**, *348*. [CrossRef] [PubMed]
11. Rasmussen, M.A.; Maslova, E.; Halldorsson, T.I.; Olsen, S.F. Characterization of dietary patterns in the Danish national birth cohort in relation to preterm birth. *PLoS ONE* **2014**, *9*, e93644. [CrossRef] [PubMed]
12. Jacka, F.N.; Ystrom, E.; Brantsaeter, A.L.; Karevold, E.; Roth, C.; Haugen, M.; Meltzer, H.M.; Schjolberg, S.; Berk, M. Maternal and early postnatal nutrition and mental health of offspring by age 5 years: A prospective cohort study. *J. Am. Acad. Child Adolesc. Psychiatry* **2013**, *52*, 1038–1047. [CrossRef] [PubMed]
13. Hoffmann, K.; Schulze, M.B.; Schienkiewitz, A.; Nothlings, U.; Boeing, H. Application of a new statistical method to derive dietary patterns in nutritional epidemiology. *Am. J. Epidemiol.* **2004**, *159*, 935–944. [CrossRef] [PubMed]
14. Vujkovic, M.; Steegers, E.A.; Looman, C.W.; Ocke, M.C.; van der Spek, P.J.; Steegers-Theunissen, R.P. The maternal Mediterranean dietary pattern is associated with a reduced risk of spina bifida in the offspring. *BJOG* **2009**, *116*, 408–415. [CrossRef] [PubMed]
15. Obermann-Borst, S.A.; Vujkovic, M.; de Vries, J.H.; Wildhagen, M.F.; Looman, C.W.; de Jonge, R.; Steegers, E.A.; Steegers-Theunissen, R.P. A maternal dietary pattern characterised by fish and seafood in association with the risk of congenital heart defects in the offspring. *BJOG* **2011**, *118*, 1205–1215. [CrossRef] [PubMed]
16. Centers for Disease Control and Prevention. National Health and Nutrition Examination Survey: Analytic Guidelines, 1999–2010. Available online: http://www.cdc.gov/nchs/data/series/sr_02/sr02_161.pdf (accessed on 29 June 2015).
17. Centers for Disease Control and Prevention. National health and nutrition examination survey: Analytic guidelines, 2011–2012. Available online: http://www.cdc.gov/nchs/data/nhanes/analytic _guidelines_11 _12.pdf (accessed on 29 June 2015).
18. Centers for Disease Control and Prevention; National Center for Health Statistics. NCHS Research Ethics Review Board (ERB) Approval. Available online: http://www.cdc.gov/nchs/nhanes/irba98.htm (accessed on 1 August 2015).
19. Moshfegh, A.J.; Rhodes, D.G.; Baer, D.J.; Murayi, T.; Clemens, J.C.; Rumpler, W.V.; Paul, D.R.; Sebastian, R.S.; Kuczynski, K.J.; Ingwersen, L.A.; *et al.* The US department of agriculture automated multiple-pass method reduces bias in the collection of energy intakes. *Am. J. Clin. Nutr.* **2008**, *88*, 324–332. [PubMed]
20. Centers for Disease Control and Prevention; National Center for Health Statistics. Dietary Interview—Total Nutrient Intakes, First Day. Available online: http://wwwn.cdc.gov/Nchs/Nhanes/2011–2012/DR1TOT_ G.htm#DR1DRSTZ (accessed on 29 June 2015).
21. Thompson, F.E.; Byers, T. Dietary assessment resource manual. *J. Nutr.* **1994**, *124*, 2245S–2317S. [PubMed]
22. Bowman, S.A.; Clemens, J.C.; Friday, J.E.; Thoerig, R.C.; Moshfegh, A.J. Food Patterns Equivalents Database 2005–06: Methodology and User Guide. Available online: http://www.ars.usda.gov/SP2UserFiles/Place/8 0400530/pdf/fped/FPED_0506.pdf (accessed on 4 April 2015).
23. U.S. Department of Agriculture. Food Patterns Equivalents Database 2011–2012. Available online: http://www.ars.usda.gov/SP2UserFiles/Place/80400530/pdf/fped/FPED_2011_12_Fact_Sheet.pdf (accessed on 29 June 2015).
24. Centers for Disease Control and Prevention; National Center for Health Statistics. Data documentation: Plasma Fasting Glucose and Insulin. Available online: http://wwwn.cdc.gov/nchs/nhanes/2005–2006/GL U_D.htm (accessed on 16 August 2014).

25. Centers for Disease Control and Prevention; National Center for Health Statistics. Data documentation: Plasma Glucose, Serum C-peptide, and Insulin. Available online: http://wwwn.cdc.gov/nchs/nhanes/2003–2004/L10AM_C.htm (accessed on 16 August 2014).

26. Matthews, D.R.; Hosker, J.P.; Rudenski, A.S.; Naylor, B.A.; Treacher, D.F.; Turner, R.C. Homeostasis model assessment: Insulin resistance and beta-cell function from fasting plasma glucose and insulin concentrations in man. *Diabetologia* **1985**, *28*, 412–419. [CrossRef] [PubMed]

27. Centers for Disease Control and Prevention; National Center for Health Statistics. Data Documentation: Glycohemoglobin. Available online: http://wwwn.cdc.gov/nchs/nhanes/2005–2006/GHB_D.htm (accessed on 16 August 2014).

28. Centers for Disease Control and Prevention; National Center for Health Statistics. Data Documentation: C-reactive Protein. Available online: http://wwwn.cdc.gov/nchs/nhanes/2005–2006/CRP_D.htm (accessed on 16 August 2014).

29. Centers for Disease Control and Prevention; National Center for Health Statistics. Data Documentation: Vitamin C. Available online: http://wwwn.cdc.gov/nchs/nhanes/2005–2006/VIC_D.htm (accessed on 16 August 2014).

30. Centers for Disease Control and Prevention; National Center for Health Statistics. Data Documentation: Vitamin D. Available online: http://wwwn.cdc.gov/nchs/nhanes/2005–2006/VID_D.htm (accessed on 16 August 2014).

31. International Association of Diabetes and Pregnancy Study Groups Consensus Panel. International association of diabetes and pregnancy study groups recommendations on the diagnosis and classification of hyperglycemia in pregnancy. *Diabetes Care* **2010**, *33*, 676–682.

32. O'Brien, R.M. A caution regarding rules of thumb for variance inflation factors. *Qual. Quant.* **2007**, *41*, 673–690. [CrossRef]

33. Centers for Disease Control and Prevention; National Center for Health Statistics. How to Create Appropriate Subsets of Data for NHANES Analyses in SAS. Available online: http://www.cdc.gov/nchs/tutorials/NHANES/SurveyDesign/Weighting/Task2b_I.htm (accessed on 9 June 2015).

34. Hoffmann, K.; Zyriax, B.C.; Boeing, H.; Windler, E. A dietary pattern derived to explain biomarker variation is strongly associated with the risk of coronary artery disease. *Am. J. Clin. Nutr.* **2004**, *80*, 633–640. [PubMed]

35. Zhang, C.; Liu, S.; Solomon, C.G.; Hu, F.B. Dietary fiber intake, dietary glycemic load, and the risk for gestational diabetes mellitus. *Diabetes Care* **2006**, *29*, 2223–2230. [CrossRef] [PubMed]

36. Bray, G.A.; Nielsen, S.J.; Popkin, B.M. Consumption of high-fructose corn syrup in beverages may play a role in the epidemic of obesity. *Am. J. Clin. Nutr.* **2004**, *79*, 537–543. [PubMed]

37. Chen, L.; Hu, F.B.; Yeung, E.; Willett, W.; Zhang, C. Prospective study of pre-gravid sugar-sweetened beverage consumption and the risk of gestational diabetes mellitus. *Diabetes Care* **2009**, *32*, 2236–2241. [CrossRef] [PubMed]

38. Montonen, J.; Järvinen, R.; Knekt, P.; Heliövaara, M.; Reunanen, A. Consumption of sweetened beverages and intakes of fructose and glucose predict type 2 diabetes occurrence. *J. Nutr.* **2007**, *137*, 1447–1454. [PubMed]

39. Palmer, J.R.; Boggs, D.A.; Krishnan, S.; Hu, F.B.; Singer, M.; Rosenberg, L. Sugar-sweetened beverages and incidence of type 2 diabetes mellitus in African American women. *Arch. Intern. Med.* **2008**, *168*, 1487–1492. [CrossRef] [PubMed]

40. Malik, V.S.; Popkin, B.M.; Bray, G.A.; Després, J.-P.; Willett, W.C.; Hu, F.B. Sugar-sweetened beverages and risk of metabolic syndrome and type 2 diabetes a meta-analysis. *Diabetes Care* **2010**, *33*, 2477–2483. [CrossRef] [PubMed]

41. Bazzano, L.A.; He, J.; Ogden, L.G.; Loria, C.M.; Vupputuri, S.; Myers, L.; Whelton, P.K. Fruit and vegetable intake and risk of cardiovascular disease in US adults: The first national health and nutrition examination survey epidemiologic follow-up study. *Am. J. Clin. Nutr.* **2002**, *76*, 93–99. [PubMed]

42. Bazzano, L.A.; Li, T.Y.; Joshipura, K.J.; Hu, F.B. Intake of fruit, vegetables, and fruit juices and risk of diabetes in women. *Diabetes Care* **2008**, *31*, 1311–1317. [CrossRef] [PubMed]

43. Radesky, J.S.; Oken, E.; Rifas-Shiman, S.L.; Kleinman, K.P.; Rich-Edwards, J.W.; Gillman, M.W. Diet during early pregnancy and development of gestational diabetes. *Paediatr. Perinat. Epidemiol.* **2008**, *22*, 47–59. [CrossRef] [PubMed]

44. Craig, W.J. Phytochemicals: Guardians of our health. *J. Am. Diet. Assoc.* **1997**, *97*, S199–S204. [CrossRef]

45. Zhang, C.; Williams, M.A.; Sorensen, T.K.; King, I.B.; Kestin, M.M.; Thompson, M.L.; Leisenring, W.M.; Dashow, E.E.; Luthy, D.A. Maternal plasma ascorbic acid (vitamin C) and risk of gestational diabetes mellitus. *Epidemiology* **2004**, *15*, 597–604. [CrossRef] [PubMed]

46. Qiu, C.; Sorensen, T.K.; Luthy, D.A.; Williams, M.A. A prospective study of maternal serum C-reactive protein (CRP) concentrations and risk of gestational diabetes mellitus. *Paediatr. Perinat. Epidemiol.* **2004**, *18*, 377–384. [CrossRef] [PubMed]

47. Wolf, M.; Sandler, L.; Hsu, K.; Vossen-Smirnakis, K.; Ecker, J.L.; Thadhani, R. First-trimester C-reactive protein and subsequent gestational diabetes. *Diabetes Care* **2003**, *26*, 819–824. [CrossRef] [PubMed]

48. Retnakaran, R.; Hanley, A.J.; Raif, N.; Connelly, P.W.; Sermer, M.; Zinman, B. C-reactive protein and gestational diabetes: The central role of maternal obesity. *J. Clin. Endocrinol. MeTable* **2003**, *88*, 3507–3512. [CrossRef] [PubMed]

49. Nettleton, J.A.; Steffen, L.M.; Schulze, M.B.; Jenny, N.S.; Barr, R.G.; Bertoni, A.G.; Jacobs, D.R., Jr. Associations between markers of subclinical atherosclerosis and dietary patterns derived by principal components analysis and reduced rank regression in the multi-ethnic study of atherosclerosis (MESA). *Am. J. Clin. Nutr.* **2007**, *85*, 1615–1625. [PubMed]

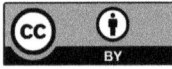

nutrients

MDPI

Article

Dietary Patterns Modulate the Risk of Non-Alcoholic Fatty Liver Disease in Chinese Adults

Chao-Qun Yang [1,†], Long Shu [2,†], Shuai Wang [1], Jia-Jia Wang [1], Yu Zhou [1], Yu-Jie Xuan [1] and Su-Fang Wang [1,*]

1   Department of Nutrition and Food Hygiene, School of Public Health, Anhui Medical University, Hefei 230032, An Hui, China; yangchaoqun9@163.com (C.-Q.Y.); wangshuai0551@126.com (S.W); wang201320103@126.com (J.-J.W.); ahykdxzy@126.com (Y.Z.); xyj209@gmail.com (Y.-J.X.)
2   Department of Nutrition, Zhejiang Hospital, Hangzhou 310000, Zhe Jiang, China; shulong19880920@126.com
*   Author to whom correspondence should be addressed; wangsufangdev@126.com; Tel.: +86-551-6516-8413; Fax: +86-551-6386-9179.
†   These authors contributed equally to this work.

Received: 13 March 2015; Accepted: 5 May 2015; Published: 15 June 2015

Abstract: Although previous studies reported the associations between the intakes of individual foods or nutrients and the risk of non-alcoholic fatty liver disease (NAFLD), the relationship between dietary patterns and NAFLD in the Chinese population has been rarely studied to date. This study aimed to investigate the associations between dietary patterns and the risk of NAFLD in a middle-aged Chinese population. The Study subjects were 999 Chinese adults aged 45–60 years in the Anhui province who participated in the Hefei Nutrition and Health Study. Dietary intake was collected by a semi-quantitative food frequency questionnaire. NAFLD was defined as the presence of moderate-severe hepatic steatosis (by B-ultrasonic examination); the absence of excessive alcohol use (>20 g day^{-1} in men and 10 g day^{-1} in women); no use of steatogenic medications within the past six months; no exposure to hepatotoxins; and no history of bariatric surgery. Log-binomial regression analysis was used to examine the association between dietary patterns and NAFLD with adjustment of potential confounding variables. Out of 999 participants, 345 (34.5%) were classified as having NAFLD. Four major dietary patterns were identified: "Traditional Chinese", "Animal food", "Grains-vegetables" and "High-salt" dietary patterns. After adjusting for potential confounders, subjects in the highest quartile of the "Animal food" pattern scores had greater prevalence ratio for NAFLD (prevalence ratio (PR) = 1.354; 95% confidence interval (CI): 1.063–1.724; $p < 0.05$) than did those in the lowest quartile. After adjustment for body mass index (BMI), compared with the lowest quartile of the "Grains-vegetables" pattern, the highest quartile had a lower prevalence ratio for NAFLD (PR = 0.777; 95% CI: 0.618–0.977, $p < 0.05$). However, the "traditional Chinese" and "high-salt" dietary patterns showed no association with the risk of NAFLD. Our findings indicated that the "Animal food" dietary pattern was associated with an increased risk of NAFLD.

Keywords: dietary patterns; factor analysis; non-alcoholic fatty liver disease; China

---

1. Introduction

Non-alcoholic fatty liver disease (NAFLD), including simple steatosis, non-alcoholic steatohepatitis (NASH) and cirrhosis, is the most common cause of chronic liver disease worldwide [1]. In China, NAFLD, parallel with increased obesity, has been recognized as a major health problem and the prevalence is increasing year by year [2,3]. In the United States, NAFLD is a significant health problem and affects 70 million adults (~30% of the adult population) [4]. A close and bi-directional relationship links NAFLD with the metabolic syndrome: not only the former is the hepatic manifestation of the latter, but also a common precursor to the development of the full-blown metabolic syndrome and its individual components [5–7].

Over the past decades, diet has been considered as an important pathogenic factor of NAFLD. Many epidemiological studies have examined the associations between the intakes of individual foods or nutrients and the risk of NAFLD [4,8,9]. Nevertheless, more commonly in reality, people do not take nutrients alone but consume meals containing many combinations of foods and nutrients [10,11]. In this context, dietary pattern analysis has emerged as a more recognizable approach to assess dietary exposures in nutritional epidemiology. Moreover, due to its ability to examine the holistic effect of diet, dietary pattern analysis also has been used to identify the associations between diet and many chronic diseases [12–14].

Recently, there has been considerable attention focused on the associations between overall dietary patterns and the risk of NAFLD. In particular, the Mediterranean diet has been reported to have beneficial effects in the prevention and the treatment of NAFLD [14]. To date, however, there is little published information on the relationship between dietary patterns and the risk of NAFLD in the Chinese population. Given this gap in knowledge, the purpose of this study was to find the association of different dietary patterns and the risk of NAFLD among Chinese adults aged 45–60 years.

2. Subjects and Methods

2.1. Study Population

This cross-sectional study was carried-out in Hefei, the capital of Anhui Province in China from December 2011 to June 2012. Hefei is composed of four areas (Shushan, Yaohai, Luyang and Baohe) and four counties (Feidong, Feixi, Lujiang and Changfeng). It is a region characterized by high intakes of fruit, pork, poultry, rice, vegetables, aquatic products and nuts in China [15]. We chose two residential communities/villages from every area/country randomly, and according to resident health records, all people aged 45–60 years, living in the selected communities/villages, were included in the study. A total of 1776 subjects, aged between 45 and 60, were invited to the Medical Center for Physical Examination. In the Anhui Province Hospital of Armed Police Forces, study participants were interviewed by a trained staff with food frequency questionnaires. After exclusion of 274 participants with missing or incomplete dietary information in their questionnaires, 1502 participants were included for the analysis of dietary pattern. In addition, we further excluded 503 participants who self-reported a history of drug usage, drinking or hereditary diseases. Finally, 999 participants remained for the analysis of the relationship between dietary patterns and NAFLD. The study was approved by the institutional review and ethics committee of Anhui medical university, China, and written informed consent was obtained from each participant.

2.2. Anthropometric and Physical Activity Measurements

Body height was measured to the nearest 0.1 cm with subjects standing without shoes. Body weight in light clothes was measured to the nearest 0.1 kg. Body mass index (BMI) was calculated as weight in kilograms divided by squared height in meters. Waist circumference (WC) was measured as the middle between the lowest rib and the superior border of the iliac crest with an inelastic measuring tape at the end of normal expiration to the nearest 1 mm and hip circumstance was measured at the maximum level over light clothing, using an inelastic plastic tape [16,17]. Information on physical activity was collected using a validated physical activity questionnaire (including the level of physical activity at work, transportation, exercise, sitting, sleeping and household activities.). The physical activity levels were measured as metabolic equivalent in hours per week (MET-h week^{-1}) in which different MET levels were ranged on a scale from sleeping (0.9 METs) to high-intensity physical activities (>6 METs). The level of physical activity was the product of time spent in each activity multiplied by specific metabolic equivalent values based on the compendium of physical activities [18].

2.3. Assessment of Dietary Intake

Dietary intake was assessed by using a 143-item (57 food groups) semi-quantitative food frequency questionnaire (FFQ). The FFQ was based on the food frequency questionnaire used in the 2010 China National Nutrition and Health Survey (CNNHS). Participants were asked to recall the frequency of each food item during the past year and the estimated portion size, using local weight units (1 Liang = 50 g) or natural units (cups). Intakes of food were converted into g day^{-1} and were used in the following analysis.

2.4. Clinical and Laboratory Examination

Blood samples were collected between 7:00 and 9:00 a.m. after fasting overnight (12 h), allowing to clot at room temperature for 1–3 h. Subsequently, a separation of serum was made via centrifugation for 15 min at 3000 rpm. The samples were analyzed in the Medical Center for Physical Examination, Anhui Province Hospital of Armed Police Forces for fasting blood glucose, serum triglycerides, total cholesterol, HDL and LDL cholesterol, and uric acid, using the Hitachi 7180 auto-analyzer (Hitachi, Tokyo, Japan).

2.5. Blood Pressure Measurement

For blood pressure measurement, participants were first asked to rest for 10 min. Then, a trained nurse measured the blood pressure twice on seated participants using a standard mercury sphygmomanometer, and the mean of two measurements was considered as the participant's blood pressure.

2.6. Definition of Other Variables

Hypertension was defined as a systolic pressure of 140 mmHg or higher and/or a diastolic pressure of 90 mmHg or higher [19]; Obesity was defined by BMI $\geq$ 28 kg m^{-2} and abdominal adiposity was defined as (male: WC $\geq$ 85 cm; female: WC $\geq$ 80 cm); Dyslipidemia was defined as presenting $\geq$ 1 of the following individual components: hypertriglyceridemia (triglycerides $\geq$ 150 mg dL^{-1} or $\geq$ 1.7 mmol L^{-1}), hypercholesterolemia (serum total cholesterol $\geq$ 200 mg dL $^{-1}$), low HDL-cholesterol (HDL-C < 50 mg dL^{-1} or <1.3 mmol L^{-1}), and high LDL-cholesterol (LDL-C $\geq$ 130 mg dL^{-1}) [20]. NAFLD was defined as the presence of moderate-severe hepatic steatosis (by B-ultrasonic examination), the absence of excessive alcohol use (>20 g day^{-1} in men and 10 g day^{-1} in women), no use of steatogenic medications within the past six months, no exposure to hepatotoxins, and no history of bariatric surgery [21].

2.7. Statistical Analyses

Factor analysis (principal component) was used to derive dietary patterns based on the frequency of consumption of 57 food groups in the FFQ. The factors were rotated using an orthogonal transformation (varimax rotation) to obtain a simpler structure with better interpretability. The eigenvalue and scree plot were applied to decide which factors remained [22]. Labeling of dietary patterns was based on the interpretation of foods with high factor loadings for each dietary pattern [23]. Only foods with a factor loading $\geq$ |0.25| were included in this study.

Factor scores were categorized into quartiles (quartile 1 represented a low intake of the food pattern; quartile 4 represented a high intake of the food pattern). The characteristics of study participants were calculated across quartiles of each dietary pattern. Data for continuous variables is presented as mean values and standard deviation. Categorical variables are presented as sum and percentages. We used Analysis of variance (ANOVA) to describe mean differences by continuous and the chi-squared test to examine the difference between categorical variables. Log-binomial regression analysis was used to evaluate the relationship between dietary patterns and the risk of NAFLD, adjusted for gender, physical activity, WC, BMI, fasting plasma glucose and blood pressure.

Two-sided *p*-values < 0.05 were considered statistically significant. All analyses were performed on the Statistical Package for Social Sciences (version 16.0, SPSS Inc., Chicago, IL, USA).

3. Results

Overall prevalence of NAFLD in our study population was 34.5%. Demographic, anthropometric, and clinical characteristics of participants with and without NAFLD are presented in Table 1 (*n* = 999). There were significant differences between participants with and without NAFLD by gender, smoking status, education economic income and central obesity.

Table 1. Demographic and lifestyle characteristics of participants in the Hefei Nutrition and Health Study.

Variables	Participants with NAFLD *n* = 345	Participants without NAFLD *n* = 654	Significance *
Demographic			
Age (years)	51.06 ± 4.45	50.92 ± 4.76	*p* = 0.651
Gender			
Male	245 (71.0)	220 (33.6)	*p* = 0.000
Female	101 (29.0)	434 (66.4)	
Smoking status (%)			
Never	226 (65.5)	561 (85.8)	*p* = 0.000
Former	10 (2.9)	4 (0.6)	
Current	109 (31.6)	89 (13.6)	
Education (%)			
<High school	72 (20.9)	181 (27.7)	*p* = 0.034
High school	105 (30.4)	201 (30.7)	
>High school	168 (48.7)	272 (41.6)	
Monthly income per person (%)			
≤1000 (RMB)	85 (24.6)	193 (29.6)	*p* = 0.036
1000–2000 (RMB)	158 (45.8)	245 (37.5)	
>2000 (RMB)	102 (29.6)	216 (32.9)	
Physical activity (%)			
Light	231 (82.8)	416 (80.5)	*p* = 0.542
Moderate	42 (15.0)	81 (15.7)	
Vigorous	6 (2.2)	18 (3.5)	
Central obesity (%)			
Yes	278 (80.6)	251 (38.4)	*p* = 0.000
No	67 (19.4)	403 (61.6)	

Categorical variables are presented as sum and percentages, and continuous variables are presented as Mean ± SD. Abbreviation: NAFLD: Non-alcoholic fatty liver disease. * *p* values for continuous variables (Analysis of variance) and for Categorical variables (chi-square test).

Four major dietary patterns were identified by factor analysis: the "traditional Chinese" pattern (high intakes of staple food, coarse grains, fruits, eggs, fish and shrimp, milk, and tea), the "animal food" pattern (high intakes of kelp/seaweed and mushroom, pork, beef, mutton, poultry, cooked meat, eggs, fish and shrimp, beans and grease); the "grains-vegetables" pattern (high intakes of coarse grains, tubers, vegetables, mushroom and kelp/seaweed, cooked meat, and beans), and the "high-salt" pattern (high intake of rice, pickled vegetables, processed meat, bacon, salted deck egg, salted fish and tea). The four factors explained 33.4% of the total variables in dietary intake (9.1%, 8.9%, 7.8% and 7.6%, respectively). In addition, the factor-loading matrixes for these dietary patterns are shown in Table 2.

Table 2. Rotated factor loading matrix for the four dietary patterns among 999 Chinese people aged 45–60 years *.

Food Groups	Dietary Patterns			
	Traditional Chinese	Animal Food	Grains-Vegetable	High-Salt
Rice	-	-	-	0.569
Steamed bun/noodles	0.440	-	-	-
Coarse grains	0.438	-	0.379	-
Tubers	-	-	0.641	-
Vegetables	-	-	0.654	-
Pickled vegetables	-	-	-	0.686
Mushroom	-	0.310	0.471	-
Fresh fruits	0.615	-	-	-
Livestock meat	-	0.660	-	-
poultry	-	0.550	-	-
Processed meat	-	0.502	0.328	-
Bacon and salted fish	-	-	-	0.594
Eggs	0.499	0.286	-	-
Fish and shrimp	0.367	0.362	-	-
Dairy products	0.609	-	-	-
Legumes	0.278	0.271	0.321	-
Fats and oils	-	0.326	-	-
Fast foods	-	-	-	0.273
Tea	0.257	-	-	0.307

* Absolute values < 0.25 were excluded for simplicity.

The characteristics of study participants across quartile categories of the dietary pattern scores are shown in Table 3. Those participants in the highest quartile of the "traditional Chinese" pattern were more likely to be females, were less likely to be smokers, and were significantly in a higher education level and income, lower prevalence of NAFLD and moderate physical activity. Conversely, compared with the lowest quartile of the "Animal food" pattern there were more likely to be male and smokers, a lower age, higher BMI, WC, and were significantly higher prevalence of obese and NAFLD. In addition, participants in the highest quartile of the "Grains-vegetables" pattern were less likely to be smokers and were more likely to be females, were significantly at a higher age, and showed a lower prevalence of NAFLD than those in the lowest quartile. Participants in the highest quartile of the "high-salt" pattern were more likely to be male, smokers, low income, higher BMI, WC and higher prevalence of NAFLD than those in the lowest quartile.

Table 3. Characteristics of the study participants by quartile (Q) categories of dietary pattern scores in the Hefei Nutrition and Health Study.

	Traditional Chinese			Animal Food			Grains-Vegetables			High-Salt		
	Q1 (n = 250)	Q4 (n = 250)	p	Q1 (n = 250)	Q4 (n = 250)	p	Q1 (n = 250)	Q4 (n = 250)	p	Q1 (n = 250)	Q4 (n = 250)	p
Age (year)	51.28 ± 4.79	50.89 ± 4.64	0.353	51.25 ± 4.75	50.22 ± 4.33	<0.05	50.54 ± 4.51	51.38 ± 4.70	<0.05	50.86 ± 4.54	51.20 ± 4.77	0.415
BMI (kg m^{-2})	24.44 ± 2.91	24.00 ± 3.02	0.098	24.06 ± 2.69	24.71 ± 2.93	<0.05	24.09 ± 3.00	24.17 ± 3.00	0.746	24.00 ± 2.94	24.75 ± 2.80	<0.01
WC (cm)	84.24 ± 9.05	82.68 ± 9.39	0.060	82.59 ± 8.55	85.59 ± 8.70	<0.001	83.80 ± 9.49	83.90 ± 9.00	0.910	81.96 ± 8.28	85.70 ± 8.80	<0.001
Obese (%)	27 (10.8)	24 (9.6)	0.406	18 (7.2)	34 (13.6)	<0.01	22 (8.8)	33 (13.2)	0.214	25 (10.0)	30 (12.0)	0.080
Hypertension (%)	75 (30.0)	58 (23.2)	0.085	67 (26.8)	72 (28.8)	0.618	74 (29.6)	68 (27.2)	0.552	65 (26.0)	81 (32.4)	0.116
NAFLD (%)	101 (40.4)	68 (27.2)	<0.01	66 (26.4)	112 (44.8)	<0.001	99 (39.6)	76 (30.4)	<0.05	70 (28.0)	94 (37.6)	<0.05
Gender												
Male	152 (60.8)	89 (35.6)	<0.001	89 (35.6)	150 (60.0)	<0.001	134 (53.6)	111 (44.4)	<0.05	70 (28.0)	155 (62.0)	<0.001
Female	98 (39.2)	161 (64.4)		161 (64.4)	100 (40.0)		116 (46.4)	139 (55.6)		180 (72.0)	95 (38.0)	
Smoking Status (%)												
Never	185 (74.0)	213 (85.2)	<0.01	212 (84.8)	171 (68.4)	<0.001	178 (71.2)	203 (81.2)	<0.05	211 (84.4)	187 (74.8)	<0.05
Former	4 (1.6)	4 (1.6)		2 (0.8)	5 (2.0)		2 (0.8)	4 (1.6)		3 (1.2)	4 (1.6)	
Current	61 (24.4)	33 (13.2)		36 (14.4)	74 (29.6)		70 (28.0)	43 (17.2)		36 (14.4)	59 (23.6)	
Education (%)												
<High school	82 (32.8)	48 (19.2)	<0.001	73 (29.2)	63 (25.2)	0.549	71 (28.4)	58 (23.2)	0.110	50 (20.0)	67 (26.8)	0.142
High school	93 (37.2)	69 (27.6)		74 (29.6)	74 (29.6)		68 (27.2)	89 (35.6)		77 (30.8)	78 (31.2)	
>High school	75 (30.0)	133 (53.2)		103 (41.2)	113 (45.2)		111 (44.4)	103 (41.2)		123 (49.2)	105 (42.0)	
Monthly Income Per Person (%)												
≤1000 (RMB)	104 (41.6)	53 (21.2)	<0.001	80 (32.0)	60 (24.0)	0.133	65 (26.0)	65 (26.0)	0.449	49 (19.6)	88 (35.2)	<0.001
1000–2000 (RMB)	94 (37.6)	97 (38.8)		89 (35.6)	97 (38.8)		114 (45.6)	102 (40.8)		98 (39.2)	106 (42.4)	
>2000 (RMB)	52 (20.8)	100 (40.0)		81 (32.4)	93 (37.2)		71 (28.4)	83 (33.2)		103 (41.2)	56 (22.4)	
Physical Activity (%)												
Light	182 (72.8)	222 (88.8)	<0.001	199 (79.6)	213 (85.2)	0.247	213 (85.2)	211 (84.4)	0.656	222 (88.8)	209 (83.6)	0.111
Moderate	54 (21.6)	26 (10.4)		40 (16.0)	30 (12.0)		33 (13.2)	32 (12.8)		26 (10.4)	34 (13.6)	
Vigorous	14 (5.6)	2 (0.8)		11 (4.4)	7 (2.8)		4 (1.6)	7 (2.8)		2 (0.8)	7 (2.8)	

Categorical variables are presented as sum and percentages, and continuous variables are presented as Mean ± SD. Abbreviation: WHR, Waist hip rate; BMI, Body mass index; WC, Waist circumference; NAFLD: Non-alcoholic fatty liver disease. * p values for continuous variables (Analysis of variance) and for Categorical variables (chi-square test).

The associations between different dietary patterns and the risk of NAFLD by Log-binomial regression were shown in Table 4. After adjusting for potential confounders, subjects in the highest quartile of the "Animal food" pattern scores had greater prevalence ratio for NAFLD (PR = 1.354; 95% CI: 1.063–1.724; $p < 0.05$) than did those in the lowest quartile. After adjustment for BMI, compared with the lowest quartile of the "Grains-vegetables" pattern, the highest quartile had a lower prevalence ratio for NAFLD (PR = 0.777; 95% CI: 0.618–0.977, $p < 0.05$). However, the "traditional Chinese" and "high-salt" dietary patterns showed no association with the risk of NAFLD.

Table 4. Multivariable models adjusted for non-alcohol fatty liver disease across the quartile (Q) categories of the dietary patterns in Anhui Province, China.

	Model 1 [1]		Model 2 [2]		Model 3 [3]	
	PR 95% CI		PR 95% CI		PR 95% CI	
Traditional Chinese						
Q1	1.000		1.000		1.000	
Q2	0.891	0.713, 1.114	0.934	0.751, 1.161	0.958	0.772, 1.188
Q3	0.855	0.681, 1.074	1.023	0.820, 1.277	0.971	0.782, 1.206
Q4	0.673	0.523, 0.867	0.861	0.674, 1.101	0.837	0.660, 1.063
P	<0.01		>0.05		>0.05	
Animal Food						
Q1	1.000		1.000		1.000	
Q2	1.152	0.871, 1.523	1.084	0.828, 1.418	1.055	0.814, 1.366
Q3	1.384	1.063, 1.802	1.192	0.922, 1.541	1.202	0.935, 1.545
Q4	1.697	1.324, 2.176	1.354	1.063, 1.724	1.255	0.991, 1.589
P	<0.01		<0.05		>0.05	
Grains-Vegetables						
Q1	1.000		1.000		1.000	
Q2	0.889	0.708, 1.116	0.974	0.782, 1.215	0.905	0.727, 1.126
Q3	0.832	0.658, 1.051	0.930	0.736, 1.176	0.860	0.683, 1.083
Q4	0.768	0.603, 0.978	0.821	0.651, 1.036	0.777	0.618, 0.977
P	<0.05		>0.05		<0.05	
High-Salt						
Q1	1.000		1.000		1.000	
Q2	1.086	0.826, 1.427	0.949	0.724, 1.244	1.011	0.771, 1.325
Q3	1.506	1.177, 1.927	1.108	0.871, 1.409	1.050	0.827, 1.331
Q4	1.343	1.041, 1.733	0.933	0.725, 1.201	0.914	0.713, 1.171
P	<0.05		>0.05		>0.05	

[1] unadjusted; [2] Further adjusted gender, age, physical activity, smoking status and blood pressure; [3] Additionally adjusted for body mass index.

4. Discussion

In this cross-sectional study of a middle-aged Chinese population, we identified four dietary patterns by means of factor analysis: "traditional Chinese", "animal food", "grains-vegetables" and "high-salt". Further analysis showed that food consumption in the "animal food" dietary pattern was associated with an increased risk of NAFLD and in the "grains-vegetables" dietary pattern was associated with an decreased risk of NAFLD, whereas "traditional Chinese" and "high-salt" dietary patterns were not associated with NAFLD. These associations were independent of gender, age, physical activity, BMI, smoking status and blood pressure. To our knowledge, this is the first study to examine the associations between different dietary patterns and the risk of NAFLD in a middle-aged Chinese population.

The "traditional Chinese" pattern, characterized by a high consumption of staple food, coarse grains, fruits, eggs, fish and shrimp, milk, and tea, is generally considered a healthy dietary pattern. However, we did not find a negative association of this pattern with NAFLD, though the prevalence of NAFLD for the highest category of this pattern was lower compared with the lowest category (27.2% *vs.* 40.4%). The complex nature of this pattern may explain this finding to some extent. On the one hand, some foods in the "traditional Chinese" pattern are a low-fat and high-carbohydrate, which have been found to promote the development of fatty liver via increased *de novo* fatty acid synthesis [24]. Additionally, fruits contain large amounts of fructose. Previous studies have found that consumption of fructose is associated with an increased risk of NAFLD [25,26]. On the other hand, some foods in the traditional Chinese dietary pattern have a low glycemic index, which have been shown to decrease total cholesterol levels, resulting in the decreased risk of NAFLD [27]. Moreover, the excess consumption of vegetable and fruits is likely to contribute to a high intake of antioxidant vitamins (e.g., vitamin A, C and E) in this pattern. It is well known that antioxidant vitamins have a protective role against oxidative stress [28], and have been reported to be associated with decreased risk of NAFLD [29–31]. Furthermore, dietary fiber intake has also been found to be inversely correlated with insulin resistance, which has been reported to be the risk factor for NAFLD [32].

The "Animal food" pattern, characterized by a high intake of kelp/seaweed and mushroom, pork, beef, mutton, poultry, cooked meat, eggs, fish and shrimp, beans and grease, was positively associated with the risk of NAFLD in the Chinese population, after adjustment for confounding factors. This association was independent of the BMI, suggesting that the association was not linked to obesity. Our finding was consistent with the present knowledge. The positive association between "animal food" pattern and NAFLD could be attributed to this pattern's unhealthy constituents (saturated, trans, and monounsaturated fat, and soft drinks). A recent study showed that saturated fatty acids have adverse effects on lipid and glucose homeostasis, which in turn worsen the progression of metabolic syndrome and NAFLD [33]. Moreover, soft drinks contain large amounts of fructose, which has been documented to be associated with increased risk of NAFLD [34]. Meanwhile, soft drinks are also rich in caramel and aspartame that potentially increase insulin resistance and inflammation [35]. Furthermore, previous studies have also indicated that fast-food consumption is positively associated with obesity and insulin resistance, major risk factors for NAFLD [36,37].

The "grains-vegetables" dietary pattern was characterized by high intakes of coarse grains, tubers, vegetables, mushroom and kelp/seaweed, cooked meat, and beans. In this study, we found a trend of an inverse association between the "grains-vegetables" dietary pattern and the risk of NAFLD (PR = 0.777, *p* < 0.05). Participants in the highest quartile of the "grains-vegetables" dietary pattern had a lower prevalence of NAFLD than those in lowest quartile (30.4% *vs.* 39.6%). In addition, dietary fiber intake has also been found to be inversely correlated with insulin resistance, which has been reported to be the risk factor for NAFLD [32]. Furthermore, fish contain a large number of unsaturated fatty acids (e.g., omega-3 polyunsaturated fatty acids (omega-3 PUFA)), which have been shown to decrease total cholesterol and triacylglycerol concentrations [38,39]. More recently, the protective role of omega-3 PUFA in NAFLD has also been reported in two pilot clinical trials [40,41]. Mushroom is a low-fat and healthy food, and constituents of this food have been reported to be associated with a reduced risk of NAFLD [29–31].

Significant association was found between the "high-salt" dietary pattern and the risk of NAFLD, the prevalence of NAFLD was higher for the highest quartile of this dietary pattern compared with the lowest quartile (37.6% *vs.* 28.0%). The "high-salt" pattern was also considered an unhealthy dietary pattern, which was characterized by a high consumption of rice, pickled vegetables, processed meat, bacon, salted deck egg, salted fish and tea. The association between this pattern and the risk of NAFLD might partly be explained by the fact that this pattern contained large amounts of meat (including saturated fat and cholesterol), vegetables (including vitamin C and E), fish (including unsaturated fatty acids) and salt. On the one hand, previous studies showed that saturated fatty acids have an adverse effect on NAFLD [33]. Additionally, animal and human studies have shown that a diet high in salt not only increases blood pressure but also deteriorates insulin metabolism [42,43]. On the other hand, vitamin C and E contained in vegetables possess antioxidant properties that protect against the development of NAFLD [29–31]. In addition, as previously reported [40,41], omega-3 PUFA contained in fish has a protective role against NAFLD. Furthermore, no association also may be related to moderate and vigorous physical activity in this pattern. A recent review by Mouzaki showed that vigorous physical activity was associated with decreased risk of developing NAFLD [9].

5. Strengths and Limitations

There are a number of strengths and limitations in this study. First, to the best of our knowledge, this is the first study investigating the relationships between different dietary patterns and the risk of NAFLD in a Chinese population. It provides evidence into the association between dietary patterns and the risk of NAFLD in the Chinese context. Second, the use of a validated semi-quantitative FFQ by a face-to-face interview ensured that the data we collected are accurate. Furthermore, for reliability, we have adjusted for potential known confounders in our analyses.

Nevertheless, several possible limitations also need to be considered in the interpretation of the present findings. It is noteworthy that the main limitation of this study is its cross-sectional nature, which prevented us from making a causal inference based on our results. Thus, our results remain to be confirmed in a future prospective study. Another limitation is principal component analysis, which requires several arbitrary decisions on the selection of included variables, the number of retained factors, the method of rotation and the labels of the factors [44].

In conclusion, our findings indicate that the "animal food" dietary pattern was significantly associated with an increased risk of NAFLD, and the "grains-vegetable" dietary pattern was significantly associated with a decreased risk of NAFLD where this association was independent of gender, age, physical activity, BMI, smoking status and blood pressure. Nevertheless, future prospective studies are required to confirm these findings. Elucidation of how diet contributes to the development of NAFLD is very important due to its high prevalence and relation to many adverse health outcomes in a Chinese population. Therefore, findings from this study could inform dietary prevention strategies as well as prognosis among subjects with high risk of NAFLD.

6. Conclusions

In conclusion, our findings indicated that the "Animal food" dietary pattern was associated with an increased risk of NAFLD.

Acknowledgments: This work was supported through the National Natural Science Foundation of China (81102125). We thank all participants from the Department of Nutrition, School of Public Health, Anhui Medical University for their assistance and support. We also gratefully acknowledge the Medical Center for Physical Examination, Anhui Province Hospital of Armed Police Forces for their important contributions to collection of data in this study.

Author Contributions: S.-F.W, C.-Q.Y and L.S conceived and designed the experiments. S.W, J.-J.W, Y.Z and Y.-J.X conducted research. C.-Q.Y and L.S analyzed data. C.-Q.Y, L.S and S.-F.W wrote the paper. All authors read and approved the final manuscript.

Conflicts of Interest: The authors declare no conflict of interest.

References

1. Colak, Y.; Tuncer, I.; Senates, E.; Ozturk, O.; Doganay, L.; Yilmaz, Y. Nonalcoholic fatty liver disease: A nutritional approach. *Metab. Syndr. Relat. Disord.* **2012**, *10*, 161–166. [CrossRef] [PubMed]
2. Hou, X.H.; Zhu, Y.X.; Lu, H.J.; Chen, H.F.; Li, Q.; Jiang, S.; Xiang, K.S.; Jia, W.P. Non-alcoholic fatty liver disease's prevalence and impact on alanine aminotransferase associated with metabolic syndrome in the chinese. *J. Gastroenterol. Hepatol.* **2011**, *26*, 722–730. [CrossRef] [PubMed]
3. Lin, Y.C.; Chang, P.F.; Chang, M.H.; Ni, Y.H. Genetic variants in GCKR and PNPLA3 confer susceptibility to nonalcoholic fatty liver disease in obese individuals. *Am. J. Clin. Nutr.* **2014**, *99*, 869–874. [CrossRef] [PubMed]
4. McCarthy, E.M.; Rinella, M.E. The role of diet and nutrient composition in nonalcoholic fatty liver disease. *J. Acad. Nutr. Diet.* **2012**, *112*, 401–409. [CrossRef] [PubMed]

5. Vernon, G.; Baranova, A.; Younossi, Z.M. Systematic review: The epidemiology and natural history of non-alcoholic fatty liver disease and non-alcoholic steatohepatitis in adults. *Aliment. Pharmacol. Ther.* **2011**, *34*, 274–285. [CrossRef] [PubMed]

6. Lonardo, A.; Ballestri, S.; Marchesini, G.; Angulo, P.; Loria, P. Nonalcoholic fatty liver disease: A precursor of the metabolic syndrome. *Dig. Liver Dis.* **2015**, *47*, 181–190. [CrossRef] [PubMed]

7. Machado, M.V.; Cortez-Pinto, H. Management of fatty liver disease with the metabolic syndrome. *Expert Rev. Gastroenterol. Hepatol.* **2014**, *8*, 487–500. [CrossRef] [PubMed]

8. Di Minno, M.N.; Russolillo, A.; Lupoli, R.; Ambrosino, P.; Di Minno, A.; Tarantino, G. Omega-3 fatty acids for the treatment of non-alcoholic fatty liver disease. *World J. Gastroenterol.* **2012**, *18*, 5839–5847. [CrossRef] [PubMed]

9. Mouzaki, M.; Allard, J.P. The role of nutrients in the development, progression, and treatment of nonalcoholic fatty liver disease. *J. Clin. Gastroenterol.* **2012**, *46*, 457–467. [CrossRef] [PubMed]

10. Cortez-Pinto, H.; Jesus, L.; Barros, H.; Lopes, C.; Moura, M.C.; Camilo, M.E. How different is the dietary pattern in non-alcoholic steatohepatitis patients? *Clin. Nutr.* **2006**, *25*, 816–823. [CrossRef] [PubMed]

11. Schulze, M.B.; Hoffmann, K. Methodological approaches to study dietary patterns in relation to risk of coronary heart disease and stroke. *Br. J. Nutr.* **2006**, *95*, 860–869. [CrossRef] [PubMed]

12. Cortez-Pinto, H.; Machado, M. Impact of body weight, diet and lifestyle on nonalcoholic fatty liver disease. *Expert Rev. Gastroenterol. Hepatol.* **2008**, *2*, 217–231. [CrossRef] [PubMed]

13. Carvalhana, S.; Machado, M.V.; Cortez-Pinto, H. Improving dietary patterns in patients with nonalcoholic fatty liver disease. *Curr. Opin. Clin. Nutr. Metab. Care* **2012**, *15*, 468–473. [CrossRef] [PubMed]

14. Abenavoli, L.; Milic, N.; Peta, V.; Alfieri, F.; De Lorenzo, A.; Bellentani, S. Alimentary regimen in non-alcoholic fatty liver disease: Mediterranean diet. *World J. Gastroenterol.* **2014**, *20*, 16831–16840. [CrossRef] [PubMed]

15. Wang, D.; He, Y.; Li, Y.; Luan, D.; Yang, X.; Zhai, F.; Ma, G. Dietary patterns and hypertension among chinese adults: A nationally representative cross-sectional study. *BMC Public Health* **2011**, *11*, 925. [CrossRef] [PubMed]

16. Esmaillzadeh, A.; Kimiagar, M.; Mehrabi, Y.; Azadbakht, L.; Hu, F.B.; Willett, W.C. Dietary patterns, insulin resistance, and prevalence of the metabolic syndrome in women. *Am. J. Clin. Nutr.* **2007**, *85*, 910–918. [PubMed]

17. Berg, C.M.; Lappas, G.; Strandhagen, E.; Wolk, A.; Toren, K.; Rosengren, A.; Aires, N.; Thelle, D.S.; Lissner, L. Food patterns and cardiovascular disease risk factors: The swedish intergene research program. *Am. J. Clin. Nutr.* **2008**, *88*, 289–297. [PubMed]

18. Zuo, H.; Shi, Z.; Yuan, B.; Dai, Y.; Hu, G.; Wu, G.; Hussain, A. Interaction between physical activity and sleep duration in relation to insulin resistance among non-diabetic Chinese adults. *BMC Public Health* **2012**, *12*, 247. [CrossRef] [PubMed]

19. Chobanian, A.V.; Bakris, G.L.; Black, H.R.; Cushman, W.C.; Green, L.A.; Izzo, J.L.; Jones, D.W.; Materson, B.J.; Oparil, S.; Wright, J.T.; *et al.* Seventh report of the joint national committee on prevention, detection, evaluation, and treatment of high blood pressure. *Hypertension* **2003**, *42*, 1206–1252. [CrossRef] [PubMed]

20. Alberti, K.G.; Eckel, R.H.; Grundy, S.M.; Zimmet, P.Z.; Cleeman, J.I.; Donato, K.A.; Fruchart, J.C.; James, W.P.; Loria, C.M.; Smith, S.C.; *et al.* Harmonizing the metabolic syndrome: A joint interim statement of the international diabetes federation task force on epidemiology and prevention; national heart, lung, and blood institute; American Heart Association; World Heart Federation; International Atherosclerosis Society; and International Association for the Study of Obesity. *Circulation* **2009**, *120*, 1640–1645. [PubMed]

21. Nascimbeni, F.; Pais, R.; Bellentani, S.; Day, C.P.; Ratziu, V.; Loria, P.; Lonardo, A. From nafld in clinical practice to answers from guidelines. *J. Hepatol.* **2013**, *59*, 859–871. [CrossRef] [PubMed]

22. Zhang, C.; Schulze, M.B.; Solomon, C.G.; Hu, F.B. A prospective study of dietary patterns, meat intake and the risk of gestational diabetes mellitus. *Diabetologia* **2006**, *49*, 2604–2613. [CrossRef] [PubMed]

23. Newby, P.K.; Tucker, K.L. Empirically derived eating patterns using factor or cluster analysis: A review. *Nutr. Rev.* **2004**, *62*, 177–203. [CrossRef] [PubMed]

24. Hudgins, L.C.; Hellerstein, M.; Seidman, C.; Neese, R.; Diakun, J.; Hirsch, J. Human fatty acid synthesis is stimulated by a eucaloric low fat, high carbohydrate diet. *J. Clin. Investig.* **1996**, *97*, 2081–2091. [CrossRef] [PubMed]

25. Mager, D.R.; Patterson, C.; So, S.; Rogenstein, C.D.; Wykes, L.J.; Roberts, E.A. Dietary and physical activity patterns in children with fatty liver. *Eur. J. Clin. Nutr.* **2010**, *64*, 628–635. [CrossRef] [PubMed]

26. Ouyang, X.; Cirillo, P.; Sautin, Y.; McCall, S.; Bruchette, J.L.; Diehl, A.M.; Johnson, R.J.; Abdelmalek, M.F. Fructose consumption as a risk factor for non-alcoholic fatty liver disease. *J. Hepatol.* **2008**, *48*, 993–999. [CrossRef] [PubMed]

27. York, L.W.; Puthalapattu, S.; Wu, G.Y. Nonalcoholic fatty liver disease and low-carbohydrate diets. *Annu. Rev. Nutr.* **2009**, *29*, 365–379. [CrossRef] [PubMed]

28. Villaca Chaves, G.; Pereira, S.E.; Saboya, C.J.; Ramalho, A. Non-alcoholic fatty liver disease and its relationship with the nutritional status of vitamin a in individuals with class III obesity. *Obes. Surg.* **2008**, *18*, 378–385. [CrossRef] [PubMed]

29. Harrison, S.A.; Torgerson, S.; Hayashi, P.; Ward, J.; Schenker, S. Vitamin E and vitamin C treatment improves fibrosis in patients with nonalcoholic steatohepatitis. *Am. J. Gastroenterol.* **2003**, *98*, 2485–2490. [CrossRef] [PubMed]

30. Foster, T.; Budoff, M.J.; Saab, S.; Ahmadi, N.; Gordon, C.; Guerci, A.D. Atorvastatin and antioxidants for the treatment of nonalcoholic fatty liver disease: The St francis heart study randomized clinical trial. *Am. J. Gastroenterol.* **2011**, *106*, 71–77. [CrossRef] [PubMed]

31. Arendt, B.M.; Allard, J.P. Effect of atorvastatin, vitamin e and c on nonalcoholic fatty liver disease: Is the combination required? *Am. J. Gastroenterol.* **2011**, *106*, 78–80. [CrossRef] [PubMed]

32. Musso, G.; Gambino, R.; De Michieli, F.; Cassader, M.; Rizzetto, M.; Durazzo, M.; Faga, E.; Silli, B.; Pagano, G. Dietary habits and their relations to insulin resistance and postprandial lipemia in nonalcoholic steatohepatitis. *Hepatology* **2003**, *37*, 909–916. [CrossRef] [PubMed]

33. Vallim, T.; Salter, A.M. Regulation of hepatic gene expression by saturated fatty acids. *Prostaglandins Leukot. Essent. Fat. Acids* **2010**, *82*, 211–218. [CrossRef] [PubMed]

34. Abid, A.; Taha, O.; Nseir, W.; Farah, R.; Grosovski, M.; Assy, N. Soft drink consumption is associated with fatty liver disease independent of metabolic syndrome. *J. Hepatol.* **2009**, *51*, 918–924. [CrossRef] [PubMed]

35. Nseir, W.; Nassar, F.; Assy, N. Soft drinks consumption and nonalcoholic fatty liver disease. *World J. Gastroenterol.* **2010**, *16*, 2579–2588. [CrossRef] [PubMed]

36. Pereira, M.A.; Kartashov, A.I.; Ebbeling, C.B.; Van Horn, L.; Slattery, M.L.; Jacobs, D.R.; Ludwig, D.S. Fast-food habits, weight gain, and insulin resistance (the cardia study): 15-year prospective analysis. *Lancet* **2005**, *365*, 36–42. [CrossRef]

37. Marchesini, G.; Brizi, M.; Morselli-Labate, A.M.; Bianchi, G.; Bugianesi, E.; McCullough, A.J.; Forlani, G.; Melchionda, N. Association of nonalcoholic fatty liver disease with insulin resistance. *Am. J. Med.* **1999**, *107*, 450–455. [CrossRef]

38. Kris-Etherton, P.M.; Pearson, T.A.; Wan, Y.; Hargrove, R.L.; Moriarty, K.; Fishell, V.; Etherton, T.D. High-monounsaturated fatty acid diets lower both plasma cholesterol and triacylglycerol concentrations. *Am. J. Clin. Nutr.* **1999**, *70*, 1009–1015. [PubMed]

39. Shapiro, H.; Tehilla, M.; Attal-Singer, J.; Bruck, R.; Luzzatti, R.; Singer, P. The therapeutic potential of long-chain omega-3 fatty acids in nonalcoholic fatty liver disease. *Clin. Nutr.* **2011**, *30*, 6–19. [CrossRef] [PubMed]

40. Tanaka, N.; Sano, K.; Horiuchi, A.; Tanaka, E.; Kiyosawa, K.; Aoyama, T. Highly purified eicosapentaenoic acid treatment improves nonalcoholic steatohepatitis. *J. Clin. Gastroenterol.* **2008**, *42*, 413–418. [CrossRef] [PubMed]

41. Capanni, M.; Calella, F.; Biagini, M.R.; Genise, S.; Raimondi, L.; Bedogni, G.; Svegliati-Baroni, G.; Sofi, F.; Milani, S.; Abbate, R.; *et al.* Prolonged *n*-3 polyunsaturated fatty acid supplementation ameliorates hepatic steatosis in patients with non-alcoholic fatty liver disease: A pilot study. *Aliment. Pharmacol. Ther.* **2006**, *23*, 1143–1151. [CrossRef] [PubMed]

42. Ogihara, T.; Asano, T.; Fujita, T. Contribution of salt intake to insulin resistance associated with hypertension. *Life Sci.* **2003**, *73*, 509–523. [CrossRef]

43. Lastra, G.; Dhuper, S.; Johnson, M.S.; Sowers, J.R. Salt, aldosterone, and insulin resistance: Impact on the cardiovascular system. *Nat. Rev. Cardiol.* **2010**, *7*, 577–584. [CrossRef] [PubMed]

44. Hu, F.B. Dietary pattern analysis: A new direction in nutritional epidemiology. *Curr. Opin. Lipidol.* **2002**, *13*, 3–9. [CrossRef] [PubMed]

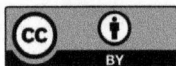

nutrients

MDPI

Article

Lifestyle Patterns Are Associated with Elevated Blood Pressure among Qatari Women of Reproductive Age: A Cross-Sectional National Study

Mohammed Al Thani [1], Al Anoud Al Thani [2], Walaa Al-Chetachi [2], Badria Al Malki [2], Shamseldin A. H. Khalifa [2], Ahmad Haj Bakri [2], Nahla Hwalla [3], Lara Nasreddine [3,†,*] and Farah Naja [3,†,*]

[1] Public Health Department, Supreme Council of Health, Doha, Al Rumaila West, 42 Doha, Qatar;
    E-Mail: malthani@sch.gov.qa
[2] Health Promotion and Non Communicable Disease Prevention Division, Supreme Council of Health,
    Doha, Al Rumaila West, 42 Doha, Qatar; E-Mails: aalthani@sch.gov.qa (A.A.A.T.);
    walchetachi@sch.gov.qa (W.A.-C.); balmalki@sch.gov.qa (B.A.M.); skhalifa1@sch.gov.qa (S.A.H.K.);
    abakri@sch.gov.qa (A.H.B.)
[3] Nutrition and Food Sciences Department, Faculty of Agriculture and Food Sciences,
    American University of Beirut, P. O. Box 11-0.236 Riad El Solh, 11072020 Beirut, Lebanon;
    E-Mail: nahla@aub.edu.lb
*   Authors to whom correspondence should be addressed;
    E-Mails: ln10@aub.edu.lb (L.N.); fn14@aub.edu.lb (F.N.);
    Tel.: +961-1-350000 (ext. 4547) (L.N.); +961-1-350000 (ext. 4504) (F.N.); Fax: +961-1-744460 (L.N. & F.N.)
†   These authors contributed equally to this manuscript.

Received: 12 June 2015 / Accepted: 27 August 2015 / Published: 9 September 2015

Abstract: Women of childbearing age are particularly vulnerable to the adverse effects of elevated blood pressure (BP), with dietary and lifestyle habits being increasingly recognized as important modifiable environmental risk factors for this condition. Using data from the National STEPwise survey conducted in Qatar in year 2012, we aimed to examine lifestyle patterns and their association with elevated BP among Qatari women of childbearing age (18–45 years). Socio-demographic, lifestyle, dietary, anthropometric and BP data were used ($n = 747$). Principal component factor analysis was applied to identify the patterns using the frequency of consumption of 13 foods/food groups, physical activity level, and smoking status. Multivariate logistic regression analyses were used to evaluate the association of the identified lifestyle patterns with elevated BP and to examine the socio-demographic correlates of these patterns. Three lifestyle patterns were identified: a "healthy" pattern characterized by intake of fruits, natural juices, and vegetables; a "fast food & smoking" pattern characterized by fast foods, sweetened beverages, and sweets, in addition to smoking; and a "traditional sedentary" pattern which consisted of refined grains, dairy products, and meat in addition to low physical activity. The fast food & smoking and the traditional & sedentary patterns were associated with an approximately 2-fold increase in the risk of elevated BP in the study population. The findings of this study highlight the synergistic effect that diet, smoking and physical inactivity may have on the risk of elevated BP among Qatari women.

Keywords: lifestyle pattern; elevated blood pressure; factor analysis; women; Qatar

1. Introduction

Globally, hypertension is the third leading cause of mortality and is a major risk factor for heart disease, stroke, and kidney failure [1,2]. According to the World Health Organization (WHO), 22.2% of the adult population in 2014 had hypertension (24% of men and 20.5% of women) [3]. This prevalence was projected to increase to 29.2% (29% of men and 29.5% of women) by year 2025 [4]. Among countries contributing significantly to this alarming increase in hypertension prevalence are countries of the Gulf Cooperation Council, where fast economic growth was accompanied by a steep rise in nutritional health problems and related disease. Qatar has recently emerged as the richest country in the world in terms of Gross Domestic Product (GDP) per capita. Though milestones have been accomplished in the betterment of life expectancy and health in the country, the WHO World Health Survey (WHS) in 2006 and later the WHO STEPwise survey in 2012 identified lifestyle-related non-communicable diseases, including obesity, diabetes and hypertension, as main health challenges, with hypertension rates increasing by 75% during this time interval [5,6].

Of all adults, women of childbearing age are particularly vulnerable to the adverse effects of elevated blood pressure (BP) and hypertension. In addition to its effect on morbidity and mortality on the mother, hypertension in women of child-bearing age has been shown to be a major risk factor during pregnancy for both mother and child, possibly due to changes in blood flow to the uterus during pregnancy [7]. One in four women with pre-existing hypertension experience superimposed preeclampsia during pregnancy, placing the mother at high risk of organ damage and often necessitating early childbirth [8]. Furthermore, rates of preterm delivery, low birth weight, neonatal unit admission, and perinatal death are around three to four times higher among mothers with hypertension [7]. A recent systematic review and meta-analysis showed significant associations between maternal hypertension and congenital heart disease risk in the offspring (Relative Risk (RR) 1.8; 95% Confidence Interval (CI) 1.5, 2.2) regardless of whether hypertension was treated or not [9]. These substantial short and long-term health risks of hypertension among women of child-bearing age make this age group an ideal target for the primary prevention of hypertension.

The escalating trend in hypertension prevalence coupled to significant downstream pathophysiological effects and enormous financial liabilities pose major public health concerns that necessitate the search for mitigating factors and strategies to address them. Prehypertension and elevated BP are recognized as frequent precursors of hypertension [10]. Dietary intake is an important modifiable environmental risk factor in the development and prevention of elevated BP and hypertension [11]. Studies on the association between dietary factors and BP have consistently shown that excess sodium and alcohol intake and inadequate intake of potassium increase BP [12]. However, the evidence for the association with other dietary factors has been less consistent. For instance, dietary protein appeared to reduce BP in a few randomized trials; however, such a relationship was not confirmed by long-term studies [13]. Furthermore, the optimal source of protein (e.g., plant or animal) implicated in BP reduction has not been also identified. It is also not clear whether the reduction of BP with a higher intake of protein is rather due to a concomitant reduction in carbohydrates [13]. Similarly, while high fiber intake has shown a modest reduction on BP [14], the benefits of dietary fiber are difficult to distinguish from the benefits of an increase in vitamins and minerals, such as potassium, coming from the same fibrous plant-based foods [12]. To overcome such inconsistencies, nutrition epidemiologists have proposed studying dietary patterns as an alternative approach to single nutrients in evaluating diet-disease relationships [15]. Several studies have investigated the association between dietary patterns and hypertension [12,16,17], consistently showing an increased risk for hypertension with higher adherence to a "Western" dietary pattern [17].

Though dietary intake is a main modulator of BP and risk of hypertension, other behavioral factors such as smoking and physical activity have also been implicated as risk factors of hypertension and are important to consider in addressing prevention. Studying a single behavioral risk factor overlooks the fact that people are exposed to a combination of risk factors which are frequently interactive and/or synergistic [18]. Recently, a few studies have addressed the association between lifestyle patterns and weight status among children [19]; dysglycemia [20] and non-communicable diseases [18]. Not only does this approach account for the collinearity or intercorrelations between risk factors, it allows for a better understanding of high-risk behaviours as they cluster in real-life and thus produces more culturally sensitive public health recommendation that can be easily interpreted and followed by the general population.

Using data from the National WHO STEPwise s survey conducted in Qatar in year 2012, this study aimed at identifying lifestyle patterns among women of reproductive age in Qatar and investigating the association of these patterns with elevated BP. A secondary objective was to examine the socio-demographic correlates of the identified lifestyle patterns. Findings of this study will pave the way for the development of culturally sensitive evidence-based interventions strategies aimed at preventing elevated BP among women of child-bearing age in Qatar.

2. Methodology

2.1. Study Design

The data presented in this paper is a secondary analysis of the National STEPwise Survey conducted in Qatar during year 2012. The survey was conducted on a nationally representative sample of Qatari adults aged between 18 and 64 years. The survey design, including sampling and data collection, was modelled based on the WHO STEPwise approach to non-communicable disease risk factor surveillance. The sample consisted of randomly selected households based on a multi-stage cluster sampling. Clusters were selected from the seven municipalities of Qatar (Doha, Al Rayyan, Al Warka, Umm Salal, Al Khor, Al Shamal, Al Daayeen). The clusters were defined as a group of contiguous blocks (between 60 and 70 blocks). Using probability proportional to size sampling, a systematic random sample of 95 clusters was selected [21]. Within each cluster, 30 households were randomly chosen. Adults of Qatari nationality between the age of 18 and 64 years were eligible to participate in the survey. In the household, in case more than one subject was eligible, using a personal digital assistant (PDA) to generate a random number, only one adult was randomly selected. Out of the 2850 households approached, 2496 participated in the study (response rate 88%). The Qatar WHO STEPwise survey protocol was granted ethical approval from the Supreme Council of Health and the Ministry of Development Planning and Statistics, Doha, Qatar. A written consent form was obtained from all study participants who were assured that all information they provided was strictly confidential, their participation is voluntary, and they have the right to refuse the participation and withdraw from the interview at any stage. Further details about the design and protocol of the Qatar STEPwise survey are found at Haj Bakri & Al-Thani (2013) [6]. The present paper focused on women of child bearing age. The selection criteria were (1) female sex; (2) age between 18 and 45; (3) healthy (no known diagnosis of hypertension, other chronic diseases, or conditions that may affect dietary intake); and (4) not pregnant. Out of 776 women who meet the inclusion criteria, 29 had missing or incomplete data for BP, dietary and/or lifestyle information and hence were excluded from the analysis.

2.2. Data Collection

The participants were visited at their household by interviewers who were trained on the methodology of the survey and protocols of data collection prior to the initiation of field work. During the interview, participants responded to the questions of the interviewers which were based on a standard multi-component questionnaire and they have also undergone physical examination. The questionnaire included information about socio-demographic (age, sex, education, marital status, job type, parental consanguinity, family history of diabetes and hypertension) and lifestyle characteristics (smoking, physical activity and dietary intake). Smoking questions addressed the smoking status of the participants as well as his/her exposure to passive smoking (days/week). As recommended by the WHO STEPwise approach, the Arabic Global Physical Activity Questionnaire (GPAQ) was used to assess physical activity. The GPAQ covers several components of physical activity, such as intensity, duration, and frequency, and it assesses three domains in which physical activity is performed (occupational physical activity, transport-related physical activity, and physical activity during discretionary or leisure time) [22]. Total physical activity was calculated by weighting each type of activity by its energy requirements defined in MET (Metabolic Equivalent of Task)-minutes. The total MET-min were computed as the sum of all MET-min/week from moderate-to-vigorous-intensity physical activities performed for each of the three domains, and was later converted to total Met-min per day [23]. Three categories of physical activity (low, moderate, high) were assigned based on METS-min per week [24]. Dietary intake was assessed using a non-quantitative (without reference to portion size) food frequency questionnaire. A total of 13 food groups were included: refined grains, fruits, vegetables, milk and dairy products, meat, poultry, fish and sea food, beans, sweets, sweetened beverages, whole grains, and natural juices. Frequency of consumption was recorded as number of days per week the food/food group was consumed. No questions on alcohol were included for cultural and religious considerations. Besides providing information on usual intakes of a particular food or food groups of interest, such non-quantitative Food Frequecy Questionnaires (FFQs) have been particularly useful in identifying dietary patterns at the population level [25]. All components of the questionnaire were tested for cultural sensitivity on a sample of Qatari adults prior to the initiation of field work.

During physical examination, the BP, weight, height and waist circumference of participants were determined. BP, both systolic and diastolic, was measured through a calibrated Omron M7 sphygmomanometer (Omron BP785; China). Three readings were obtained for both systolic and diastolic BP at 5 minutes intervals. The average of the second and the third readings were used. Elevated BP was defined as either systolic pressure ⩾ 130 or diastolic pressure ⩾ 85 mm Hg [26,27].

Weight and height measurements were taken using standardized techniques and calibrated equipment. Subjects were weighed to the nearest 0.1 kg in light indoor clothing and with bare feet or stockings. Using a stadiometer, height was measured without shoes and recorded to the nearest 0.5 cm. Body mass index (BMI) was calculated as the ratio of weight (kilograms) to the square of height (meters).

2.3. Lifestyle Patterns Derivation

Using the exploratory Principal Component Factor Analysis (PCFA), lifestyle patterns were identified based on the frequency of consumption of the 13 foods/food groups, physical activity (in Mets-Minutes), and smoking status (non-smoker, past smoker and current smoker). Prior to running the PCFA, the correlation matrix between all the variables was visually and statistically examined to justify undertaking the analysis. The chi square for Bartlett test of sphericity was significant at a *p*-value less than 0.05, and the Kaiser-Meyer-Olkin test (KMO) was greater than 0.6, indicating that the correlation among the variables was sufficiently strong for a factor analysis. The number of factors retained was based on three criteria: (1) the Kaiser criterion (eigenvalues > 1); (2) inflection point of the scree plot (3) and the interpretability of factors. The factors were rotated by a Varimax rotation (orthogonal transformation). Factor loadings indicated the strength and direction of the association between the patterns and the lifestyle variables. Factor scores were calculated by multiple regression approach with each participant possessing a score on each of the three factors. These scores indicated the degree to which each subject's diet adheres to the identified pattern. For each pattern, participants were grouped into tertiles of pattern scores.

2.4. Statistical Analyses

In order to correct for the selection probabilities, the sample distribution was calibrated to the Qatari population totals using geographical and 5 year-age distributions. Data analysis was weighted using sampling weights calculated as the inverse of the sampling fractions. In weighting, the distribution of the 2010 Qatari population by municipality and 5 year age group was used as the reference [21]. Socio-demographic, lifestyle characteristics, eating habits and anthropometric measurements were described using means ± standard deviations (SD) and proportions for continuous and categorical variables, respectively. The chi-square test, *t*-test and ANOVA were used to chart comparisons between groups. Multiple logistic regression analyses were applied to identify the socio-demographic and lifestyle correlates of adherence to the identified patterns. Adherence was defined as belonging to the third tertile of the pattern score. The associations of the lifestyle patterns with elevated BP were evaluated by means of multivariate logistic regression models, with tertiles of dietary patterns' scores as independent variables and elevated BP as the outcome variables. Belonging to the third tertile of a certain pattern's score indicated that the participants had higher adherence to this pattern when compared to other participants who belonged to the first and second tertiles. The multivariate logistic regression models were adjusted for variables found to be associated with either BP or the lifestyle patterns and these included age, education, marital status, parental consanguinity, family history BP, number of meals not eaten at home, exposure to passive smoking and BMI. The Statistical Package for the Social Sciences (SPSS, version 14.1, Chicago, IL, USA) was used for all computations [28] and a *p*-value < 0.05 was considered significant.

3. Results

Socio-demographics, lifestyle and anthropometric characteristics of study participants by BP status are presented in Table 1. Out of the 747 women study participants, 105 (14%) had an elevated BP. Study participants' mean age was 31.0 ± 7.0 years. Eighty % of subjects had high school or higher education level with almost 52% working (either government (47.7%) or private (4%) employment), 29.6% were housewives. A considerable proportion (35.1%) reported parental consanguinity. Family history of diabetes and hypertension were reported among 68% and 64.3% of participants, respectively. The majority of subjects were non-smokers (97.7%) with only 1.5% being current smokers. Over 50% of subjects belonged to the low physical activity category, with walking constituting 55.5% of total physical activity. This percentage was higher than work (26.2%) and leisure time (18.3%) related activities. Thirty eight percent of subjects were obese (BMI $\geq$ 30 kg/m^2). Comparisons between subjects with elevated *versus* those with normal BP showed that subjects with elevated BP were older (33.5 ± 6.9 *vs.* 30.5 ± 6.9, *p* < 0.01), more likely to be married (73.6% *vs.* 63.7%; *p* < 0.05); and have a family history of BP (77.4% *vs.* 62.1%; *p* < 0.05). Furthermore, obesity was more prevalent among subjects with elevated BP compared to those with normal BP (50.0% *vs.* 35.2%, *p* < 0.05).

Table 1. Weighted socio-demographics, lifestyle and anthropometric characteristics of study participants by blood pressure status [a] (*n* = 747).

Variable Name	Total n = 747	Normal Blood Pressure n = 642	Elevated Blood [†] Pressure n = 105	Significance [††]
Age (years)	31.0 ± 7.0	30.5 ± 6.9	33.5 ± 6.9	*p* = 0.000 **
Education				
Up to intermediate level [b]	140 (20)	113 (17.6)	24 (22.9)	
Finished high school	280 (40)	248 (38.7)	35 (33.3)	*p* = 0.36
University/graduate level	326 (43.7)	280 (43.7)	46 (43.8)	
Marital Status				
Not married	261 (34.9)	233 (36.3)	28 (26.4)	*p* = 0.05 *
Married	486 (65.1)	409 (63.7)	78 (73.6)	
Job type				
Governmental employee	356 (47.7)	309 (48.1)	47 (44.8)	
Non-governmental employee [c]	30 (4.0)	26 (4.0)	4 (3.8)	*p* = 0.42
Not working	140 (18.7)	124 (19.3)	16 (15.2)	
Housewife	221 (29.6)	183 (28.5)	38 (36.2)	
Parental Consanguinity				
No	485 (64.9)	417 (65.0)	68 (64.8)	*p* = 0.97
Yes	262 (35.1)	225 (35.0)	37 (35.2)	

Table 1. *Cont.*

Variable Name	Total $n = 747$	Normal Blood Pressure $n = 642$	Elevated Blood [†] Pressure $n = 105$	Significance [††]
Family history of diabetes				
No	240 (32.1)	207 (32.2)	33 (31.4)	$p = 0.87$
Yes	507 (67.9)	435 (67.8)	72 (68.6)	
Family history of High blood pressure				
No	267 (35.7)	243 (37.9)	24 (22.6)	$p = 0.002$ *
Yes	480 (64.3)	399 (62.1)	82 (77.4)	
Oil type used in cooking				
Vegetable oil	714 (96.4)	613 (96.2)	101 (97.1)	$p = 0.66$
Animal oil	27 (3.6)	24 (3.8)	3 (2.9)	
Number of Meals not prepared at home (per week)	2.4 ± 2.3	2.5 ± 2.4	2.1 ± 2.0	$p = 0.10$
Smoking Status				
Non smoker	730 (97.7)	628 (97.8)	102 (97.1)	
Past smoker	6 (0.8)	6 (0.9)	0 (0.0)	$p = 0.28$
Current smoker	11 (1.5)	8 (1.2)	3 (2.9)	
Exposure to passive Smoking [d] (days/week)	1.2 ± 2.9	1.2 ± 2.9	1.3 ± 3.0	$p = 0.71$
Physical Activity Level				
Low	416 (55.8)	352 (54.9)	64 (61.0)	
Moderate	162 (21.7)	144 (22.5)	18 (17.1)	$p = 0.41$
High	168 (22.5)	145 (22.6)	23 (21.9)	
Total physical activity (Met-minutes per day)	389.9 ± 761.9	394.5 ± 772.7	369.2 ± 701.5	$p = 0.75$
Percent activity from work (%) ($n = 551$)	26.2 ± 37.7	25.5 ± 37.2	31.7 ± 40.6	$p = 0.22$
Percent activity from walking (%)	55.5 ± 40.8	55.6 ± 41.1	54.3 ± 39.8	$p = 0.80$
Percent activity form free time (%)	18.3 ± 30.8	18.9 ± 31.7	14.1 ± 23.9	$p = 0.15$
Sedentary time (minutes/day)	183.6 ± 168.3	183.0 ± 164.4	189.5 ± 191.2	$p = 0.71$
Body mass index(BMI) (kg/m^2)	29.1 ± 7.2	28.7 ± 7.1	30.9 ± 6.9	$p = 0.004$ *
Obese($\geqslant$30 kg/m^2)	279 (37.3)	226 (35.2)	53 (50.0)	$p = 0.007$ *

[†] Elevated blood pressure in this study was defined as either systolic pressure $\geqslant$130 or diastolic pressure $\geqslant$85 mm Hg; [††] *p*-values were derived from *t* test and Chi Square test for continuous and categorical variables respectively; [a] Percentages are within column; [b] This category includes: no schooling, elementary and intermediate schooling; [c] This category includes: private and own business; [d] This includes passive smoking from family members and at work; * $p \leqslant 0.05$; ** $p \leqslant 0.001$.

Figure 1 is the scree plot showing eigenvalues for the 15 components derived from the lifestyle and dietary data using PCFA. Examination of the scree plot revealed a clear inflection at the third component (Figure 1). Taken together with the Kaiser criterion of an eigenvalue >1, it was deduced that three components/factors ought to be retained.

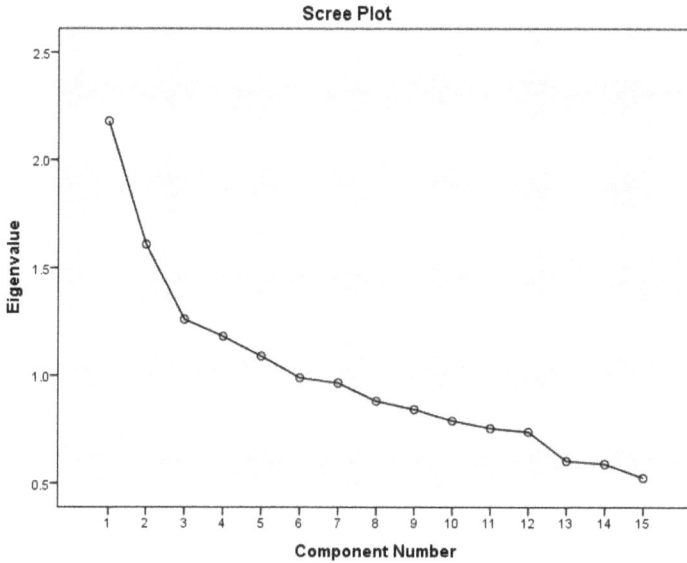

Figure 1. Scree plot showing eigenvalues for the 15 components, extracted in weighted factor analysis of lifestyle and dietary data of study participants (*n* = 747).

Factor loadings and the variance explained by each of the retained three patterns are shown in Table 2 (loadings greater than 0.3 are bolded). Together these patterns explained 34.1% of the variance ("Healthy": 12.4%; "Fast food & smoking": 12.1% and "Traditional sedentary": 9.6%). The "Healthy" pattern wascharacterized by a high intake of fruits, beans, natural juices, vegetables, fish, and whole grains. In addition to smoking, the "Fast food & smoking" pattern was characterized by fast foods, sweetened beverages, sweets and poultry. The "Traditional sedentary" pattern consisted mainly of refined grains, meat and low physical activity. It is important to note that beans loaded on the "Traditional sedentary" pattern (0.26) in addition to the "Fast food & smoking" pattern (0.56). Whole grains had a high negative loading on the "Traditional sedentary" pattern (−0.55).

Table 2. Weighted factor loading matrix of the three identified lifestyle patterns among a nationally representative sample of Qatari women [a] (*n* = 747).

	Lifestyle Patterns		
	Healthy	Fast Food & Smoking	
Fruits	0.68	−0.20	
Beans	0.56		0.27
Natural juices	0.55		
Vegetables	0.44		
Fish	0.44		−0.21
Dairy	0.24		0.21
Fast foods		0.78	
Sweetened beverages		0.63	

Table 2. *Cont.*

	Lifestyle Patterns		
	Healthy	Fast Food & Smoking	
Sweets		0.54	
Smoking		0.39	
Poultry		0.34	
Refined grains		0.22	0.74
Whole grains	0.32	−0.21	−0.55
Physical activity (Mets/day)			−0.43
Meat			0.30
Percent variance explained	12.4	12.1	9.6

[a] Factor loadings of less than |0.2| were not listed in the table for simplicity. Loadings ⩾ 0.3 are bolded.

To further characterize the identified patterns, the dietary intakes, physical activity, smoking characteristics of study participants were described for the first and third tertiles of each of the patterns' scores (Table 3). Compared to participants in the first tertile of the "Healthy" pattern, those belonging to the third tertile had significantly higher frequencies (days/week) of consumption of fruits, beans, natural juices, vegetables, fish and sea food, dairy products, and whole grains, and had lower frequencies of consumption of sweetened beverages and poultry. As for the "Fast food & smoking" pattern, frequencies of consumption of beans, fast food, sweetened beverages, sweets, poultry, refined grains, and meat were higher among subjects in the third tertile compared to those in the first tertile. Fruits, vegetables and whole grains frequencies of consumption were lower among subjects in the third compared to the first tertile of this pattern. Furthermore, a higher proportion of smokers was found among subjects in the third tertile of the "Fast food & smoking" pattern. Foods/food groups with higher frequency of consumption among subjects in the third as compared to the first tertile of the "Traditional sedentary" pattern were beans, dairy products, sweetened beverages, sweets, poultry, refined grains, and meat. In contrast, lower frequency of consumption was noted for fruits, natural juices, vegetables, fish and sea food, fast food and whole grains. Though no difference in physical activity was noted for any of the first two patterns, subjects belonging to third tertile of the "Traditional sedentary" pattern had significantly lower levels of physical activity compared to those belonging to the first tertile (Table 3).

Table 4 displays the association of the derived lifestyle patterns with elevated BP as evaluated by multivariate logistic regression analyses. After adjustment for socio-demographic characteristics and BMI, the results showed that subjects belonging to the second tertile of the "Fast food & smoking" pattern had a two-fold increase in the odds of elevated BP compared to those in the first tertile (Odds Ratio (OR): 2.1, 95% CI: 1.4–3.3). A similar association was observed for subjects in the third compared to the first tertile of this pattern however the odds did not reach significance. The small number of smokers in the study sample may not have provided enough power to detect a significant association in the third tertile. Furthermore, a gradual increase in the odds of elevated BP was observed with a higher adherence to the "Traditional sedentary" pattern reaching OR: 2.2, 95% CI 1.3–3.7 for the third compared to the first tertile of this pattern (*p* for trend <0.05) (Table 4).

Table 3. Weighted dietary intake, smoking, and physical activity of study participants by tertiles of the three identified patterns' scores [a] (n = 747).

Factor Items	Healthy		Fast Food & Smoking		Traditional Sedentary	
	1st Tertile	3rd Tertile	1st Tertile	3rd Tertile	1st Tertile	3rd Tertile
	Mean ± SD					
Fruits (days/week)	1.2 ± 1.4	5.1 ± 2.4 **	3.6 ± 2.7	2.3 ± 2.3 **	3.5 ± 2.7	2.7 ± 2.3 *
Beans (days/week)	0.8 ± 0.9	2.7 ± 2.1 **	1.3 ± 1.4	2.0 ± 2.1 **	1.2 ± 1.4	2.1 ± 2.0 **
Natural juice(days/week)	1.9 ± 2.0	5.3 ± 2.3 **	3.4 ± 2.7	3.5 ± 2.7	3.8 ± 2.8	3.0 ± 2.5 *
Vegetables (days/week)	4.0 ± 2.7	6.5 ± 1.4 **	5.7 ± 2.2	5.0 ± 2.5 *	5.5 ± 2.3	5.4 ± 2.3
Fish and sea food (days/week)	0.8 ± 0.8	2.2 ± 1.6 **	1.6 ± 1.3	1.3 ± 1.3 *	1.7 ± 1.5	1.1 ± 1.1 **
Dairy products (days/week)	5.4 ± 2.5	6.2 ± 1.8 **	5.9 ± 2.1	5.9 ± 2.2	5.5 ± 2.4	6.3 ± 1.7 **
Fast food (days/week)	1.7 ± 1.9	1.9 ± 2.0	0.6 ± 0.8	3.6 ± 2.3 **	1.9 ± 2.2	1.3 ± 1.4 **
Sweetened beverages(days/week)	2.9 ± 2.9	2.2 ± 2.7 *	0.6 ± 1.2	5.1 ± 2.6 **	2.2 ± 2.7	2.4 ± 2.7 *
Sweets (days/week)	4.3 ± 2.8	4.2 ± 2.6	2.4 ± 2.3	5.9 ± 1.9 **	3.9 ± 2.7	4.7 ± 2.6 *
Smoking Status [b]						
Non smoker	239 (97.2)	229 (99.1)	259 (100.0)	205 (94.0) **	233 (94.7)	248 (100.0) **
Past smoker	1 (0.4)	2 (0.9)	0 (0.0)	10 (4.6)	3 (1.2)	0 (0)
Current smoker	6 (2.4)	0 (0.0)	0 (0.0)	3 (1.4)	10 (4.1)	0 (0)
Poultry(days/week)	5.4 ± 2.2	4.7 ± 2.1 *	4.0 ± 2.3	5.9 ± 1.8 **	4.4 ± 2.3	5.6 ± 2.0 **
Refined grains (days/week)	5.6 ± 2.4	5.2 ± 2.5	4.7 ± 2.8	5.8 ± 2.1 **	2.9 ± 2.5	7.0 ± 0.2 **
Whole grains (days/week)	0.9 ± 1.9	2.8 ± 2.9 **	2.6 ± 2.9	1.4 ± 2.3 **	4.0 ± 3.0	0.4 ± 1.1 **
Total physical activity (Met-minutes per day)	450 ± 770	372.3 ± 672.9	386.0 ± 677.9	463.5 ± 844.9	627.5 ± 1054.0	203.4 ± 429.0 **
Meat (days/week)	1.3 ± 1.4	2.0 ± 1.6 **	1.4 ± 1.3	1.9 ± 1.8 *	1.2 ± 1.4	2.1 ± 1.8 **

[a] Intake of the various food groups referred to frequency of consumption as expressed by number of days per week the food/food group was consumed;
[b] For smoking the numbers represent *n* (%); * $p \leq 0.05$; ** $p \leq 0.001$.

Table 4. Weighted odds ratio and their 95% Confidence Interval (CI) for the association of the identified lifestyle patterns with elevated blood pressure in the study population ($n = 747$).

	Dietary Patterns		
	Healthy	**Fast Food & Smoking**	**Traditional Sedentary**
	Age adjusted model		
1st tertile	Ref.	Ref.	Ref.
2nd tertile	1.3 (0.8–2.1)	**2.1 (1.3–3.2)**	2.1 (1.2–3.5)
3rd tertile	1.6 (0.9–2.5)	1.2 (0.7–2.0)	**2.2 (1.3–3.7)**
	Multivariate model 2 [a]		
1st tertile	Ref.	Ref.	Ref.
2nd tertile	1.3 (0.8–2.2)	**2.1 (1.4–3.3)**	2.0 (1.2–3.5)
3rd tertile	1.4 (0.9–2.2)	1.1 (0.7–2.0)	**2.2 (1.3–3.7)**

[a] This model is adjusted for age, education, marital status, parental consanguinity, family history of blood pressure, number of meals not eaten at home, exposure to passive smoking and Body mass index (BMI).

Multivariate logistic regression models were used in order to determine the correlates of each of the lifestyle patterns. In each of the models, adherence to the lifestyle pattern (belonging to the third tertile *vs.* second and first tertiles) was the outcome with all socio-demographic and lifestyle characteristics as independent variables. Results showed that a higher education level was associated with the "Healthy" pattern (OR: 2.0, 95% CI: 1.2–3.2). Adherence to the "Fast food & smoking" pattern was associated with a consumption of a higher number of meals outside home (OR: 1.5, 95% CI: 1.4–1.7) and a higher exposure to passive smoking (OR: 1.10, 95% CI: 1.04–1.16). Furthermore, older subjects were less likely to adhere to this pattern (OR: 0.97, 95% CI: 0.94–0.98). While parental consanguinity was associated with a greater adherence to the "Traditional sedentary" pattern in the study sample (OR: 1.4, 95% CI: 1.0–1.9), a higher level of education was associated with a lower adherence to this pattern (OR: 0.6, 95% CI: 0.4–1.0).

4. Discussion

To our knowledge, this is the first study to investigate lifestyle patterns and their association with elevated BP. Using data stemming from the National STEPwise survey conducted in Qatar in year 2012, we identified three lifestyle patterns amongst Qatari women of reproductive age, with only the "Fast food & smoking" and "Traditional sedentary" patterns being associated with increased risk of raised BP. Together, the identified patterns explained 33.7% of the variance, which falls within the range reported in the literature (23.5%–45%) [18,20,29]. Only a few studies have adopted the lifestyle pattern approach and aimed at investigating the combined effects of food intake and other health-related lifestyle characteristics on disease risk [18,20,29]. A brief description of these studies is presented in the table below (Table 5).

Table 5. Summary of studies investigating lifestyle factors and their associations with disease among adults.

Authors's Name	Study Population	Disease Outcome	Lifestyle Factors	Main Findings
Navarro Silvera et al. (2011) [29] USA	n: 1782 Age: 30–79 years	Subtypes of Esophageal and Gastric Cancer[a]	1. Meat & nitrate; 2. Fruit & vegetable; 3. Smoking & alcohol; 4. Legume & meat alternate; 5. Gastroesophageal reflux disease (GERD) & body mass index (BMI); 6. Fish & vitamin C	<ul><li>"Meat & nitrate" intake associated with increased risk of EA, GCA, and OGA</li><li>"Fruit & vegetable" associated with reduced risk of EA, ESCC and GCA</li><li>"Smoking & alcohol" associated with increased risk of ESCC and ESCC</li><li>"GERD & obesity" associated with increased risk of EA</li><li>Fish & vitamin C" associated with increased risk of ESCC</li></ul>
Steele et al. (2014) [18] Brazil	n: 108,706 Age: >18 years Sex: 61.3% female	N/A	1 Prudent pattern: regular consumption of fruit and vegetables, daily fresh-fruit juice, and fat-reduced milk; physical activity practice, protection against UV radiation, reduced soft drink consumption; 2 Risky pattern: fat-rich meat consumption, excessive alcoholic beverage intake, current smoking, excess TV watching (especially in men), regular soft drink consumption (especially in women)	N/A
Waidyatilaka et al. (2014) [20] Sri Lanka	n: 617 Age: 30–45 years Sex: 100% females	Cardiometabolic risk variables[b]	1 Pattern 1: rice and rice flour-based products, pulses, seafood, fruits, vegetables and green leafy vegetables; 2 Pattern 2: wheat, wheat-based products and tubers, red meat, and processed meat; 3 Pattern 3: snacks dairy products and poultry, low physical activity	<ul><li>Pattern 1 has no association with dysglycaemic risk</li><li>Pattern 2 and 3 positively associated with dysglycaemic risk</li><li>Pattern 1 associated with increased HbA1c and reduced WC</li><li>Pattern 2 associated with increased WC, BMI, FM%, FM% and hs-CRP and TAG</li><li>Pattern 3 associated with increased WC, BMI, FM%, HbA1c, FBS, TC, TAG, and hs-CRP and reduced FFM% and HDL</li></ul>

[a] Subtypes of Esophageal and Gastric Cancer: Esophageal adenocarcinoma (EA), esophageal squamous cell carcinoma (ESCC), gastric cardia adenocarcinoma (GCA), other gastric cancers (OGA); [b] Cardiometabolic risk variables: dysglycaemic risk, waist circumference (WC), fat mass percentage (FM%), fat-free mass percentage (FFM%), (HbA1c), fasting blood sugar (FBS), total cholesterol (TC), high sensitivity C-reactive protein (hs-CRP), High Density Lipoproteins (HDL); TriAcylGlycerids (TAG).

As not only diet but also other lifestyle characteristics such as smoking and physical activity are known to increase the risk for elevated BP and other non-communicable diseases (NCDs), the measurement of the combined effect of these variables on disease risk provides valuable information for evidence-based and culturally sensitive primary prevention and health promotion. It was in fact suggested that disease risk increases with the number of unhealthy behaviors such as smoking, unhealthy diet and sedentary behavior [18] and that some of these unhealthy behaviors may interact to produce an even greater risk than if the individual risks are added together [30].

The findings of this study showed that the "Healthy" pattern, characterized by the consumption of plant-based foods (fruits, natural juices, vegetables, beans, whole grains) and fish, was not associated with increased risk of elevated BP in the study population. The "Healthy" pattern of this study shares many characteristics of what is usually described in the literature, as the "Prudent" or "Healthy" dietary pattern [17]. Some of the studies investigating dietary patterns in relation to the risk of hypertension have reported a protective effect from the "Prudent" or "Healthy" pattern [31,32], while others, and in accordance with our findings, have reported a lack of association [33–35]. Available evidence suggests that plant-based dietary patterns, including diets rich in fruits, vegetables, and combination diets such as the DASH (Dietary Approaches to Stop Hypertension), may be associated with BP reductions in both hypertensive and normotensive individuals [36,37]. Plant-based foods are in fact good sources of potassium, magnesium, dietary fiber and anthocyanins, all of which have been suggested to exert beneficial effects on BP regulation [12]. The "Healthy" pattern was also characterized by a higher frequency of fish consumption, which may imply a higher intake of omega 3 fatty acids. Available evidence suggests that high intakes of fish oils from supplements may be associated with BP reduction, while evidence on naturally occurring omega 3 fatty acids from fatty fish is less convincing [12]. This highlights, once more, the importance of adopting a holistic pattern dietary analysis approach, rather than investigating the consumption of individual foods, when looking at factors associated with disease risk [12]. In this context, it is important to note that the fact that the "Healthy" pattern did not load on physical activity may have diluted the protective effects of its dietary components, thus explaining the lack of association between the "Healthy" pattern and BP. In fact, substantial evidence links higher levels of physical to lower risks of hypertension and underlines a dose-dependent inverse relationship between levels of physical activity and BP [11]. The recent guidelines of the American College of Cardiology and the American Heart Association for the reduction of cardiovascular risk, including elevated BP, stress a combination of lifestyle intervention strategies that incorporate higher physical activity levels with healthy dietary patterns emphasizing vegetables, fruits, whole grains, fish, and legumes [11].

The "Fast food & smoking" pattern, which is characterized by smoking and the consumption of fast foods, sweetened beverages, and sweets, was associated with a two-fold increase in the risk of elevated BP amongst Qatari women of reproductive age, even after adjustment for potential confounders including BMI. As such, our findings demonstrate the synergistic effects of smoking with dietary habits on disease risk. Available evidence suggests that smoking is associated with increased BP, even though a clear causal relationship has not yet been documented. In a prospective cohort study based on the Women's Health Study, smoking was found to be associated with an increased risk of developing hypertension, with the strongest effect being documented among women smoking at least 15 cigarettes per day [38]. The increase in BP in smokers may depend on several factors including (1) the toxic effects of carbon monoxide and other smoking-related chemical compounds on the arterial wall; (2) the increase in red blood cell number and blood viscosity-secondary to carbon monoxide exposure [39] and (3) sympathetic and adrenergic stimulation, which is mainly caused by nicotine and its metabolites [40]. In addition to smoking, the "Fast food & smoking" pattern is also characterized by the consumption of fast food, which may imply a higher intake of salt, saturated fatty acids (SFA) and trans fatty acids (TFA). While high salt intake has been established as a risk factor for hypertension and elevated BP, the relationship between BP and the intakes of SFA and TFA is less conclusive [41–43]. It has been suggested that high SFA intakes may adversely affect vascular function and increase BP by

Nutrients **2015**, 7, 7593–7615

proinflammatory mechanisms within the endothelium [43], while TFA consumption was associated with an impairment of endothelial function, as reflected by a reduction in brachial artery flow-mediated vasodilatation [44]. Higher frequency of consumption of sweets and sugar sweetened beverages (SSBs) was another characteristic of the "Fast food & smoking" pattern, thus implying a higher intake of sugar. Even though available evidence is conflicting, a recent systematic review and meta-analysis of randomized controlled trials showed that higher intakes of sugars are associated with increased BP levels [45]. High glucose intakes and postprandial hyperglycemia were suggested to impair vascular endothelial function by inducing lipid peroxidation and decreasing Nitric Oxide bioavailability [46]. High fructose intakes have been also mechanistically linked to an impairment of insulin signaling [47], increased lipogenesis [48] and disruption of vascular homeostasis [46,49]. Interestingly, it has been postulated that increased dietary fructose and salt may exert an additive effect on BP elevation [50]. Recent studies have in fact shed new light on the role of dietary fructose in enhancing salt absorption at the levels of the intestine and the kidney, highlighting a possible synergistic effect between fructose and salt in the development of hypertension [50]. Taken together, it can be noted that even though controversy characterizes the associations between individual dietary components and BP, our study shows that a lifestyle pattern in Qatar characterized by smoking coupled with dietary habits that may increase the intake of SFA, TFA, salt and sugar is associated with a two fold increase in elevated BP risk.

In this study, women who were predominantly physically inactive and consumed more meat and refined grains ("Traditional sedentary") had also a significant increase in the risk of elevated BP. Physical inactivity has been repetitively identified as a risk factor for elevated BP and hypertension, with the protective effects of physical activity being documented in prehypertensive as well as hypertensive individuals [51–53]. A recent meta-analysis of 13 prospective cohort studies confirmed an inverse, dose–response association between levels of recreational physical activity and risk for developing hypertension [51,52]. Mechanistically, it was shown that physical activity significantly improves vascular function [54] and that habitual aerobic exercise training improves arterial stiffness [55] as well as endothelium-dependent vasorelaxation through increasing nitric oxide release [54]. The high prevalence of physical inactivity amongst Qatari women does not bode well for the future health profile of the population of Qatar. A higher frequency of red meat consumption was another characteristic of the "Traditional sedentary" pattern. The evidence on the association between meat and BP is controversial. In a prospective cohort of female US health professionals, red meat intake was positively associated with the risk of hypertension [56], while in a cross-sectional study on Dutch adults, meat protein was not found to be associated with incident hypertension [57]. In contrast, Ahhmed and Muguruma (2010) reported that meat protein may play a protective role against hypertension, a role that is mainly mediated by the angiotension-converting enzyme inhibitory activity of some of its protein hydorlysates [58]. A recent large prospective cohort of French women showed that while there was no association of unprocessed red meat consumption with hypertension, the consumption of processed red meat was significantly associated with a risk for hypertension [59]. Red meat in general, and processed meat in particular, are major sources of saturated fat and cholesterol, which have been suggested to have detrimental effects on BP control [56,60]. In addition, processed red meat is usually high in salt and contains various preservatives, additives, and other chemicals arising from food processing [56]. The advanced glycation and lipoxidation end products formed during the processing or cooking of red meat may impair insulin activity [61], induce inflammatory mediators [62] and may therefore impact BP regulation [56]. Qatar's STEPwise survey did not differentiate between the intake of processed *vs.* unprocessed meat.

The "Traditional sedentary" pattern is also characterized by a more frequent consumption of refined grains, while loading negatively on whole grains. These characteristic point towards a high glycemic index (GI) dietary pattern. Even though the evidence on the association between GI and BP is conflicting, it is suggested that high GI diets lead to postprandial hyperglycemia, which in turn increases reactive oxygen species and lowers antioxidant concentrations. These changes are associated with increased BP and reduced endothelium-dependent blood flow [63]. It is important to note that the "Traditional sedentary" pattern has also loaded on dairy products, a food group that has been associated with protective effects against hypertension [64], given its unique micronutrient composition (vitamin D, calcium, phosphorous and potassium), its rich array of bioactive lactotripeptides and its low sodium content [64]. However, several large prospective cohort studies reported benefits from consuming low-fat *versus* whole-fat dairy products [65,66]. Dairy fat is primarily saturated fat, including medium and longer chain fatty acids that are atherogenic, which may potentially counter the benefits of dairy consumption [64]. The STEPwise survey conducted in Qatar did not allow differentiation between whole versus low fat varieties of dairy products.

This study has also examined the socio-demographic determinants of the identified lifestyle patterns. Adherence to the "Healthy" pattern was found to be associated with a higher education level. In line with these findings, Steele *et al.* (2014) showed that, amongst Brazilian adults, the prudent lifestyle pattern was positively associated with the number of schooling years. Higher education levels may in fact be associated with higher nutrition knowledge, an essential precursor to healthy dietary and lifestyle habits [67]. In our study, adherence to the "Fast food & smoking" pattern was associated with a higher consumption of meals outside home, while older and married women were less likely to adhere to this pattern. Similarly, Steele *et al.* (2014) showed that adherence to what they termed the "risky pattern", characterized by the consumption of fat-rich meat, excessive alcohol and current smoking habits, was also found to be inversely associated with age. A possible explanation may be that older subjects tend to maintain traditional dietary and lifestyle habits as compared to younger generations who have greater exposure to "fashionable" foods and are more vulnerable to emerging marketing trends [68]. The inverse association between age and adherence to the "Fast food & smoking" pattern might also reflect a state of nutrition transition, from a "traditional" to a "western" lifestyle pattern, a phenomenon that typically manifests itself in younger age groups as is currently experienced by many countries of the Eastern Mediterranean region [69,70]. As for adherence to the "Traditional sedentary" pattern, it was found to be positively associated with parental consanguinity, which suggests that this pattern may be the closest to the traditional Qatari lifestyle pattern.

The present study had several strengths. Using the standardized WHO STEPwise survey approach in data collection and analysis, this study is the first to report on the association between lifestyle patterns and the risk of elevated BP. Its findings are stemming from a nationally representative sample of women of reproductive age, and weighting was performed to correct for the sample distribution. Interviewer errors and inter-observer measurement error in anthropometric assessment and BP measurement were minimized by extensive training of all interviewers to maintain quality of measurements and data collection The Arabic Global Physical Activity Questionnaire (GPAC) was used to assess physical activity, and its scoring followed a standardized approach, as recommended by the WHO. The derivation of lifestyle patterns provides a broader picture of food consumption and lifestyle components as they relate to disease risk, and may thus have more practical applications than the analysis of single foods, nutrients or behaviors.

Findings of this study should, however, be considered in light of the following limitations. First, the study had a cross-sectional design, and thus its findings can mainly be used to infer associations rather than assessing causal relationships. However, to eliminate possible reverse causation, we have excluded participants who reported having hypertension or those who reported dietary changes at the time of BP examinations (including patients with Diabetes). The rationale for the exclusion of participants with known diagnosis of hypertension was based on the fact that these participants might have received lifestyle consultations and have consequently changed their diet, exercise and smoking habits. These changes may dilute the effect of diet on elevated blood pressure and lead to a type II error.

Second, information on portion size was not collected. However, it is important to note that the complex cognitive process of portion size estimation may pose additional challenges to study participants who consume varying portion sizes across meals [71] and may not be always aware of the portion size [72]. Although quantification skills may improve with training and the use of food photograph aids [73], inclusion of portion size questions may increase respondent burden and lead to data omission, and hence contribute only marginally beyond frequency data in improving validity of the dietary assessment tool [74]. Therefore, recent research in this area has focused on the development of non-quantitative dietary questionnaires (without collection of portion size information) as targeted dietary assessment tools to rank individuals by intake of specific food groups or dietary patterns rather than providing absolute values for foods and/or nutrients [75]. Besides providing information on usual intakes of a particular food or food groups of interest, such questionnaires are particularly useful in identifying dietary patterns at the population level [76]. Third, salt intake, which is an important factor influencing BP, was not assessed in the present study. Most studies investigating the association between dietary patterns and BP did not examine salt intake, since valid assessment of salt intake necessitates the collection of 24-hour urine samples or the adoption of robust dietary assessment tools [77]. Lastly, it remains important to note that no information on alcohol intake was obtained, the latter being a possible risk factor for elevated BP. For culture-specific reasons, this information was not collected in the Qatar STEPwise survey.

5. Conclusions

This study documented a significant positive association between elevated BP and specific Qatari lifestyle patterns amongst women of reproductive age. More specifically, the "Fast food & smoking" pattern (smoking, and consumption of fast foods, sweetened beverages, and sweets) and the "Traditional sedentary" pattern (physical inactivity and the consumption of meat and refined grains) were associated with an approximately two-fold increase in the risk of elevated BP in this age group. These findings highlight the synergistic effects that diet and other lifestyle components may have on disease risk.

The results of this study therefore support the recommendations of the Eighth Report of the Joint National Committee on Prevention, Detection, Evaluation, and Treatment of High Blood Pressure (JNC 8) and the European Society of Hypertension/European Society of Hypertension of Cardiology, which state that appropriate lifestyle interventions, including increased physical activity and the adoption of healthy dietary patterns, should be fostered for the prevention and treatment of hypertension [51]. Qatar launched, in April 2015, the Qatar Dietary Guidelines, which aim at directing both individual behavior change and the development of health and food policies in Qatar [78]. It would be of value to revisit the guidelines in light of the information provided in this study and investigate the impact of these guidelines on dietary habits of the population in general and of Qatari women in particular.

Acknowledgments: The study was funded by the Supreme Council of Health, Doha, Qatar. The authors wish to thank the Ministry of Development Planning and Statistics, Hamad Medical Corporation (HMC), Primary Health Care Corporation (PHCC) and Qatar Diabetes Association (QDA) for their firm commitment and work. The authors express their deep gratitude to all survey team members as well as to all the subjects who participated in this study.

Author Contributions: M.A.T. conceptualized the study, supervised all related activities and evaluated its significance to Qatar; A.A.T. contributed to study design and, in her capacity as a WHO focal point, coordinated various aspects of the study; W.A.C. supervised data collection and contributed to the interpretation of the data; B.A.M. managed and supervised data collection and coordinated field work; S.H.K. supervised data management and coding; A.H.B. led the narrative reporting of the 2012 Qatar WHO STEPwise survey; N.H. contributed to the conceptualization of the study and to the interpretation of the data; L.N and F.N conducted data analysis and wrote the manuscript. All authors read and approved the final manuscript and critically reviewed the manuscript.

Conflicts of Interest: The authors declare no conflict of interest.

References

1. Lim, S.S.; Vos, T.; Flaxman, A.D.; Danaei, G.; Shibuya, K.; Adair-Rohani, H.; AlMazroa, M.A.; Amann, M.; Anderson, H.R.; Andrews, K.G. A comparative risk assessment of burden of disease and injury attributable to 67 risk factors and risk factor clusters in 21 regions, 1990–2010: A systematic analysis for the Global Burden of Disease Study 2010. *Lancet* **2013**, *380*, 2224–2260. [CrossRef]
2. World Health Organization. *A Global Brief on Hypertension: Silent Killer, Global Public Health Crisis*; World Health Organization: Geneva, Switzerland, 2013.
3. Raised Blood Pressure (SBP ≥ 140 or DBP ≥ 90): Data by WHO Region. Available online: http://apps.who.int/gho/data/view.main.2540?lang=en (accessed on 5 May 2015).
4. Kearney, P.M.; Whelton, M.; Reynolds, K.; Muntner, P.; Whelton, P.K.; He, J. Global burden of hypertension: Analysis of worldwide data. *Lancet* **2005**, *365*, 217–223. [CrossRef]
5. World Health Organization. *World Health Survey*; World Health Organization: Geneva, Switzerland, 2006.
6. Haj Bakri, A.; Al-Thani, A. *Chronic Disease Risk Factor Surveillance: Qatar STEPS Report 2012*; Supreme Council of Health: Doha, Qatar, 2013.
7. Bramham, K.; Parnell, B.; Nelson-Piercy, C.; Seed, P.T.; Poston, L.; Chappell, L.C. Chronic hypertension and pregnancy outcomes: Systematic review and meta-analysis. *BMJ* **2014**, *348*. Available online: http://www.bmj.com/content/348/bmj.g2301 (accessed on 4 May 2015). [CrossRef] [PubMed]
8. Lovgren, T.R.; Galan, H.L. Preeclampsia: The Compromised Fetus, the Compromised Mother. In *Anesthesia and the Fetus*; Wiley-Blackwell: Oxford, UK, 2013; pp. 303–314.
9. Ramakrishnan, A.; Lee, L.J.; Mitchell, L.E.; Agopian, A.J. Maternal Hypertension during Pregnancy and the Risk of Congenital Heart Defects in Offspring: A Systematic Review and Meta-analysis. *Pediatr. Cardiol.* **2015**. Available online: http://link.springer.com/article/10.1007%2Fs00246-015-1182-9 (accessed on 11 May 2015). [CrossRef] [PubMed]
10. De Marco, M.; de Simone, G.; Roman, M.J.; Chinali, M.; Lee, E.T.; Russell, M.; Howard, B.V.; Devereux, R.B. Cardiovascular and metabolic predictors of progression of prehypertension into hypertension: The Strong Heart Study. *Hypertension* **2009**, *54*, 974–980. [CrossRef] [PubMed]
11. Eckel, R.H.; Jakicic, J.M.; Ard, J.D.; de Jesus, J.M.; Houston Miller, N.; Hubbard, V.S.; Lee, I.M.; Lichtenstein, A.H.; Loria, C.M.; Millen, B.E.; *et al.* 2013 AHA/ACC guideline on lifestyle management to reduce cardiovascular risk: A report of the American College of Cardiology/American Heart Association Task Force on Practice Guidelines. *J. Am. Coll. Cardiol.* **2014**, *63*, 2960–2984. [CrossRef]
12. Bazzano, L.A.; Green, T.; Harrison, T.N.; Reynolds, K. Dietary approaches to prevent hypertension. *Curr. Hypertens. Rep.* **2013**, *15*, 694–702. [CrossRef] [PubMed]
13. Teunissen-Beekman, K.F.; van Baak, M.A. The role of dietary protein in blood pressure regulation. *Curr. Opin. Lipidol.* **2013**, *24*, 65–70. [CrossRef] [PubMed]
14. Streppel, M.T.; Arends, L.R.; van't Veer, P.; Grobbee, D.E.; Geleijnse, J.M. Dietary fiber and blood pressure: A meta-analysis of randomized placebo-controlled trials. *Arch. Intern. Med.* **2005**, *165*, 150–156. [CrossRef] [PubMed]
15. Jacques, P.F.; Tucker, K.L. Are dietary patterns useful for understanding the role of diet in chronic disease? *Am. J. Clin. Nutr.* **2001**, *73*, 1–2. [PubMed]
16. Jiang, J.; Liu, M.; Parvez, F.; Wang, B.; Wu, F.; Eunus, M.; Bangalore, S.; Ahmed, A.; Islam, T.; Rakibuz-Zaman, M. Association of major dietary patterns and blood pressure longitudinal change in Bangladesh. *J. Hypertens.* **2015**, *33*, 1193–1200. [CrossRef] [PubMed]
17. Shi, Z.; Taylor, A.W.; Atlantis, E.; Wittert, G.A. Empirically derived dietary patterns and hypertension. *Curr. Nutr. Rep.* **2012**, *1*, 73–86. [CrossRef]
18. Steele, E.M.; Claro, R.M.; Monteiro, C.A. Behavioural patterns of protective and risk factors for non-communicable diseases in Brazil. *Public Health Nutr.* **2014**, *17*, 369–375. [CrossRef] [PubMed]
19. Gubbels, J.S.; Kremers, S.P.; Stafleu, A.; Goldbohm, R.A.; de Vries, N.K.; Thijs, C. Clustering of energy balance-related behaviors in 5-year-old children: Lifestyle patterns and their longitudinal association with weight status development in early childhood. *Int. J. Behav. Nutr. Phys. Act.* **2012**, *9*, 77. Available online: http://www.ncbi.nlm.nih.gov/pmc/articles/PMC3441251/pdf/1479-5868-9-77.png (accessed on 6 May 2015). [CrossRef] [PubMed]

20. Waidyatilaka, I.; de Silva, A.; de Lanerolle-Dias, M.; Wickremasinghe, R.; Atukorala, S.; Somasundaram, N.; Lanerolle, P. Lifestyle patterns and dysglycaemic risk in urban Sri Lankan women. *Br. J. Nutr.* **2014**, *112*, 952–957. [CrossRef] [PubMed]

21. Final Results of Census 2010. Available online: http://www.qsa.gov.qa/qatarcensus/Census_Results.aspx (accessed on 8 May 2015).

22. Global Physical Activity Surveillance. Available online: http://www.who.int/chp/steps/GPAQ/en/ (accessed on 20 March 2015).

23. World Health Organization. In *Global Physical Activity Questionnaire (GPAQ) Analysis Guide*; World Health Organization: Geneva, Switzerland, 2012.

24. Hallal, P.C.; Andersen, L.B.; Bull, F.C.; Guthold, R.; Haskell, W.; Ekelund, U. Global physical activity levels: Surveillance progress, pitfalls, and prospects. *Lancet* **2012**, *380*, 247–257. [CrossRef]

25. Wong, J.E.; Parnell, W.R.; Black, K.E.; Skidmore, P.M. Reliability and relative validity of a food frequency questionnaire to assess food group intakes in New Zealand adolescents. *Nutr. J.* **2012**, *11*. [CrossRef] [PubMed]

26. Expert Panel on Detection Evaluation and Treatment of High Blood Cholesterol in Adults. Executive summary of the third report of the national cholesterol education program (NCEP) expert panel on detection, evaluation, and treatment of high blood cholesterol in adults (adult treatment panel III). *JAMA* **2001**, *285*, 2486–2497.

27. Alberti, K.G.; Eckel, R.H.; Grundy, S.M.; Zimmet, P.Z.; Cleeman, J.I.; Donato, K.A.; Fruchart, J.C.; James, W.P.; Loria, C.M.; Smith, S.C., Jr. Harmonizing the metabolic syndrome: A joint interim statement of the International Diabetes Federation Task Force on Epidemiology and Prevention; National Heart, Lung, and Blood Institute; American Heart Association; World Heart Federation; International Atherosclerosis Society; and International Association for the Study of Obesity. *Circulation* **2009**, *120*, 1640–1645. [PubMed]

28. IBM Corp. *IBM SPSS Statistics for Windows, 14.1*; IBM Corp.: Armonk, NY, USA, 2010.

29. Navarro Silvera, S.A.; Mayne, S.T.; Risch, H.A.; Gammon, M.D.; Vaughan, T.; Chow, W.H.; Dubin, J.A.; Dubrow, R.; Schoenberg, J.; Stanford, J.L.; *et al.* Principal component analysis of dietary and lifestyle patterns in relation to risk of subtypes of esophageal and gastric cancer. *Ann. Epidemiol.* **2011**, *21*, 543–550. [CrossRef] [PubMed]

30. Meng, L.; Maskarinec, G.; Lee, J.; Kolonel, L.N. Lifestyle factors and chronic diseases: Application of a composite risk index. *Prev. Med.* **1999**, *29*, 296–304. [CrossRef] [PubMed]

31. Wang, D.; He, Y.; Li, Y.; Luan, D.; Yang, X.; Zhai, F.; Ma, G. Dietary patterns and hypertension among Chinese adults: A nationally representative cross-sectional study. *BMC Public Health* **2011**, *11*, 1–10. Available online: http://www.biomedcentral.com/1471-2458/11/925 (accessed on 8 May 2015). [CrossRef] [PubMed]

32. Sadakane, A.; Tsutsumi, A.; Gotoh, T.; Ishikawa, S.; Ojima, T.; Kario, K.; Nakamura, Y.; Kayaba, K. Dietary patterns and levels of blood pressure and serum lipids in a Japanese population. *J. Epidemiol.* **2008**, *18*, 58–67. [CrossRef] [PubMed]

33. Oliveira, A.; Rodriguez-Artalejo, F.; Gaio, R.; Santos, A.C.; Ramos, E.; Lopes, C. Major habitual dietary patterns are associated with acute myocardial infarction and cardiovascular risk markers in a southern European population. *J. Am. Diet. Assoc.* **2011**, *111*, 241–250. [CrossRef] [PubMed]

34. Villegas, R.; Kearney, P.M.; Perry, I.J. The cumulative effect of core lifestyle behaviours on the prevalence of hypertension and dyslipidemia. *BMC Public Health* **2008**, *8*, 210. [CrossRef] [PubMed]

35. Qin, Y.; Melse-Boonstra, A.; Pan, X.; Zhao, J.; Yuan, B.; Dai, Y.; Zhou, M.; Geleijnse, J.M.; Kok, F.J.; Shi, Z. Association of dietary pattern and body weight with blood pressure in Jiangsu Province, China. *BMC Public Health* **2014**, *14*, 948. [CrossRef] [PubMed]

36. Berkow, S.E.; Barnard, N.D. Blood pressure regulation and vegetarian diets. *Nutr. Rev.* **2005**, *63*, 1–8. [CrossRef] [PubMed]

37. Wang, L.; Manson, J.E.; Gaziano, J.M.; Buring, J.E.; Sesso, H.D. Fruit and vegetable intake and the risk of hypertension in middle-aged and older women. *Am. J. Hypertens.* **2012**, *25*, 180–189. [CrossRef] [PubMed]

38. Bowman, T.S.; Gaziano, J.M.; Buring, J.E.; Sesso, H.D. A prospective study of cigarette smoking and risk of incident hypertension in women. *J. Am. Coll. Cardiol.* **2007**, *50*, 2085–2092. [CrossRef] [PubMed]

39. Levenson, J.; Simon, A.C.; Cambien, F.A.; Beretti, C. Cigarette smoking and hypertension. Factors independently associated with blood hyperviscosity and arterial rigidity. *Arteriosclerosis* **1987**, *7*, 572–577. [CrossRef] [PubMed]

40. Leone, A. Smoking and hypertension: Independent or additive effects to determining vascular damage? *Curr. Vasc. Pharmacol.* **2011**, *9*, 585–593. [CrossRef] [PubMed]

41. World Health Organization. *Guideline: Sodium Intake for Adults and Children*; World Health Organization: Geneva, Switzerland, 2012.

42. European Food Safety Authority. Opinion of the scientific panel on dietetic products, nutrition and allergies on a request from the commission related to the presence of trans fatty acids in foods and the effect on human health of the consumption of trans fatty acids. *EFSA J.* **2004**, *81*, 1–49.

43. Hall, W.L. Dietary saturated and unsaturated fats as determinants of blood pressure and vascular function. *Nutr. Res. Rev.* **2009**, *22*, 18–38. [CrossRef] [PubMed]

44. De Roos, N.M.; Bots, M.L.; Katan, M.B. Replacement of dietary saturated fatty acids by trans fatty acids lowers serum HDL cholesterol and impairs endothelial function in healthy men and women. *Arterioscler. Thromb. Vasc. Biol.* **2001**, *21*, 1233–1237. [CrossRef] [PubMed]

45. Te Morenga, L.A.; Howatson, A.J.; Jones, R.M.; Mann, J. Dietary sugars and cardiometabolic risk: Systematic review and meta-analyses of randomized controlled trials of the effects on blood pressure and lipids. *Am. J. Clin. Nutr.* **2014**, *100*, 65–79. [CrossRef] [PubMed]

46. Mah, E.; Noh, S.K.; Ballard, K.D.; Matos, M.E.; Volek, J.S.; Bruno, R.S. Postprandial hyperglycemia impairs vascular endothelial function in healthy men by inducing lipid peroxidation and increasing asymmetric dimethylarginine:arginine. *J. Nutr.* **2011**, *141*, 1961–1968. [CrossRef] [PubMed]

47. Stanhope, K.L.; Schwarz, J.M.; Keim, N.L.; Griffen, S.C.; Bremer, A.A.; Graham, J.L.; Hatcher, B.; Cox, C.L.; Dyachenko, A.; Zhang, W. Consuming fructose-sweetened, not glucose-sweetened, beverages increases visceral adiposity and lipids and decreases insulin sensitivity in overweight/obese humans. *J. Clin. Investig.* **2009**, *119*, 1322–1334. [CrossRef] [PubMed]

48. Samuel, V.T. Fructose induced lipogenesis: From sugar to fat to insulin resistance. *Trends Endocrinol. Metab.* **2011**, *22*, 60–65. [CrossRef] [PubMed]

49. Siervo, M.; Montagnese, C.; Mathers, J.C.; Soroka, K.R.; Stephan, B.C.; Wells, J.C. Sugar consumption and global prevalence of obesity and hypertension: An ecological analysis. *Public Health Nutr.* **2014**, *17*, 587–596. [CrossRef] [PubMed]

50. Madero, M.; Perez-Pozo, S.E.; Jalal, D.; Johnson, R.J.; Sanchez-Lozada, L.G. Dietary fructose and hypertension. *Curr. Hypertens. Rep.* **2011**, *13*, 29–35. [CrossRef] [PubMed]

51. Kokkinos, P. Cardiorespiratory fitness, exercise, and blood pressure. *Hypertension* **2014**, *64*, 1160–1164. [CrossRef] [PubMed]

52. Huai, P.; Xun, H.; Reilly, K.H.; Wang, Y.; Ma, W.; Xi, B. Physical activity and risk of hypertension: A meta-analysis of prospective cohort studies. *Hypertension* **2013**, *62*, 1021–1026. [CrossRef] [PubMed]

53. Brook, R.D.; Appel, L.J.; Rubenfire, M.; Ogedegbe, G.; Bisognano, J.D.; Elliott, W.J.; Fuchs, F.D.; Hughes, J.W.; Lackland, D.T.; Staffileno, B.A.; et al. Beyond medications and diet: Alternative approaches to lowering blood pressure. *Hypertension* **2013**, *61*, 1360–1383. [CrossRef] [PubMed]

54. Pal, S.; Radavelli-Bagatini, S.; Ho, S. Potential benefits of exercise on blood pressure and vascular function. *J. Am. Soc. Hypertens.* **2013**, *7*, 494–506. [CrossRef] [PubMed]

55. Seals, D.R.; Moreau, K.L.; Gates, P.E.; Eskurza, I. Modulatory influences on ageing of the vasculature in healthy humans. *Exp. Gerontol.* **2006**, *41*, 501–507. [CrossRef] [PubMed]

56. Wang, L.; Manson, J.E.; Buring, J.E.; Sesso, H.D. Meat intake and the risk of hypertension in middle-aged and older women. *J. Hypertens.* **2008**, *26*, 215–222. [CrossRef] [PubMed]

57. Altorf-van der Kuil, W.; Engberink, M.F.; Geleijnse, J.M.; Boer, J.M.; Monique Verschuren, W.M. Sources of dietary protein and risk of hypertension in a general Dutch population. *Br. J. Nutr.* **2012**, *108*, 1897–1903. [CrossRef] [PubMed]

58. Ahhmed, A.M.; Muguruma, M. A review of meat protein hydrolysates and hypertension. *Meat Sci.* **2010**, *86*, 110–118. [CrossRef] [PubMed]

59. Lajous, M.; Bijon, A.; Fagherazzi, G.; Rossignol, E.; Boutron-Ruault, M.C.; Clavel-Chapelon, F. Processed and unprocessed red meat consumption and hypertension in women. *Am. J. Clin. Nutr.* **2014**, *100*, 948–952. [CrossRef] [PubMed]

60. Stamler, J.; Liu, K.; Ruth, K.J.; Pryer, J.; Greenland, P. Eight-year blood pressure change in middle-aged men: Relationship to multiple nutrients. *Hypertension* **2002**, *39*, 1000–1006. [CrossRef] [PubMed]

61. Peppa, M.; Goldberg, T.; Cai, W.; Rayfield, E.; Vlassara, H. Glycotoxins: A missing link in the "relationship of dietary fat and meat intake in relation to risk of type 2 diabetes in men". *Diabetes Care* **2002**, *25*, 1898–1899. [CrossRef] [PubMed]

62. Vlassara, H.; Cai, W.; Crandall, J.; Goldberg, T.; Oberstein, R.; Dardaine, V.; Peppa, M.; Rayfield, E.J. Inflammatory mediators are induced by dietary glycotoxins, a major risk factor for diabetic angiopathy. *Proc. Natl. Acad. Sci. USA* **2002**, *99*, 15596–15601. [CrossRef] [PubMed]

63. Title, L.M.; Cummings, P.M.; Giddens, K.; Nassar, B.A. Oral glucose loading acutely attenuates endothelium-dependent vasodilation in healthy adults without diabetes: An effect prevented by vitamins C and E. *J. Am. Coll. Cardiol.* **2000**, *36*, 2185–2191. [CrossRef]

64. McGrane, M.M.; Essery, E.; Obbagy, J.; Lyon, J.; MacNeil, P.; Spahn, J.; van Horn, L. Dairy consumption, blood pressure, and risk of hypertension: An evidence-based review of recent literature. *Curr. Cardiovasc. Risk Rep.* **2011**, *5*, 287–298. [CrossRef] [PubMed]

65. Toledo, E.; Delgado-Rodriguez, M.; Estruch, R.; Salas-Salvado, J.; Corella, D.; Gomez-Gracia, E.; Fiol, M.; Lamuela-Raventos, R.M.; Schroder, H.; Aros, F.; *et al.* Low-fat dairy products and blood pressure: Follow-up of 2290 older persons at high cardiovascular risk participating in the PREDIMED study. *Br. J. Nutr.* **2009**, *101*, 59–67. [CrossRef] [PubMed]

66. Alonso, A.; Beunza, J.J.; Delgado-Rodriguez, M.; Martinez, J.A.; Martinez-Gonzalez, M.A. Low-fat dairy consumption and reduced risk of hypertension: The Seguimiento Universidad de Navarra (SUN) cohort. *Am. J. Clin. Nutr.* **2005**, *82*, 972–979. [PubMed]

67. Darmon, N.; Drewnowski, A. Does social class predict diet quality? *Am. J. Clin. Nutr.* **2008**, *87*, 1107–1117. [PubMed]

68. Hu, E.A.; Toledo, E.; Diez-Espino, J.; Estruch, R.; Corella, D.; Salas-Salvado, J.; Vinyoles, E.; Gomez-Gracia, E.;Aros, F.; Fiol, M.; *et al.* Lifestyles and risk factors associated with adherence to the Mediterranean diet: A baseline assessment of the PREDIMED trial. *PLoS ONE* **2013**, *8*, e60166. Available online: http://journals.plos.org/plosone/article?id=10.1371/journal.pone.0060166 (accessed on 15 May 2015). [CrossRef] [PubMed]

69. Naja, F.; Nasreddine, L.; Itani, L.; Chamieh, M.C.; Adra, N.; Sibai, A.M.; Hwalla, N. Dietary patterns and their association with obesity and sociodemographic factors in a national sample of Lebanese adults. *Public Health Nutr.* **2011**, *14*, 1570–1578. [CrossRef] [PubMed]

70. Nasreddine, L.; Hwalla, N.; Sibai, A.; Hamze, M.; Parent-Massin, D. Food consumption patterns in an adult urban population in Beirut, Lebanon. *Public Health Nutr.* **2006**, *9*, 194–203. [CrossRef] [PubMed]

71. Watanabe, M.; Yamaoka, K.; Yokotsuka, M.; Adachi, M.; Tango, T. Validity and reproducibility of the FFQ (FFQW82) for dietary assessment in female adolescents. *Public Health Nutr.* **2011**, *14*, 297–305. [CrossRef] [PubMed]

72. Livingstone, M.B.; Robson, P.J. Measurement of dietary intake in children. *Proc. Nutr. Soc.* **2000**, *59*, 279–293. [CrossRef] [PubMed]

73. Foster, E.; Matthews, J.N.; Nelson, M.; Harris, J.M.; Mathers, J.C.; Adamson, A.J. Accuracy of estimates of food portion size using food photographs—The importance of using age-appropriate tools. *Public Health Nutr.* **2006**, *9*, 509–514. [CrossRef] [PubMed]

74. Schlundt, D.G.; Buchowski, M.S.; Hargreaves, M.K.; Hankin, J.H.; Signorello, L.B.; Blot, W.J. Separate estimates of portion size were not essential for energy and nutrient estimation: Results from the Southern Community Cohort food-frequency questionnaire pilot study. *Public Health Nutr.* **2007**, *10*, 245–251. [CrossRef] [PubMed]

75. Magarey, A.; Watson, J.; Golley, R.K.; Burrows, T.; Sutherland, R.; McNaughton, S.A.; Denney-Wilson, E.; Campbell, K.; Collins, C. Assessing dietary intake in children and adolescents: Considerations and recommendations for obesity research. *Int. J. Pediatr. Obes.* **2011**, *6*, 2–11. [CrossRef] [PubMed]

76. Magarey, A.; Golley, R.; Spurrier, N.; Goodwin, E.; Ong, F. Reliability and validity of the Children's Dietary Questionnaire; a new tool to measure children's dietary patterns. *Int. J. Pediatr. Obes.* **2009**, *4*, 257–265. [CrossRef] [PubMed]

77. Bentley, B. A review of methods to measure dietary sodium intake. *J. Cardiovasc. Nurs.* **2006**, *21*, 63–67. [CrossRef] [PubMed]

78. Supreme Council of Health (Qatar).   *Qatar Dietary Guidelines*; Supreme Council of Health: Doha, Qatar, 2015. Available online: http://eservices.sch.gov.qa/qdg/En/download.jsp (accessed on 2 August 2015).

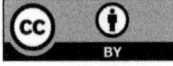

nutrients

MDPI

Article

A Western Dietary Pattern Is Associated with Poor Academic Performance in Australian Adolescents

Anett Nyaradi [1,2,*], Jianghong Li [2,3,4], Siobhan Hickling [1], Jonathan K. Foster [2,5,6,7], Angela Jacques [1], Gina L. Ambrosini [1,2] and Wendy H. Oddy [2]

[1] School of Population Health, The University of Western Australia, Perth 6009, Australia; Siobhan.Hickling@uwa.edu.au (S.H.); Gina.Ambrosini@uwa.edu.au (G.L.A.); Angela.Jacques@uwa.edu.au (A.J.)
[2] Telethon Kids Institute, The University of Western Australia, Perth 6008, Australia; jianghong.li@wzb.eu (J.L.); J.Foster@curtin.edu.au (J.K.F.); Wendy.Oddy@telethonkids.org.au (W.H.O.)
[3] WZB Berlin Social Research Center, Reichpietschufer 50 D-10785 Berlin, Germany
[4] Centre for Population Health Research, The Faculty of Health Sciences, Curtin University, Perth 6102, Australia
[5] School of Psychology & Speech Pathology, Curtin University; Perth 6102, Australia
[6] Neurosciences Unit, Health Department of Western Australia; Perth 6010, Australia
[7] School of Paediatrics & Child Health, The University of Western Australia, Perth 6008, Australia
* Author to whom correspondence should be addressed; Anett.Nyaradi@telethonkids.org.au; Tel.: +61-8-9489-7777; Fax: +61-8-9489-7700.

Received: 12 March 2015; Accepted: 10 April 2015; Published: 17 April 2015

Abstract: The aim of this study was to investigate cross-sectional associations between dietary patterns and academic performance among 14-year-old adolescents. Study participants were from the Western Australian Pregnancy Cohort (Raine) Study. A food frequency questionnaire was administered when the adolescents were 14 years old, and from the dietary data, a 'Healthy' and a 'Western' dietary pattern were identified by factor analysis. The Western Australian Literacy and Numeracy Assessment (WALNA) results from grade nine (age 14) were linked to the Raine Study data by The Western Australian Data Linkage Branch. Associations between the dietary patterns and the WALNA (mathematics, reading and writing scores) were assessed using multivariate linear regression models adjusting for family and socioeconomic characteristics. Complete data on dietary patterns, academic performance and covariates were available for individuals across the different analyses as follows: $n = 779$ for mathematics, $n = 741$ for reading and $n = 470$ for writing. Following adjustment, significant negative associations between the 'Western' dietary pattern and test scores for mathematics ($\beta = -13.14$; 95% CI: -24.57; -1.76); $p = 0.024$) and reading ($\beta = -19.16$; 95% CI: -29.85; -8.47; $p \leq 0.001$) were observed. A similar trend was found with respect to writing ($\beta = -17.28$; 95% CI: -35.74; 1.18; $p = 0.066$). ANOVA showed significant trends in estimated means of academic scores across quartiles for both the Western and Healthy patterns. Higher scores for the 'Western' dietary pattern are associated with poorer academic performance in adolescence.

Keywords: diet; academic performance; adolescence; Raine Study

1. Introduction

Adolescence is a period of life when major psychosocial and biological changes occur, resulting in the highest nutrient requirement at any time across the lifecycle [1]. Adolescence is also an important stage for brain development, characterized by synaptic pruning, myelination and a growing number of neural connections, especially in the prefrontal cortex [2,3]. Adolescence is a vulnerable period of the life course with regard to nutrition because, with increasing independence from parents, food choices are more frequently made by adolescents. During this time of development, peer pressure and media promotion exert a relatively greater influence on food purchases, often in favour of less healthy nutritional choices [1].

The academic performance of children and adolescents has been a focus for public health researchers. School performance influences future education, which ultimately shapes an individuals' socioeconomic status; in which in turn, is associated with health and health behaviour [4]. Nutrition is one of the most important and modifiable environmental factors that may affect brain development, and therefore cognition and academic performance [5].

Relatively little research has reported the effect of diet on academic performance in adolescents. Having regular lunch and dinner were negatively associated, while higher consumption of soft drinks, pizza, hot dogs, sweets and snacks that indicated poor diet were positively associated with self-reported learning difficulties in mathematics in Norwegian adolescents. Moreover, regular breakfast in the same study was negatively linked with learning difficulties in mathematics, reading and writing [6]. In Korea, regular meals have been linked with higher academic performance in adolescents [7]. A study in Iceland reported lower academic achievement in adolescents with increased consumption of French fries, hamburgers and hot dogs indicating poor dietary habits and higher academic scores in adolescents with positive dietary habits, consuming more fruits and vegetables [8]. In Sweden, adolescents who consumed more fish during the week, had higher academic grades [9]. Researchers showed positive associations between higher fruits, vegetables and milk consumption and academic achievement in Canadian adolescents [10].

In the present study, based on the findings reported in the extant literature, we hypothesised that a healthier diet would be associated with higher academic achievement (specifically mathematics, reading and writing achievement) and conversely a western type diet with poorer academic performance in Australian adolescents at 14 years of age.

2. Methods

2.1. Study Population

The study utilised data from the Western Australian Pregnancy Cohort (Raine) Study. In the original study, 2900 pregnant women from Perth, Western Australia, were serially recruited between 1989 and 1991 into a randomised controlled trial to study the effects of pregnancy ultrasounds on the newborn [11]. The women, enrolled in the study at between 16 to 20 weeks' pregnant when they presented at King Edward Memorial Hospital, the major tertiary maternity facility in Perth, Western Australia and surrounding private practices. A total of 2868 babies (born between 1989 and 1992) and their families were followed up at regular intervals. Ethics approval was granted by The Human Ethics Committee at King Edward Memorial Hospital and Princess Margaret Hospital for children. The current study was approved by the University of Western Australia Human Research Ethics Committee.

Access to the educational data through a data linkage process was approved by the Western Australian Department of Health Human Research Ethics Committee. Parents and participants provided informed consent at each follow-up. At aged 18 years Raine Study participants consented to future follow-up investigations. For this analysis, we included data collected at the one, eight and 14-year cohort follow-ups (*i.e.*, core data collected at age 14 plus data for potential confounders collected at earlier time points).

2.2. Dietary Patterns

Dietary data were collected using a semi-quantitative food frequency questionnaire (FFQ) developed by the Commonwealth Scientific and Industrial Research Organisation (CSIRO), Adelaide, Australia [12,13]. This questionnaire was administered and evaluated at 14 years of age in the Raine cohort [14]. The FFQ was mailed to study families; primary caregiver completed the FFQ, in consultation with the adolescent participant and 1631 questionnaires were returned for analysis. Information on the usual frequency of consumption and typical serve size over the past 12 months for 212 foods was collected by the FFQ. Intakes of these foods were then grouped into 38 major food groups, measured as grams per day of intake [15].

Dietary patterns were derived by factor analysis (sample size = 1613) from the major food groups; this process was limited to factors with an eigenvalue >1, and varimax rotation was undertaken to improve the separation and interpretability of the factors [15]. Two major dietary patterns were identified where factor 1 explained 50% of the common variance shared by food group intakes (13% of total variance) and factor 2 explained 34% of the common variance in food intakes (8.5% of the total variance); these patterns were named 'Healthy' (factor 1: high in fruits, vegetables, whole grains, legumes and fish) and 'Western' (factor 2: high intake of take-away foods, red and processed meat, soft drinks, fried and refined food) [15]. Each subject received a dietary pattern score, measured as a z-score for each pattern (one dietary pattern does not exclude the other pattern in an individual because a combination of foods are eaten). Total energy intake was estimated by linking the recorded food intakes for each individual from the FFQ with the Australian Food Composition Tables by the CSIRO [15]. Total energy intake was included in our analysis as a covariate. Details of the methodology, the reliability and the validity of the FFQ have been previously published [14–16]. The dietary patterns with factor loadings are shown in Supplementary Table 1.

2.3. Western Australian Literacy and Numeracy Assessment (WALNA) Score

The Western Australian Literacy and Numeracy Assessment (WALNA) was administered and collected by the Western Australian Department of Education to all students in Western Australia annually in grades three (age eight years), five (age ten years), seven (age 12 years) and nine (age 14 years) between 1998–2007. This was part of an Australia-wide program, such that the findings are comparable with similar assessment programs undertaken in other Australian states and their results were reported against nationally agreed benchmarks. The WALNA data include test results for mathematics, reading, writing (in grades three, five, seven and nine) and spelling (in grades three, five and seven). These educational data were obtained from a combination of multiple-choice, open-response and short-response questions, and only year nine data are reported here. The standardized raw scores for each of the mathematics, reading, writing and spelling scores were summed via an ordinal scale and converted into an interval scale. This process was completed using a Rasch measurement model [17] for easier understanding and interpretation of results. In the Rasch score all subjects are placed on a common scale, and it is a standard practice in the analysis of educational data as shown in previous studies [18,19].

With respect to the interval scale for all four areas of assessment (mathematics, reading, writing and spelling), higher scores represent higher levels of achievement. Educational professionals assessed the content and construct validity of the WALNA measures each year; these analyses demonstrate an internal reliability of 0.8 [18].

In our study, we used the grade nine (age 14 years) WALNA data that included mathematics, reading and writing scores. A probabilistic method of matching at the individual level (based on a full name, date of birth, gender and address) was used by The Western Australian Data Linkage Branch to link the WALNA to the Raine study has an accuracy of >99% (18). Once the links were created, only deidentified data from both sources were provided to the researchers for analysis, ensuring that no individual level data were accessed as part of the 'separation principle' [20].

2.4. Covariates

Sociodemographic characteristics identified as maternal education, maternal race, family income, family functioning and the presence of the biological father in the family were included in the analyses as potential confounders. Maternal education (collected at the eight year follow-up in the Raine Study) was considered in eight categories: (i) did not finish high school; (ii) finished high school and completed the tertiary entrance exam; (iii) trade/apprentice certificate; (iv) college/TAFE (Technical and Further Education) certificate; (v) diploma; (vi) bachelor degree; (vii) postgraduate degree; and (viii) 'other'. Maternal race was characterized into three categories (Caucasian; Aboriginal; "other"), while family income (collected at the 14 year follow-up) was classified according to four levels: ≤$25,000; $25,001–$50,000; $50,001–$78,000; and >$78,000 per annum. Family functioning (14 years follow-up) was included in the analysis as a continuous variable (higher scores represented better functioning) and was measured by the McMaster Family Assessment Device [21]. This measure collected information about family communication, problem solving, affective responsiveness and behaviour control. The presence of the biological father in the family when the child was 14 years of age was dichotomised as 'yes' or 'no'.

Characteristics of adolescents including gender, body mass index ((BMI) (kg/m^2) weights and heights) and the level of physical activity (outside of school hours) were obtained. We included these variables in the statistical models, because both BMI and physical activity have been associated with cognitive performance and academic achievement in adolescents [22,23]. BMI was grouped into four categories defined by Cole [24]: underweight, normal weight, overweight and obese. Participants were assigned to three categories of physical activity using a questionnaire, as per previous studies using Raine data [15]: <1 time/week; 1–3 times/week; and 4+ times/week.

The diet score at one year of age was based on the infants' dietary intake over the previous 24 h. Data from more than 2000 foods were collapsed into food groups and a continuous score was developed that provided a score between 0–70 (higher score representing better diet) [25]. This diet score was included in the analyses, as it was previously found in the Raine Study that diet during infancy was associated with cognitive development in middle childhood and may be a predictor for later academic performance [26,27].

2.5. Statistical Analysis

The data were initially analysed to generate descriptive statistics. We then built three models using multivariable linear regression to evaluate the relationship between diet and the WALNA scores at age 14. In model one, we minimally adjusted for total energy intake to ensure that outcomes were independent of total energy consumption. In model two, we additionally adjusted for maternal education and race, family income and functioning, the presence of biological father in the family, diet score at one year and child gender. In model three, we adjusted for all variables that had been included in models one and two, but additionally included adolescent BMI and physical activity level to determine if these covariates modified our results. Finally, we examined 21 key food groups identified as the main contributors to the dietary patterns (as continuous variables, measured by grams/day intake) with factor loadings ≥0.30 across both 'Healthy' and 'Western' dietary patterns (Table 1) in order to identify those food groups specifically associated with academic scores. All analyses were performed using IBM SPSS Statistics 22. Results are reported using a significance level (*i.e.*, alpha) of 0.05.

3. Results

Table 1 lists the characteristics of the Raine cohort included in this study. Complete data for mathematics, reading and writing scores were available for *n* = 779, *n* = 741 and *n* = 470 adolescents, respectively. The descriptive statistics did not differ significantly across all three samples according to the academic subjects.

Table 1. Descriptive characteristics of the Western Australian Pregnancy Cohort (Raine) Study at age 14 by educational outcomes, mathematics, reading and writing at 14 years.

Continuous Variables	Sample 1—Mathematics n = 779	Sample 2—Reading n = 741	Sample 3—Writing n = 470
	Mean (SD)	Mean (SD)	Mean (SD)
Mathematics (grade nine)	541.14 (86.75)	497.75 (78.46)	574.77 (104.91)
Reading (grade nine)			
Writing (grade nine)			
Healthy dietary pattern	−0.08 (0.88)	−0.07 (0.88)	−0.09 (0.80)
Western dietary pattern	−0.07 (0.81)	−0.08 (0.81)	−0.07 (0.74)
Total energy intake (KJ)	9298.89(2792.38)	9267.44 (2790.26)	8949.42 (2541.27)
Diet quality score (age one follow-up)	42.52 (9.97)	42.67 (9.83)	42.84 (9.80)
Family functioning score	1.79 (0.44)	1.79 (0.45)	1.79 (0.45)
Categorical Variables	n (%)	n (%)	n (%)
Maternal education (age eight follow-up)			
not finished high school	199 (25.5)	183 (24.7)	112 (23.8)
finished high school, tertiary entry exam	138 (17.7)	134 (18.1)	80 (17.0)
trade/apprentice certificate	26 (3.3)	22 (3.0)	15 (3.2)
collage/TAFE certificate	157 (20.2)	146 (19.7)	90 (19.1)
diploma	92 (11.8)	92 (12.4)	58 (12.3)
bachelor degree	83 (10.7)	83 (11.2)	59 (12.6)
postgraduate degree	57 (7.3)	56 (7.5)	42 (9.0)
other	27 (3.5)	25 (3.4)	14 (3.0)
Maternal race			
Caucasian	719 (92.3)	683 (92.2)	433 (92.1)
Aboriginal	6 (0.8)	6 (0.8)	3 (0.6)
other (*i.e.*, Asian)	54 (6.9)	52 (7.0)	34 (7.3)
Family income			
≤AUS$25,000	94 (12.1)	87 (11.7)	54 (11.5)
AUS$25,001–AUS$50,000	240 (30.8)	228 (30.8)	117 (24.9)
AUS$50,001–AUS$78,000	217 (27.9)	207 (27.9)	133 (28.3)
>AUS$78,000 per annum	228 (29.2)	219 (29.6)	166 (35.3)
Father presence in the family			
yes	498 (63.9)	481 (64.9)	316 (67.2)
no	281 (36.1)	260 (35.1)	154 (32.8)
BMI			
normal	544 (69.8)	518 (69.9)	325 (69.2)
underweight	46 (5.9)	47 (6.3)	31 (6.6)
overweight	129 (16.6)	120 (16.2)	73 (15.5)
obese	60 (7.7)	56 (7.6)	41 (8.7)
Physical activity			
≥4 times per week	279 (35.8)	266 (35.9)	187 (39.8)
1–3 times per week	416 (53.4)	396 (53.4)	228 (48.5)
<1 time per week	84 (10.8)	79 (10.7)	55 (11.7)
Gender of the child			
female	390 (50.1)	372 (50.2)	238 (50.6)
male	389 (49.9)	369 (49.8)	232 (49.4)

Nutrients **2015**, *7*, 2961–2982

Table 2 shows the results of the multivariate linear regression models for each academic performance score in relation to dietary patterns (both as continuous variables and quartiles). In model one, one standard deviation higher z-score for the 'Western' dietary pattern (continuous variable) at 14 years of age was associated with lower test scores for mathematics (β = −29.05; 95% CI: −39.50; −18.61; $p \leq 0.001$), reading (β = −26.47; 95% CI: −6.00; −16.93; $p \leq 0.001$) and writing (β = −27.71; 95% CI: −44.00; −11.43; p = 0.001). Further, a one standard deviation higher z-score on the 'Healthy' dietary pattern (continuous variable) was associated with higher scores in mathematics (β = 9.28; 95% CI: 2.83; 15.72; p = 0.005), reading (β = 12.74; 95% CI: 6.84; 18.64; $p \leq 0.001$) and writing (β =18.87; 95% CI: 8.12; 29.62; p = 0.001).

In model two, these results remained significant with respect to the 'Western' dietary pattern (continuous variable) (mathematics (β = −14.95; 95% CI: −25.87; −4.04; p = 0.007), reading (β =−19.38; 95% CI: −29.53; −9.23; $p \leq 0.001$) and writing (β = −18.16; 95% CI: −35.51; −0.82; p = 0.040)), but were no longer significant for the 'Healthy' dietary pattern (continuous variable).

With respect to model three, the associations with the Western dietary pattern (continuous variable) were not altered by BMI and physical activity for mathematics (β = −13.14; 95% CI: −24.57; −1.76); p = 0.024) or reading (β = −19.16; 95% CI: −29.85; −8.47; $p \leq 0.001$). However, the association with writing scores was attenuated from −18.16 (β = −17.28; 95% CI: −35.74; 1.18; p = 0.066). This difference in outcome for writing between model two and model three may be due to a Type II statistical error due to the lower sample size for the writing scores (n = 470) compared with the mathematics (n = 779) and reading (n = 741) scores. Higher BMI was associated with a lower mathematics score (F = 3.81, p = 0.010) in model three, but there were no associations between BMI and reading or writing. Physical activity was not associated with any of the WALNA scores in model three. The final model explained 19%–20% of variance (adjusted R squared) in academic performance. More detail concerning the associations between 'Western' and 'Healthy' dietary patterns (as continuous variables) and mathematics, reading and writing scores and covariates at age 14 are provided in Table 3. When dividing the 'Healthy' and 'Western' dietary patterns into quartiles, the results of the multivariate linear regression models were similar to the previously described associations between the continuous dietary pattern scores and academic outcomes (results are presented in Table 2).

Table 4 presents the estimated adjusted means for mathematics, reading and writing scores for the quartiles of 'Western' and 'Healthy' dietary pattern scores (estimated according to the predicted values derived from the fitted models). There was an estimated 46 point decrease in mathematics score, 59 point decrease in reading score and 57 point decrease in writing score, comparing adolescents in the first quartile of the 'Western' dietary pattern (the lowest level) to the fourth quartile (highest level) and 9 points increase in mathematics, 28 points increase in reading and 42 points increase in writing scores when comparing the 'Healthy' dietary pattern first and fourth quartiles. Although ANOVA for trend was significant for both the 'Western' and 'Healthy' dietary patterns regarding the estimated means of academic outcome scores, the multivariate regression analysis did not show significant associations between the 'Healthy' pattern and academic outcomes after adjusting for the covariates.

Table 2. Multivariate regression models between WALNA scores at grade nine (age 14) and dietary patterns (both as continuous variables and as quartiles) at age 14 in the Western Australian Pregnancy Cohort (Raine) Study.

WALNA Scores (Grade Nine)	Dietary Patterns (Continuous and Quartiles) [*]	Model 1 [**] β (95% CI)	p	Model 2 [**] β (95% CI)	p	Model 3 [****] β (95% CI)	p
Mathematics n = 779	Healthy	9.28 (2.83; 15.72)	0.005	3.14 (−3.68; 9.97)	0.366	4.37 (−2.78; 11.51)	0.231
	Western	−29.05 (−39.50; −18.61)	0.001	−14.95 (−25.87; −4.04)	0.007	−13.14 (−24.57; −1.76)	0.024
Reading n = 741	Healthy	12.74 (6.84; 18.64)	0.001	3.88 (−2.42; 10.17)	0.227	5.47 (−1.15; 12.09)	0.105
	Western	−26.47 (−36.00; −16.93)	0.001	−19.38 (−29.53; −9.23)	0.001	−19.16 (−29.85; −8.47)	0.001
Writing n = 470	Healthy	18.87 (8.12; 29.62)	0.001	3.67 (−8.06; 15.41)	0.539	4.84 (−7.57; 17.25)	0.444
	Western	−27.71 (−44.00; −11.43)	0.001	−18.16 (−35.51; −0.82)	0.040	−17.28 (−35.74; 1.18)	0.066
Mathematics n = 779	Healthy						
	4st Quartile	28.72 (12.90; 44.54)	<0.001	8.39 (−8.75; 25.52)	0.337	12.25 (−5.74; 30.24)	0.182
	3nd Quartile	9.90 (−5.49; 25.29)	0.207	3.35 (−12.91; 19.62)	0.686	5.63 (−11.52; 22.77)	0.520
	2rd Quartile	4.21 (−11.42; 19.84)	0.597	2.18 (−13.95; 18.31)	0.791	4.69 (−12.36; 21.75)	0.589
	1th Quartile	0		0		0	
	Western						
	4st Quartile	−50.77 (−72.28; −29.25)	<0.001	−23.24 (−45.79; −0.69)	0.043	−22.40 (−45.62; 0.82)	0.059
	3nd Quartile	−30.41 (−49.31; −11.52)	0.002	−16.80 (−36.30; 2.70)	0.091	−17.83 (−37.94; 2.28)	0.082
	2rd Quartile	−13.49 (−29.88; 2.91)	0.107	−5.62 (−22.42; 11.19)	0.512	−5.25 (−12.36; 21.75)	0.558
	1th Quartile	0		0		0	
Reading n = 741	Healthy						
	4st Quartile	37.20 (22.59; 51.82)	<0.001	13.86 (−2.14; 29.86)	0.089	17.93 (0.95; 34.90)	0.038
	3nd Quartile	21.20 (7.07; 35.34)	0.003	6.68 (−8.48; 21.84)	0.387	8.83 (−7.27; 24.93)	0.282
	2rd Quartile	19.51 (5.17; 33.86)	0.008	13.79 (−1.22; 28.81)	0.072	14.04 (−1.96; 30.03)	0.085
	1th Quartile	0		0		0	
	Western						
	4st Quartile	−45.11 (−64.95; −25.27)	0.000	−29.52 (−50.60; −8.44)	0.006	−30.45 (−52.34; −8.57)	0.006
	3nd Quartile	−28.68 (−46.10; −11.26)	0.001	−21.92 (−40.07; −13.77)	0.018	−20.36 (−39.26; −1.45)	0.035
	2rd Quartile	−13.76 (−28.90; 1.39)	0.075	−15.05 (−30.83; 0.73)	0.062	−13.56 (−30.28; 3.17)	0.112
	1th Quartile	0		0		0	
Writing n = 470	Healthy						
	4st Quartile	47.43 (22.33; 72.53)	0.000	15.77 (−11.91; 43.45)	0.264	21.96 (−7.17; 51.09)	0.139
	3nd Quartile	22.50 (−0.59; 45.58)	0.056	5.85 (−19.38; 31.08)	0.649	11.85 (−14.77; 38.46)	0.382
	2rd Quartile	19.63 (−4.07; 43.33)	0.104	18.91 (−6.33; 44.16)	0.142	20.51 (−6.20; 47.22)	0.132
	1th Quartile	0		0		0	
	Western						
	4st Quartile	−50.64 (−84.10; −17.17)	0.003	−31.20 (−67.02; 4.62)	0.088	−29.90 (−67.28; 7.48)	0.117
	3nd Quartile	−31.64 (−61.13; −2.16)	0.035	−21.86 (−67.02; 4.62)	0.165	−20.59 (−52.94; 11.75)	0.212
	2rd Quartile	−8.63 (−34.64; 17.39)	0.515	1.68 (−25.79; 29.14)	0.904	2.12 (−27.48; 31.72)	0.888
	1th Quartile	0		0		0	

[*] 1st quartile = lowest level; 4th quartile = highest level. [**] Model 1 includes: Healthy and Western dietary pattern, total energy intake. [***] Model 2 includes: all variables in model 1 plus maternal education, maternal race, family income, the presence of biological father in the family, family functioning, diet quality at age one and gender. [****] Model 3 includes: all variables in model 2 plus BMI and physical activity.

Table 3. Detailed multivariate regression analysis associations between Western and Healthy dietary patterns and mathematics, reading and writing scores and covariates at age 14 in the Western Australian Pregnancy Cohort (Raine) Study.

	Mathematics		Reading		Writing	
	β (95% CI)	p	β (95% CI)	p	β (95% CI)	p
Healthy dietary pattern	4.37 (−2.78; 11.51)	0.231	5.47 (−1.15; 12.09)	0.105	4.84 (−7.57; 17.25)	0.444
Western dietary pattern	−13.14 (−24.57; −1.76)	0.024	−19.16 (−29.85; −8.47)	0.001	−17.28 (−35.74; 1.18)	0.066
Total energy intake	−0.002 (−0.005; 0.002)	0.386	−0.001 (−0.004; 0.003)	0.684	0 (−0.006; 0.006)	0.985
Diet quality score (age one follow-up)	0.59 (−0.002; 1.18)	0.051	0.27 (−0.29; 0.83)	0.348	0.74 (−0.19; 1.67)	0.117
Family functioning	−6.99 (−19.72; 5.75)	0.282	−8.71 (−20.51; 3.09)	0.148	−10.57 (−30.37; 9.22)	0.294
Maternal education (age eight follow-up)						
not finished high school	−36.95 (−68.75; −5.16)	0.023	−30.52 (−60.70; −0.34)	0.047	−02.09 (−55.40; 51.21)	0.938
finished high school, tertiary entry exam	−22.67 (−55.18; 9.84)	0.171	−26.50 (−57.12; 4.12)	0.090	−5.57 (−60.06; 48.91)	0.841
trade/apprentice certificate	−20.28 (−62.54; 21.97)	0.346	4.80 (−36.19; 45.79)	0.818	29.07 (−40.54; 98.67)	0.412
college/TAFE certificate	−22.34 (−54.43; 9.75)	0.172	−18.11 (−48.53; 12.31)	0.243	−6.13 (−60.10; 47.84)	0.824
diploma	4.76 (−28.96; 38.49)	0.782	−14.85 (−46.54; 16.83)	0.358	29.45 (−26.38; 85.28)	0.300
bachelor degree	3.46 (−30.77; 37.70)	0.843	1.51 (−30.67; 33.68)	0.927	28.52 (−27.82; 84.86)	0.320
postgraduate degree	45.29 (9.03; 81.56)	0.014	26.80 (−7.33; 60.92)	0.124	64.14 (5.49; 122.79)	0.032
other	0		0		0	
Maternal race						
Caucasian	−39.51 (−61.52; −17.51)	<0.001	−23.06 (−43.50; −2.63)	0.027	−55.95 (−89.83; −22.06)	0.001
Aborigines	4.44 (−62.12; 70.99)	0.896	−23.51 (−84.40; 37.39)	0.449	−11.30 (−124.74; 102.13)	0.845
Other (i.e., Asian)	0		0		0	
Family income						
≤AUS$25,000	−33.50 (−55.49; −11.61)	0.003	−28.95 (−49.49; −8.42)	0.006	−52.52 (−87.31; −17.79)	0.003
AUS$25,001–AUS$50,000	−20.04 (−35.90; −4.19)	0.013	−19.49 (−34.27; −4.70)	0.010	−27.26 (−52.98; −1.53)	0.038
AUS$50,001–AUS$78,000	−11.18 (−26.33; 3.97)	0.148	−2.42 (−16.57; 11.74)	0.737	−2.33 (−25.34; 20.69)	0.843
>AUS$78,000 per annum	0		0		0	
Father presence in the family						
no	−8.50 (−21.85; 4.84)	0.211	−4.74 (−17.21; 7.74)	0.456	5.51 (−16.29; 27.30)	0.620
yes	0		0		0	
BMI						
normal	26.60 (5.19; 48.01)	0.015	14.47 (−5.67; 34.60)	0.159	16.85 (−15.80; 49.50)	0.311
underweight	37.05 (6.36; 67.73)	0.018	17.78 (−10.39; 45.94)	0.216	20.90 (024.96; 66.75)	0.371
overweight	8.02 (−16.19; 32.23)	0.516	4.33 (−18.47; 27.13)	0.709	−4.17 (−41.28; 32.94)	0.825
obese	0		0		0	
Physical activity						
≥4 times per week	−0.97 (−20.83; 18.89)	0.924	2.26 (−16.34; 20.87)	0.811	7.22 (−22.54; 36.98)	0.634
1–3 times per week	−4.31 (−22.90; 14.28)	0.649	4.02 (−13.47; 21.51)	0.652	4.39 (−24.12; 32.90)	0.762
<1 time per week	0		0		0	
Gender of the child						
male	17.80 (5.81; 29.79)	0.004	−17.38 (−28.59; −6.17)	0.002	−46.40 (−65.43; 027.31)	<0.001
female	0		0		0	

Table 4. Estimated means (from predicted values of multivariable regression models) of academic scores for the quartiles of Western and Healthy dietary patterns scores in the Western Australian Pregnancy Cohort (Raine) Study at 14 years of age.

Estimated Mean for the Whole Sample with SD	Estimated Mean Mathematics Score *	Estimated Mean Reading Score *	Estimated Mean Writing Score *
	541.14 (41.42)	497.75 (36.52)	574.77 (50.87)
Healthy dietary pattern			
1st quartiles	524.99	480.94	551.22
2nd quartiles	540.55	498.72	574.68
3rd quartiles	548.94	505.22	583.79
4th quartiles	554.44 **	509.61 **	593.18 **
Western dietary pattern			
1st quartiles	562.35	525.49	601.79
2nd quartiles	544.86	504.56	576.99
3rd quartiles	536.67	487.65	560.26
4th quartiles	516.30 **	466.15 **	545.04 **

* Adjusted for Healthy and Western dietary patterns, total energy intake, maternal education, maternal race, family income, the presence of the biological father in the family, family functioning, diet quality at one year, gender, BMI and physical activity. ** *p* Values for trend in ANOVAs are all <0.001.

Further, we examined the difference in the predicted adjusted academic scores between adolescents in the 5th percentile (lowest level) and 95th percentile (highest level) of the 'Western' dietary pattern score. We found that the estimated mean mathematics score for the 5th percentile of the 'Western' dietary pattern score was 563.64 compared with the whole sample (mean 541.14; SD = 41.42), with a difference of 22.5 points (*i.e.*, 0.54 SD above the sample estimate), while for the 95th percentile the mean mathematics score was 495.91 (*i.e.*, 45.23 points (1.09 SD) below the whole sample mean). Similarly, the estimated mean reading score at the 5th percentile was 536.18 compared with the whole sample (mean 497.75; SD = 36.52) with a difference of 38.43 points (1.05 SD above the sample estimate), while at the 95th percentile the estimated mean was 436.44 with a difference of 61.31 points (1.68 SD below the sample mean). The estimated mean writing score at the 5th percentile was 620.49, which was 45.72 points (0.90 SD) above the whole sample mean (574.77; SD = 50.87); the mean writing score for the 95th percentile was 525.62, which was 49.15 points (0.97 SD) below the whole sample mean. Figure 1 illustrates these findings.

We also analysed the intake of 21 key food groups of the 'Western' and 'Healthy' dietary patterns in association with mathematics, reading and writing scores in the fully adjusted model. (This is equivalent to 'model three' in the previously described analyses, except dietary patterns were not adjusted for). We found that higher intake of confectionery and soft drink were associated with lower scores in mathematics (confectionary: (β = −0.182; 95% CI: −0.328; −0.035; p = 0.015; soft drink: (β = −0.032; 95% CI: −0.051; −0.012; p = 0.001) and reading (confectionary: (β = −0.246; 95% CI: −0.384; −0.108; $p \leq 0.001$; soft drink: (β = −0.022; 95% CI: −0.041; −0.003; p = 0.023). We also found that a higher intake of processed meat (β = −0.307; 95% CI: −0.520; −0.093; p = 0.005) and fried potato (β = −0.497; 95% CI: −0.937; −0.058; p = 0.027) were associated with lower scores in reading. Higher intake of yellow and red vegetables were associated with higher scores in mathematics (β = 0.292; 95% CI: 0.038; 0.546; p = 0.024) and reading (β = 0.284; 95% CI: 0.048; 0.520; p = 0.018), while higher intake of fresh fruit was associated with higher scores in mathematics (β = 0.034; 95% CI: 0.001; 0.067; p = 0.044). Higher intake of wholegrain was associated with higher scores in reading (β = 0.102; 95% CI: 0.015; 0.188; p = 0.022). The small β values reflect 1gram difference in food group intake. None of the specific food groups showed significant associations with writing. Significant results are illustrated in Figure 2.

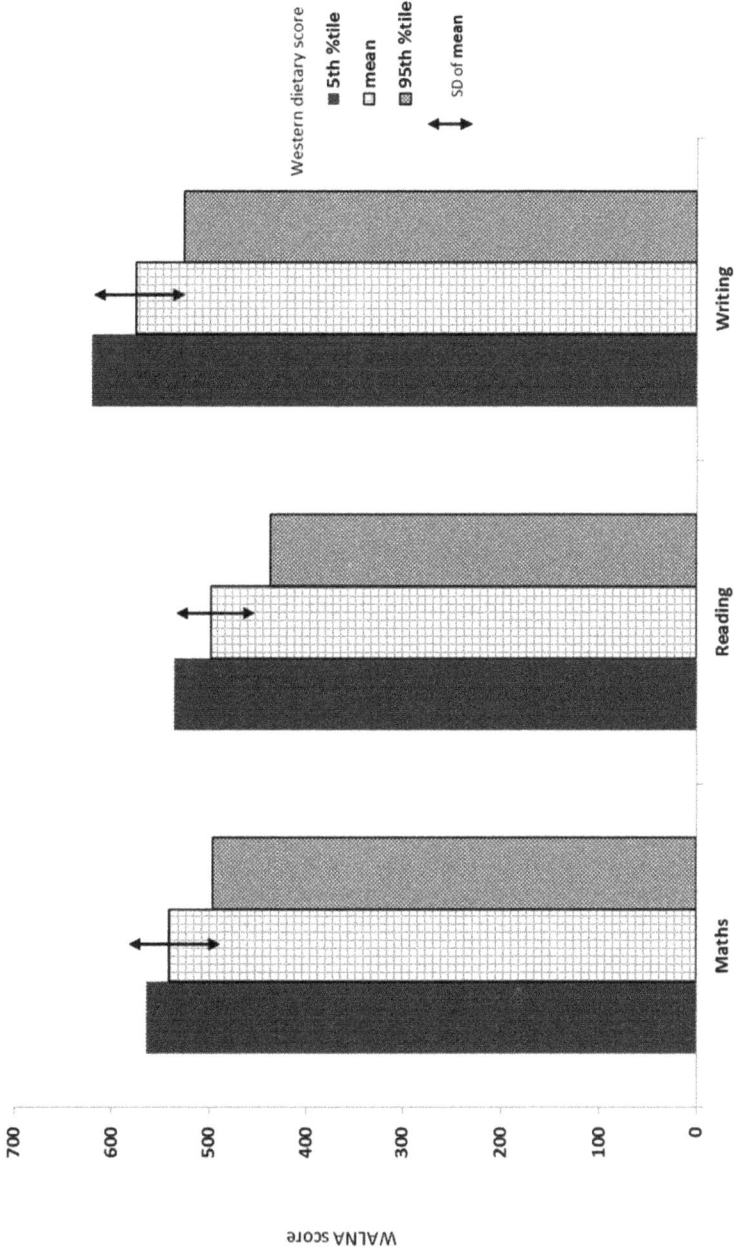

Figure 1. The differences in the predicted adjusted academic scores between the 5th percentile (lowest level) and 95th percentile (highest level) of the Western dietary pattern score in the Western Australian Pregnancy Cohort (Raine) Study at 14 years of age.

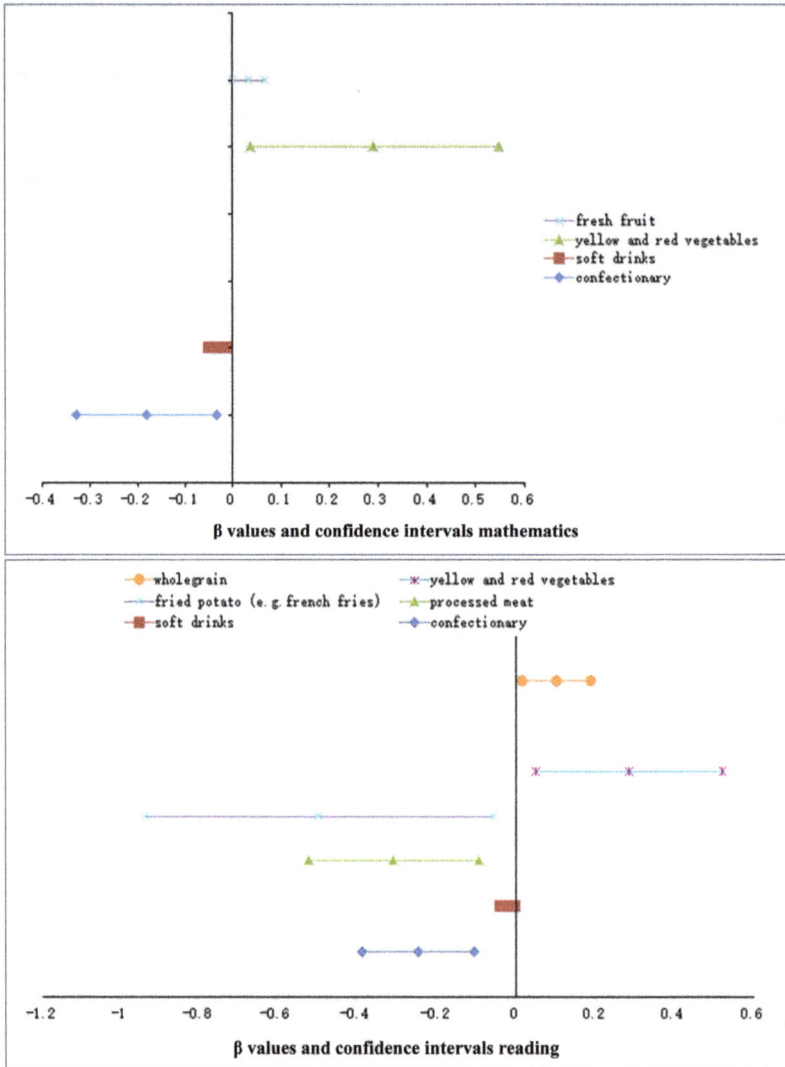

Figure 2. Significant associations in multivariable regression models between food groups and academic outcomes (mathematics and reading) in the Raine Study illustrated in forest plots by β values and 95% confidence intervals.

4. Discussion

We examined the associations between adolescents' dietary pattern intake and academic performance in the Raine cohort at age 14 and found that a higher z-score for the 'Western' dietary pattern was associated with significantly poorer academic performance (specifically, poorer scores in mathematics, reading and writing) independent of maternal education and race, family income, functioning and structure. These results showed an average of 1SD difference to the means of the academic scores for those children who had the 5th percentile (lowest level) and 95th percentile (highest level) of the 'Western' dietary pattern score. The inclusion of adolescent BMI and physical activity level in the analyses did not alter these results. We found positive associations between academic performance and consumption of fruit, yellow and red vegetables and whole grains. Negative associations between academic performance and consumption of confectionary, soft drink, fried potato and processed meat, were observed.

4.1. Diet and Academic Performance during Adolescence

Academic performance of adolescents has been shown to be influenced by meal patterns (breakfast, lunch and dinner) and both poor (e.g., consuming French fries, hot dogs, soft drinks), and good (e.g., consuming fruits, vegetables, fish) diets [6–10,28]. These previous reports are consistent with our current findings that show associations between a higher intake of the 'Western' dietary pattern and its food components with lower academic performance.

Only one study to date has reported on the positive association between whole diet quality and academic performance in children in grade five [29]. In another study undertaken by our research group in the same cohort, the 'Western' dietary pattern at age 14 had a negative influence on 17 year old adolescents' cognitive performance, specifically with respect to their psychomotor and executive functioning [30]. It is known that cognitive performance is a significant predictor for academic achievement [31].

We showed in the current study that BMI manifested significant associations with educational attainment in mathematics but not with reading and writing, and that physical activity was not associated with academic performance. However, our results were not modified by including BMI and physical activity in the multivariate regression modelling with academic performance as the outcome. This is in contrast with other studies that have found associations between physical activity, BMI, dietary factors and academic performance in children and adolescents [8,32,33].

4.2. Mechanisms Underlying the Association between Diet and Academic Performance during Adolescence

Adolescence is a sensitive developmental time period for the brain, particularly with respect to the prefrontal cortex and other important brain structures, including the hippocampus which is critically involved in learning and memory [34]. It is plausible that diet could be a significant environmental factor influencing brain plasticity during this sensitive time period.

The 'Western' dietary pattern (which includes a high intake of 'take away' foods, red and processed meat, soft drinks, and fried and refined food) correlates with overall intake of total fat, saturated fat, refined sugar and sodium [15]. Moreover, this 'Western' dietary pattern has been associated with increased biomarkers predictive of the metabolic syndrome in the same cohort [35]. Further, high fat and refined carbohydrate consumption and metabolic syndrome and its biomarkers have all been linked with cognitive dysfunction (and possibly lower academic performance) through hippocampal and frontal lobe volume loss and dysfunction [36,37]. This dysfunction may be due to neuroinflammation, oxidative stress, damaged blood-brain barrier and/or abnormal brain lipid metabolism [36,37].

The 'Western' dietary pattern is not only high in saturated fat, refined sugar and sodium but is also poor in micronutrients. Micronutrients are necessary for brain function. Specifically, folate has been positively associated with academic achievement in 15 year old adolescents [38], while iron deficiency has been linked to poorer mathematics scores in both children and adolescents [39]. Conversely, associations between higher intake of fruit and yellow red vegetables and better mathematics and reading scores may be due to increased levels of micronutrient content in these foods.

Another possible explanation for our findings is that adolescents who scored higher on the 'Western' dietary pattern may have been less likely to eat breakfast regularly. Children who regularly eat breakfast tend to have better overall diet quality [40] (and possibly *vice versa*). In another study in the Raine cohort, a positive correlation was observed between breakfast quality and overall diet quality [41]. A good quality (*i.e.*, low glycaemic index) breakfast has been linked to better academic performance, while poor quality breakfast or no breakfast has been linked to poorer academic scores in children and adolescents [6,40,42]. Breakfast provides the brain with fuel (glucose) after an overnight fast, which is important in preserving brain functions. In addition, those children who eat breakfast generally have higher micronutrient intake compared to those who skip breakfast [42].

4.3. Strengths and Limitations

One of the strengths of our study is that academic performance scores including mathematics, reading and writing were uniformly obtained by an independent organization via national testing. Further, we were able to adjust for a range of maternal and family socioeconomic covariates and adolescent characteristics that may have represented confounding.

A limitation of our study was that, since this was a cross- sectional analysis, we are not able to claim cause and effect in the observed relationships. Another limitation is that we were not able to adjust for maternal intelligence. However, we were able to adjust for maternal education, which is a valid proxy measure for maternal intelligence [43]. Finally, we acknowledge that we cannot rule out the possibility of other confounding factors that we were not able to adjust for in our analyses and which may have been significant drivers of academic performance.

5. Conclusions

We have identified a 'Western' dietary pattern as a risk factor for poorer academic performance during adolescence. Adolescence is a sensitive period for brain development and a vulnerable time of life with respect to nutrition. Therefore, public health policies and health promotion programs should rigorously target the issue of food intake during this stage of individual development. To date, this is one of the few studies to report on the associations between dietary patterns and academic performance; therefore, more prospective studies are required to support our findings.

Acknowledgments: We would like to thank: Raine Study participants and their families for their ongoing participation in the study; the Raine Study Team for co-ordination and the collection of data presented here; We acknowledge the University of Western Australia (UWA), the Raine Medical Research Foundation, the UWA Faculty of Medicine, Dentistry and Health Sciences, the Women's and Infant's Research Foundation, the Telethon Kids Institute, Curtin University and Edith Cowan University for providing core funding for the Raine Study. The 14 year follow-up of the Raine Study was supported by the Commonwealth Scientific and Industrial Research Organisation (CSIRO), Healthway and the National Health and Medical Research Council. We would like to thank the Developmental Pathway Project and Rebecca Glauert, the Western Australian Department of Health Data Linkage Branch and the Western Australian Government Department of Education for their contribution, in particular with respect to the academic performance data evaluated in this study.

Anett Nyaradi is supported by an Australian Postgraduate Award and a Western Australian Pregnancy Cohort (Raine) Scholarship. Jonathan Foster is supported by a Curtin University Senior Research Fellowship and the Health Department of Western Australia. Wendy Oddy is funded by a National Health and Medical Research Council Population Health Research Fellowship and leads the program of nutrition research on the Raine Study.

Financial Disclosure: The authors have no financial relationships relevant to this article to disclose.

Author Contributions: Anett Nyaradi conceptualized this project, analysed the data and wrote the first draft of the manuscript. Jianghong Li, Siobhan Hickling, Siobhan Hickling and Wendy H. Oddy contributed to the statistical analysis and drafts of the manuscript. Angela Jacques contributed to the statistical analysis and to the review of the manuscript. Gina L. Ambrosini was responsible for the development of dietary patterns, contributed to the interpretation of dietary data, and reviewed the final draft of the manuscript.

Conflicts of Interest: The authors declare no conflict of interest.

References

1. Gidding, S.S.; Dennison, B.A.; Birch, L.L.; Daniels, S.R.; Gilman, M.W.; Lichtenstein, A.H.; Rattay, K.T.; Steinberger, J.; Stettler, N.; van Horn, L. Dietary recommendations for children and adolescents: A guide for practitioners. *Pediatrics* **2006**, *117*, 544–559. [CrossRef] [PubMed]

2. Lenroot, R.K.; Giedd, J.N. Brain development in children and adolescents: Insights from anatomical magnetic resonance imaging. *Neurosci. Biobehav. Rev.* **2006**, *30*, 718–729. [CrossRef] [PubMed]

3. Steinberg, L. Cognitive and affective development in adolescence. *Trends Cogn. Sci.* **2005**, *9*, 69–74. [CrossRef] [PubMed]

4. Cutler, D.M.; Lleras-Muney, A. *Education and Health: Insights from International Comparisons*; National Bureau of Economic Research: Cambridge, MA, USA, 2012.

5. Nyaradi, A.; Li, J.; Hickling, S.; Foster, J.; Oddy, W.H. The role of nutrition in children's neurocognitive development, from pregnancy through childhood. *Front. Hum. Neurosci.* **2013**, *7*. [CrossRef]

6. Øverby, N.C.; Lüdemann, E.; Høigaard, R. Self-reported learning difficulties and dietary intake in norwegian adolescents. *Scand. J. Public Health* **2013**, *41*, 754–760. [CrossRef] [PubMed]

7. Kim, H.; Frongillo, E.; Han, S.; Oh, S.; Kim, W.; Jang, Y.; Won, H.; Lee, H.; Kim, S. Academic performance of korean children is associated with dietary behaviours and physical status. *Asia Pac. J. Clin. Nutr.* **2003**, *12*, 186–192. [PubMed]

8. Kristjánsson, L.; Sigfúsdóttir, D.; John, A. Health behavior and academic achievement among adolescents: The relative contribution of dietary habits, physical activity, body mass index, and self-esteem. *Health Educ. Behav.* **2010**, *37*, 51–64. [CrossRef] [PubMed]

9. Kim, J.L.; Winkvist, A.; Åberg, M.A.; Åberg, N.; Sundberg, R.; Torén, K.; Brisman, J. Fish consumption and school grades in Swedish adolescents: A study of the large general population. *Acta Paediatr.* **2010**, *99*, 72–77. [PubMed]

10. MacLellan, D.; Taylor, J.; Wood, K. Food intake and academic performance among adolescents. *Can. J. Diet. Pract. Res.* **2008**, *69*, 141–144. [CrossRef] [PubMed]

11. Newnham, J.P.; Evans, S.F.; Michael, C.A.; Stanley, F.J.; Landau, L.I. Effects of frequent ultrasound during pregnancy: A randomised controlled trial. *Lancet* **1993**, *342*, 887–891. [CrossRef] [PubMed]

12. Baghurst, K.; Record, S. Intake and sources in selected Australian subpopulations of dietary constituents implicated in the etiology of chronic diseases. *J. Food Nutr.* **1983**, *40*, 1–15.

13. Baghurst, K.I.; Record, S.J. A computerised dietary analysis system for use with diet diaries or food frequency questionnaires. *Commun. Health Stud.* **1984**, *8*, 11–18. [CrossRef]

14. Ambrosini, G.L.; de Klerk, N.H.; O'Sullivan, T.A.; Beilin, L.J.; Oddy, W.H. The reliability of a food frequency questionnaire for use among adolescents. *Eur. J. Clin.Nutr.* **2009**, *63*, 1251–1259. [CrossRef] [PubMed]

15. Ambrosini, G.L.; Oddy, W.H.; Robinson, M.; O'Sullivan, T.A.; Hands, B.P.; de Klerk, N.H.; Silburn, S.R.; Zubrick, S.R.; Kendall, G.E.; Stanley, F.J.; *et al.* Adolescent dietary patterns are associated with lifestyle and family psycho-social factors. *Public Health Nutr.* **2009**, *12*, 1807–1815. [CrossRef] [PubMed]

16. Ambrosini, G.L.; O'Sullivan, T.A.; de Klerk, N.H.; Mori, T.A.; Beilin, L.J.; Oddy, W.H. Relative validity of adolescent dietary patterns: A comparison of a FFQ and 3 d food record. *Br. J. Nutr.* **2011**, *105*, 625–633. [CrossRef] [PubMed]

17. Doig, B.; Groves, S. Easier analysis and better reporting: Modelling ordinal data in mathematics education research. *Math. Educ. Res. J.* **2006**, *18*, 56–76. [CrossRef]

18. Malacova, E.; Li, J.; Blair, E.; Leonard, H.; de Klerk, N.; Stanley, F. Association of birth outcomes and maternal, school, and neighborhood characteristics with subsequent numeracy achievement. *Am. J. Epidemiol.* **2008**, *168*, 21–29. [CrossRef] [PubMed]

19. Paracchini, S.; Ang, Q.W.; Stanley, F.J.; Monaco, A.P.; Pennell, C.E.; Whitehouse, A.J.O. Analysis of dyslexia candidate genes in the Raine cohort representing the general Australian population. *Genes Brain Behav.* **2011**, *10*, 158–165. [CrossRef] [PubMed]

20. Kelman, C.W.; Bass, A.J.; Holman, C.D. Research use of linked health data—A best practice protocol. *Aust. N. Z. J. Public Health* **2002**, *26*, 251–255. [CrossRef] [PubMed]

21. Epstein, N.; Baldwin, L.; Bishop, D. The Mcmaster family assessment device. *J. Marital Fam. Ther.* **1983**, *9*, 171–180. [CrossRef]

22. Li, Y.; Dai, Q.; Jackson, J.C.; Zhang, J. Overweight is associated with decreased cognitive functioning among school-age children and adolescents. *Obesity* **2008**, *16*, 1809–1815. [CrossRef] [PubMed]

23. Ardoy, D.N.; Fernandez-Rodriguez, J.M.; Jimenez-Pavon, D.; Castillo, R.; Ruiz, J.R.; Ortega, F.B. A physical education trial improves adolescents' cognitive performance and academic achievement: The Edufit Study. *Scand. J. Med. Sci. Sports* **2013**, *24*, 52–61. [CrossRef]

24. Cole, T.J.; Flegal, K.M.; Nicholls, D.; Jackson, A.A. Body mass index cut offs to define thinness in children and adolescents: International survey. *BMJ* **2007**, *335*, 194–202. [CrossRef] [PubMed]

25. Meyerkort, C.E.; Oddy, W.H.; O'Sullivan, T.A.; Henderson, J.; Pennell, C.E. Early diet quality in a longitudinal study of Australian children: Associations with nutrition and body mass index later in childhood and adolescence. *J. Dev. Orig. Health Dis.* **2012**, *3*, 21–31. [CrossRef] [PubMed]

26. Nyaradi, A.; Li, J.; Hickling, S.; Whitehouse, A.J.O.; Foster, J.K.; Oddy, W.H. Diet in the early years of life influences cognitive outcomes at 10 years: A prospective cohort study. *Acta Paediatr.* **2013**, *102*, 1165–1173. [CrossRef] [PubMed]

27. Nyaradi, A.; Oddy, W.H.; Hickling, S.; Li, J.; Foster, J. The relationship between nutrition in infancy and cognitive performance during adolescence. *Front. Nutr.* **2015**, *2*. [CrossRef]

28. Park, S.; Sherry, B.; Foti, K.; Blanck, H.M. Self-reported academic grades and other correlates of sugar-sweetened soda intake among us adolescents. *J. Acad. Nutr. Diet.* **2012**, *112*, 125–131. [CrossRef] [PubMed]

29. Florence, M.D.; Asbridge, M.; Veugelers, P.J. Diet quality and academic performance. *J. Sch. Health* **2008**, *78*, 209–215. [CrossRef] [PubMed]

30. Nyaradi, A.; Foster, J.K.; Hickling, S.; Li, J.; Ambrosini, G.L.; Jacques, A.; Oddy, W.H. Prospective associations between dietary patterns and cognitive performance during adolescence. *J. Child Psychol. Psychiatry* **2014**, *9*, 1017–1024. [CrossRef]

31. Tramontana, M.G.; Hooper, S.R.; Selzer, S.C. Research on the preschool prediction of later academic achievement: A review. *Dev. Rev.* **1988**, *8*, 89–146. [CrossRef]

32. Edwards, J.U.; Mauch, L.; Winkelman, M.R. Relationship of nutrition and physical activity behaviors and fitness measures to academic performance for sixth graders in a Midwest city school district. *J. Sch. Health* **2011**, *81*, 65–73. [CrossRef] [PubMed]

33. Sigfúsdóttir, I.D.; Kristjánsson, Á.L.; Allegrante, J.P. Health behaviour and academic achievement in Icelandic school children. *Health Educ. Res.* **2007**, *22*, 70–80. [CrossRef] [PubMed]

34. Giedd, J.N. The teen brain: Insights from neuroimaging. *J. Adolesc. Health* **2008**, *42*, 335–343. [CrossRef] [PubMed]

35. Ambrosini, G.L.; Huang, R.C.; Mori, T.A.; Hands, B.P.; O'Sullivan, T.A.; de Klerk, N.H.; Beilin, L.J.; Oddy, W.H. Dietary patterns and markers for the metabolic syndrome in Australian adolescents. *Nutr. Metab. Cardiovasc. Dis.* **2010**, *20*, 274–283. [CrossRef] [PubMed]

36. Yates, K.F.; Sweat, V.; Yau, P.L.; Turchiano, M.M.; Convit, A. Impact of metabolic syndrome on cognition and brain: A selected review of the literature. *Arterioscler. Thromb. Vasc. Biol.* **2012**, *32*, 2060–2067. [CrossRef] [PubMed]

37. Kanoski, S.E.; Davidson, T.L. Western diet consumption and cognitive impairment: Links to hippocampal dysfunction and obesity. *Physiol. Behav.* **2011**, *103*, 59–68. [CrossRef] [PubMed]

38. Nilsson, T.K.; Yngve, A.; Böttiger, A.K.; Hurtig-Wennlöf, A.; Sjöström, M. High folate intake is related to better academic achievement in Swedish adolescents. *Pediatrics* **2011**, *128*, e358–e365. [CrossRef] [PubMed]

39. Halterman, J.; Kaczorowski, J.; Szilagyi, P.; Aligne, C.; Andrew, A. Iron deficiency and cognitive achievement among school-ages children and adolescents in the unites states. *Pediatrics* **2001**, *107*, 1381. [CrossRef] [PubMed]

40. Lien, L. Is breakfast consumption related to mental distress and academic performance in adolescents? *Public Health Nutr.* **2007**, *10*, 422–428. [CrossRef] [PubMed]

41. O'Sullivan, T.A.; Robinson, M.; Kendall, G.E.; Miller, M.; Jacoby, P.; Silburn, S.R.; Oddy, W.H. A good quality breakfast is associated with better mental health in adolescence. *Public Health Nutr.* **2009**, *12*, 249–258. [CrossRef] [PubMed]

42. Rampersaud, G.C.; Pereira, M.A.; Girard, B.L.; Adams, J.; Metzl, J.D. Breakfast habits, nutritional status, body weight, and academic performance in children and adolescents. *J. Am. Diet. Assoc.* **2005**, *105*, 743–760. [CrossRef] [PubMed]

43. Deary, I.J.; Strand, S.; Smith, P.; Fernandes, C. Intelligence and educational achievement. *Intelligence* **2007**, *35*, 13–21. [CrossRef]

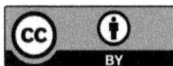

nutrients

MDPI

Article

Dietary Patterns Derived by Cluster Analysis are Associated with Cognitive Function among Korean Older Adults

Jihye Kim [1], Areum Yu [1], Bo Youl Choi [2], Jung Hyun Nam [3], Mi Kyung Kim [2], Dong Hoon Oh [3] and Yoon Jung Yang [4],*

[1] Department of clinical nutrition, Graduate School of Health Sciences, Dongduk Women's University, 23-1 Wolgok-dong, Sungbuk-gu, Seoul 136-714, Korea; eluzai81@gmail.com (J.K.); arreumnew@naver.com (A.Y.)

[2] Department of Preventive Medicine, College of Medicine, Hanyang University, 17 Haengdang Dong, Sungdong Gu, Seoul 133-791, Korea; bychoi@hanyang.ac.kr (B.Y.C.); kmkkim@hanyang.ac.kr (M.K.K.)

[3] Department of Psychiatry, College of Medicine, Hanyang University, 17 Haengdang Dong, Sungdong Gu, Seoul 133-791, Korea; jhnama@hanyang.ac.kr (J.H.N.); odh@hanyang.ac.kr (D.H.O.)

[4] Department of Foods and Nutrition, College of Natural Sciences, Dongduk Women's University, 23-1 Wolgok-dong, Sungbuk-gu, Seoul 136-714, Korea

* Author to whom correspondence should be addressed; yjyang@dongduk.ac.kr; Tel.: +82-2-940-4465; Fax: +82-2-940-4610.

Received: 10 February 2015; Accepted: 12 May 2015; Published: 29 May 2015

Abstract: The objective of this study was to investigate major dietary patterns among older Korean adults through cluster analysis and to determine an association between dietary patterns and cognitive function. This is a cross-sectional study. The data from the Korean Multi-Rural Communities Cohort Study was used. Participants included 765 participants aged 60 years and over. A quantitative food frequency questionnaire with 106 items was used to investigate dietary intake. The Korean version of the MMSE-KC (Mini-Mental Status Examination–Korean version) was used to assess cognitive function. Two major dietary patterns were identified using K-means cluster analysis. The "MFDF" dietary pattern indicated high consumption of Multigrain rice, Fish, Dairy products, Fruits and fruit juices, while the "WNC" dietary pattern referred to higher intakes of White rice, Noodles, and Coffee. Means of the total MMSE-KC and orientation score of the participants in the MFDF dietary pattern were higher than those of the WNC dietary pattern. Compared with the WNC dietary pattern, the MFDF dietary pattern showed a lower risk of cognitive impairment after adjusting for covariates (OR 0.64, 95% CI 0.44–0.94). The MFDF dietary pattern, with high consumption of multigrain rice, fish, dairy products, and fruits may be related to better cognition among Korean older adults.

Keywords: dietary pattern; older adults; cluster analysis; cognitive impairment

1. Introduction

The proportion of the world's population aged ≥ 60 years was 12% in 2013 and is expected to reach 21% by 2050 [1]. Along with the increase in the aging population, the prevalence of dementia has also been increasing rapidly [2], and cost for the care of dementia will also be increased with its prevalence [3]. In 2011, the cost of caring for dementia alone was approximately US $7.1 billion in Korea, and it was estimated that this would increase to about US $100.6 billion by 2050 [3]. Therefore, the social and economic burden is expected to increase significantly.

Mild cognitive impairment (MCI) can be defined as an intermediate state of cognitive function between cognitive decline, seen in normal aging and dementia [4]. Several studies reported MCI to be a great risk factor for developing dementia [5,6]. As a result, it is important to prevent MCI in order to reduce the risk of dementia.

Many studies have investigated the association between specific nutrients and cognitive function, but the associations of specific nutrients such as antioxidant vitamins, B-vitamins, and n-3 polyunsaturated fatty acids with cognitive function have not been consistent [7–13]. People consume various foods with complex combinations of nutrients. Therefore, dietary pattern analysis may be a useful tool to consider overall diet, and can be used to investigate the association between overall diet and cognitive function.

Several studies conducted in western countries have reported that "whole food" [14], "healthy" [15,16], and "Mediterranean-style" [17] dietary patterns were related to better cognitive function. In addition, "processed food" dietary patterns were related to a higher risk of cognitive impairment [14,18]. In Asian countries, a "vegetables-fruits" dietary pattern (higher intake of vegetables, fruits, soy products and legumes) and a "snacks-drinks-milk products" dietary pattern (higher intake of fast food, sweets and desserts, nuts, and milk products) were related to a lower risk of cognitive impairment in older Chinese people [19]. Koreans have distinct dietary patterns, but few studies have been conducted on the association between Korean dietary patterns and MCI. Thus, the objective of this study was to investigate major dietary patterns by using cluster analysis, and to determine an association between the dietary patterns and cognitive function among Korean older adults.

2. Materials and Methods

2.1. Study Population

The Korean Multi-Rural Communities Cohort Study (MRCohort), which is a part of the Korean Genome Epidemiology Study (KoGES), has been conducted since 2004 to determine risk factors for cardiovascular disease in the Korean population. The target population of this community-based cohort is residents aged 40 years and over living in rural areas (Yangpyeong, Gyeonggi, South Korea). Cognitive function has been assessed in the participants aged 60 years and over since 2009. Thus, the participants included in the present study were the participants aged 60 years and over for which data were collected between July 2009 and August 2010 ($n = 808$). Participants with implausible self-reports on energy intake of <500 kcal/day ($n = 2$) were excluded. Since our study is a cross-sectional design study, older people already having cognitive impairment lose their ability to prepare or purchase healthy foods, thus the possibility of reverse causality can exist. Therefore, to reduce the influence of inaccuracy conferred by participants with cognitive impairment, participants with the lowest 5% of cognitive function score (3–14; mean $\pm$ SD = 11.6 $\pm$ 2.8) were eliminated [20]. Thus, the final subjects were 765 participants aged 60 years and over (331 men and 434 women). The Declaration of Helsinki was upheld, and all procedures involving human participants were approved by the Institutional Review Board of Hanyang University. Written informed consent was obtained from all participants.

2.2. General Characteristics and Anthropometrics Variables

All procedures were conducted according to standardized protocols developed for examination and questionnaire procedures. A structured questionnaire was conducted by trained interviewers to obtain information on demographic characteristics (age, sex, education, and marital status), medical history (hypertension, hyperlipidemia, diabetes, cardiovascular disease, or stroke), and lifestyle factors (smoking, alcohol consumption, regular exercise, and intake of dietary supplements). Participants were asked to report whether they had smoked or had consumed alcoholic drinks in their entire life. If they had smoked or consumed alcoholic drinks in their entire life, they were additionally asked whether they were former smokers/drinkers or current smokers/drinkers. The proportions of current smokers/drinkers were presented in the results. If participants reported that they had exercised regularly, they were classified into regular exercisers.

Nutrients **2015**, *7*, 4154–4169

Anthropometric measurements were acquired by using standardized methods. Height was measured using a standard height scale to within 0.1 cm. Participants were weighed using a metric weight scale to the nearest 0.01 kg in light clothing without shoes. Body mass index (BMI) was calculated as weight (kg)/height (m^2).

2.3. Cognitive Function Examination

The Mini-Mental State Examination (MMSE) is one of the most frequently used screening tools for the assessment of cognitive function [21]. In this study, the MMSE-KC (Mini-Mental Status Examination-Korean version) was used to assess cognitive function. The MMSE-KC was developed as a part of the Korean version of the Consortium to Establish a Registry of Alzheimer's Disease (CERAD) Assessment, and it has been proven to be as equally valid and reliable as the English version of the CERAD [22]. The MMSE-KC was administrated by trained interviewers using a standard protocol. Scores can range from 0 to 30, with higher scores indicating better cognitive function. The MMSE-KC consists of the following areas: orientation (10 points), memory (3 points), attention and calculation (5 points), memory recall (3 points), language function (6 points), visuospatial construction (1 points), and understanding and judgment (2 point). Since MMSE is affected by socio-demographic characteristics, the participants were diagnosed as having mild cognitive impairment (MCI) using the criteria of the MMSE-KC according to age, sex, and education [23]. Participants with scores less than 1.5 standard deviations from the mean were categorized as "MCI". Among items from the MMSE-KC, orientation and memory evaluation were used to identify a relationship between dietary patterns and cognitive function with the total score of the MMSE-KC. The MMSE-KC has been applied in several studies to assess the cognitive function of Koreans [24–26].

2.4. Dietary Data

The quantitative food frequency questionnaire (FFQ), with 106 food items, was administrated by trained interviewers to assess dietary intake. The validity and reproducibility of the FFQ have been reported in detail elsewhere [27]. Daily intakes of specific nutrients were calculated by multiplying the frequency of consumption per day, portion size of the 106 food items in grams, and nutrients per gram. Nutrients per gram were acquired using CAN-PRO 4.0 (Computer Aided Nutritional Analysis Program, the Korea Nutrition Society).

2.5. Statistical Analysis

The 106 food items were consolidated into 23 food groups depending on the similarity of intakes and nutrient profiles: white rice, multigrain rice, noodles, rice cakes, cereals, breads, sweet foods, nuts, beans, eggs, potatoes, salty vegetables, vegetables, meats, soups, fish, seafood, dairy products, soymilk, coffee, green tea, soft drinks, and fruits and fruit juices.

Factor analysis is commonly used to detect a dietary pattern by finding factors that are composed of correlated dietary variables. Individuals cannot be classified into distinct groups by factor analysis. Unlike factor analysis, cluster analysis classifies individuals into relatively homogeneous groups, thus, cluster analysis enables us to compare distinct groups directly. Cluster analysis was performed to derive dietary patterns and to divide participants based on the similarity of their diets using the FASTCLUS procedure. This procedure sorts participants into relatively homogeneous groups through use of the K-means method. The K-means cluster analysis, a non-hierarchical cluster technique, is done on the basis of Euclidean distances; therefore, the centers of cluster are grounded on least squares estimation. This analysis requires the number of clusters to be specified prior to analysis. The FASTCLUS procedure was initially run with 20 clusters, and then participants in clusters with fewer than 5 participants were temporarily removed [28]. From this sample, the number of clusters was varied (from 2 to 6) to determine the optimal number of clusters to provide a solution of reasonable size, with the interpretable clusters. Through this process, two cluster solutions were selected as the representation of the dietary patterns in this population. To evaluate the stability of the clusters,

K-means cluster analysis was conducted repeatedly with two cluster solutions in random samples of 50% of the participants, and similar results were identified as those in the original analysis. Once the specified number of clusters was settled, the participants were reassigned to the nearest cluster [28].

Nutrient Adequacy Ratios (NAR) and Mean Adequacy Ratio (MAR) were computed for protein and micronutrients (Vitamin A, Vitamin C, thiamine, riboflavin, niacin, Vitamin B_6, folate, Vitamin B_{12}, calcium, phosphorus, magnesium, iron, and zinc) on the basis of the recommended nutritional intake (RNI) from the Dietary Reference Intakes for Koreans (KDRIs) to evaluate the nutrient adequacy of the diet depending on the dietary pattern [29]. The NAR is defined as the ratio of a certain nutrient intake to its RNI. The MAR was computed by calculating the average of the NAR values. A MAR value of 100% shows that dietary intake is equal to the RNI.

Characteristics of the participants and food intakes were compared between the dietary patterns using the Chi-square test for categorical variables and *t*-test for continuous variables, and the variables which showed significantly different distributions between the dietary patterns were considered as potential confounders. Nutrient intakes and MMSE-KC scores were tested by the general linear model compared between the dietary patterns after adjusting potential confounders (age, sex, education, alcohol consumption, regular exercise, and history of diabetes). Multivariate logistic regression analysis was conducted to investigate the association between major dietary patterns and cognitive function after adjusting for potential confounders. All statistical analyses were performed using SAS software (version 9.3; SAS Institute, Cary, NC, USA).

3. Results

A total of 36% of the participants were categorized into the cognitive impairment group. Two major dietary patterns were identified using the K-means cluster analysis in the study population. Group names were assigned based on the foods and food groups with high consumption. Mean intakes (g/day) of foods and food groups of the two dietary patterns are presented in Table 1. The Cluster 1 dietary pattern had higher mean intakes of Multigrain rice, Fish, Dairy products, and Fruits and fruit juices. Consequently, this pattern was named the "MFDF dietary pattern". The Cluster 2 dietary pattern was characterized by significantly higher mean intakes of White rice, Noodles, and Coffee, for which it was named the "WNC dietary pattern".

Table 1. Means of food and food groups intakes in the two dietary patterns.

Foods & food groups	MFDF (*n* = 589)	WNC (*n* = 176)	*p* [1]
White rice (g/day)	0.2 ± 5.6	254.4 ± 78.6	<0.0001
Multigrain rice (g/day)	251.8 ± 75.1	1.0 ± 3.4	<0.0001
Noodles (g/day)	19.4 ± 23.1	24.9 ± 30.4	0.027
Rice cakes (g/day)	2.6 ± 5.2	2.6 ± 8.9	0.994
Cereals (g/day)	0.05 ± 0.5	0.1 ± 1.1	0.615
Breads (g/day)	8.1 ± 18.0	8.3 ± 20.2	0.909
Sweet foods (g/day)	3.1 ± 8.0	3.5 ± 9.4	0.564
Nuts (g/day)	1.0 ± 3.3	0.6 ± 1.9	0.075
Beans (g/day)	22.7 ± 28.9	23.8 ± 29.8	0.664
Eggs (g/day)	9.3 ± 17.3	11.0 ± 19.9	0.309
Potatoes (g/day)	18.8 ± 25.6	14.6 ± 27.5	0.065
Salty vegetables (g/day)	154.6 ± 114.3	161.8 ± 106.0	0.455
Vegetables (g/day)	63.4 ± 58.2	60.1 ± 62.3	0.516
Meats (g/day)	16.2 ± 24.6	20.0 ± 24.4	0.073
Soups (g/day)	4.0 ± 10.2	3.6 ± 6.6	0.554
Fish (g/day)	43.9 ± 55.0	34.8 ± 44.1	0.025
Seafood (g/day)	4.5 ± 8.2	6.5 ± 14.5	0.090
Dairy products (g/day)	92.8 ± 127.4	67.7 ± 113.1	0.019
Soymilk (g/day)	17.7 ± 45.9	27.2 ± 83.8	0.149
Coffee (g/day)	8.2 ± 8.1	10.5 ± 9.2	0.004
Green tea (g/day)	22.9 ± 44.6	20.9 ± 46.4	0.605
Soft drinks (g/day)	21.1 ± 40.9	24.2 ± 45.7	0.388
Fruits & fruit juices (g/day)	172.6 ± 155.8	135.4 ± 116.3	0.001

MFDF: Multigrain rice, Fish, Dairy products, and Fruits & fruit juices; WNC: White rice, Noodles, and Coffee; Values are the Mean ± SD; [1] *t*-test for continuous variables.

General characteristics of the participants by dietary pattern are shown in Table 2. A total of 589 participants (77.0%) were classified into the MFDF dietary pattern, while 176 participants (23.0%) were classified into the WNC dietary pattern. Mean ages of the MFDF and WNC dietary patterns were 67.5 (SD = 5.0) years and 67.9 (SD = 5.7) years, respectively. The proportion of men was significantly higher in the WNC dietary pattern (60.2%, $p < 0.0001$). There were no significant differences in the proportions of educational levels between the two dietary patterns. "Farmer" was the major job of the participants in both dietary patterns. Significant differences existed between the two dietary patterns in regards to current alcohol drinkers, regular exercise, and diabetes. The proportion of current alcohol drinkers was higher in the WNC dietary pattern than the MFDF dietary pattern ($p = 0.001$). Conversely, the proportions of those who exercised regularly ($p < 0.0001$) and were diagnosed with diabetes ($p = 0.002$) were higher in the MFDF dietary pattern than the WNC dietary pattern. No significant differences in age, BMI (Body Mass Index), educational level, occupation, marital status, smoking status, dietary supplement use, or medical history, except for diabetes, were found between the two dietary patterns.

Table 2. General characteristics of the participants in the two dietary patterns.

Characteristics	MFDF (n = 589)	WNC (n = 176)	p [1]
Age (years)	67.5 ± 5.0 [2]	67.9 ± 5.7	0.311
Height (cm)	156.3 ± 8.4	158.2 ± 8.6	0.008
Weight (kg)	59.8 ± 9.3	60.3 ± 9.0	0.513
BMI	24.5 ± 3.2	24.1 ± 3.1	0.172
Men (%)	38.2	60.2	<0.0001
Education (%)			0.355
Uneducated	17.8	22.9	
Elementary	53.1	45.7	
Middle school	12.2	12.6	
High school	11.4	14.3	
College or Higher	5.4	4.6	
Occupation			0.279
Office work	5.3	7.4	
Non-office work	2.0	1.7	
Service industry	4.6	4.0	
Farmer	52.8	56.8	
Housework	13.8	8.5	
Unemployed	19.7	17.6	
Others	1.9	4.0	
Marital status			0.226
Currently married, or cohabiting (%)	78.8	83.0	
Alone (%)	21.2	17.1	
Current alcohol drinker (%)	36.8	50.6	0.001
Current smoker (%)	2.2	4.0	0.197
Regular exerciser (%)	34.1	15.3	<0.0001
Dietary supplement user (%)	12.1	8.0	0.129
Disease			
Cardiovascular disease (%)	7.1	5.7	0.503
Hypertension (%)	36.0	28.4	0.063
Hyperlipidemia (%)	3.2	2.3	0.516
Diabetes (%)	13.9	5.1	0.002
Stroke (%)	2.0	3.4	0.292

MFDF: Multigrain rice, Fish, Dairy products, and Fruits & fruit juices; WNC: White rice, Noodles, and Coffee; BMI: Body Mass Index; [1] t-test for continuous variables and Chi-square test for categorical variables; [2] Mean ± SD.

Dietary intakes of the participants are presented in Table 3 after adjusting for sex. The total energy intake was not different between the two dietary patterns, but the mean percentages of energy intake from carbohydrate, protein, and fat were significantly different. No significant differences in carbohydrate intake were observed between the two groups. However, protein and fat consumption were higher in the MFDF dietary pattern than the WNC dietary pattern. Consumption of β-carotene and B vitamins (vitamin$_6$ and folate) was also higher in the MFDF dietary pattern. The same tendency was observed for *n*-3 polyunsaturated fatty acid. The consumptions of potassium and calcium were significantly higher in the MFDF dietary pattern. There were no significant differences in the intakes of sodium, magnesium, iron, zinc, and selenium between the two dietary patterns. The MAR score, representing diet quality, was also higher in the MFDF dietary pattern than in the WNC dietary pattern.

Analysis of the MMSE-KC scores revealed significant differences between the MFDF and the WNC dietary patterns. The mean of the total MMSE-KC score of the participants in the MFDF dietary pattern was higher than that of the WNC dietary pattern after adjusting for sex, alcohol consumption, regular exercise, and diabetes ($p = 0.040$). In addition, the mean of orientation score from the MMSE-KC was also higher in the MFDF group after adjusting for sex, alcohol consumption, regular exercise, and diabetes ($p = 0.047$). (Figure 1).

The association between the dietary patterns and cognitive impairment was explored through logistic regression analysis (Table 4). Compared with the WNC dietary pattern, the MFDF dietary pattern showed lower risk of cognitive impairment after adjusting for age, sex, educational level, alcohol consumption, regular exercise, and diabetes (OR 0.64, 95% CI 0.44–0.94).

Table 3. Nutrient intake of participants in the two dietary patterns.

Dietary intakes	MFDF (*n* = 589)	WNC (*n* = 176)	*p* [1]
Total energy (kcal)	1464.6 ± 18.2 [2]	1422.9 ± 32.7	0.270
Percentage of energy			
From carbohydrate (%)	76.1 ± 0.3	78.1 ± 0.5	0.0002
From protein (%)	11.8 ± 0.1	11.1 ± 0.2	<0.0001
From fat (%)	12.4 ± 0.2	10.3 ± 0.4	0.0003
Carbohydrate (g)	275.9 ± 3.2	274.4 ± 5.7	0.815
Protein (g)	46.1 ± 0.8	40.3 ± 1.4	0.0004
Fat (g)	20.2 ± 0.5	17.5 ± 1.0	0.015
Total fatty acid (g)	10.1 ± 0.3	9.0 ± 0.6	0.102
Saturated fatty acid (g)	4.3 ± 0.2	3.8 ± 0.3	0.151
Monounsaturated fatty acid (g)	4.5 ± 0.2	4.1 ± 0.3	0.269
Polyunsaturated fatty acid (g)	2.4 ± 0.1	2.1 ± 0.1	0.091
n-3 polyunsaturated fatty acid (g)	0.4 ± 0.02	0.3 ± 0.03	0.040
β-carotene (μg)	2567.9 ± 79.9	2219.8 ± 143.8	0.036
Vitamin C (mg)	78.9 ± 2.1	71.8 ± 3.8	0.104
Vitamin E (mg)	6.6 ± 0.1	6.1 ± 0.3	0.115
Vitamin D (μg)	2.0 ± 0.1	1.7 ± 0.2	0.051
Vitamin B_6 (mg)	1.2 ± 0.02	1.0 ± 0.03	0.001
Vitamin B_{12} (μg)	2.2 ± 0.1	2.2 ± 0.2	0.837
Folate (μg)	417.0 ± 7.1	363.2 ± 12.8	0.0003
Sodium	2861.4 ± 68.0	2806.4 ± 122.3	0.697
Potassium	2072.6 ± 39.1	1754.3 ± 70.3	<0.0001
Calcium	368.8 ± 9.7	302.8 ± 17.4	0.001
Magnesium	39.7 ± 1.1	35.1 ± 2.0	0.051
Iron(mg)	37.4 ± 2.3	33.8 ± 4.2	0.455
Zinc(mg)	7.9 ± 0.1	7.5 ± 0.2	0.197
Selenium(μg)	64.8 ± 1.0	64.0 ± 1.8	0.703
MAR	0.7 ± 0.01	0.6 ± 0.01	<0.0001

MFDF: Multigrain rice, Fish, Dairy products, and Fruits & fruit juices; WNC: White rice, Noodles, and Coffee; MAR: mean adequacy ratio; [1] *p* values for differences across two dietary patterns were obtained using the general linear model after adjusting for sex; [2] Least Squares Mean ± SE.

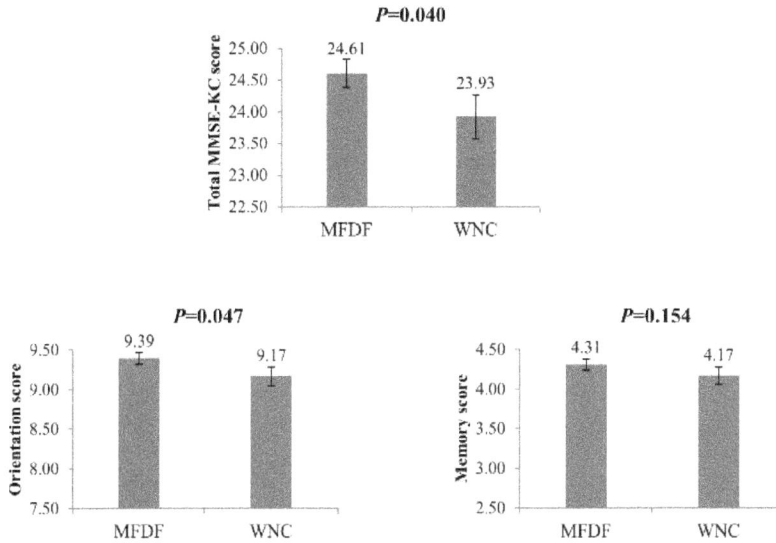

Figure 1. Means of the total MMSE-KC, orientation, and memory scores across the two dietary patterns. MFDF: Multigrain rice, Fish, Dairy products, and Fruits & fruit juices; WNC: White rice, Noodles, and Coffee. All dietary patterns were adjusted for sex, alcohol consumption, regular exercise, and diabetes.

Table 4. Odds ratio with 95% confidence interval for cognitive impairment according to dietary patterns.

	Model 1 [1]	Model 2 [2]	Model 3 [3]
WNC	1.00(reference)	1.00	1.00
MFDF	0.67 (0.47, 0.95)	0.62 (0.43, 0.90)	0.64 (0.44, 0.94)

MFDF: Multigrain rice, Fish, Dairy products, and Fruits & fruit juices; WNC: White rice, Noodles, and Coffee; [1] Model 1 was not adjusted; [2] Model 2 was adjusted by age, sex, and education; [3] Model 3 was adjusted by age, sex, education, alcohol consumption, regular exercise, and diabetes.

4. Discussion

Two distinct dietary patterns were identified by cluster analysis in older Korean adults residing in rural areas. The participants (77.0%) with high consumption of multigrain rice, fish, dairy foods, and fruits and fruit juices were assigned to the MFDF dietary pattern, while the remaining 23.0% with higher intakes of white rice, noodles, and coffee were assigned to the WNC dietary pattern. The MFDF pattern was associated with lower risk of cognitive impairment than the WNC dietary pattern.

Several studies have reported the association between chronic diseases and dietary pattern [30–32], but limited studies have been done on the relationship between dietary patterns and cognitive function. Among some of the studies reporting relations between dietary patterns and cognitive function, the "healthy" dietary pattern reported in a middle-aged French population [15] and "whole food" dietary pattern in Australians aged 65 years of age or over [18] were similar to the MFDF dietary pattern observed in this study. No similar pattern to the WNC dietary pattern was present among Western studies.

The MFDF and WNC dietary patterns were similar to the dietary patterns of previous studies carried out among Koreans [33–35]. The MFDF dietary pattern (high consumption of multigrain rice, fish, dairy products, and fruits and fruit juices) was generally similar to the "Korean Healthy" dietary pattern (higher consumption of whole grains, legumes, vegetables, and fruits) [34] and the "modified traditional" dietary pattern (lower consumption of white rice and higher consumption of fruits, dairy products, and legumes) [33]. On the other hand, the WNC dietary pattern was analogous to the "Traditional Korean" dietary pattern (higher consumption of white rice and lower consumption of milk products) [35], "Rice-oriented" dietary pattern (higher consumption of white rice and lower consumption of vegetables, fruits, meat, and dairy products) [36], and "Traditional" dietary pattern (higher consumption of white rice) [33].

The proportion of participants who exercised regularly was higher in the MFDF dietary pattern than in the WNC dietary pattern. Recent research has identified physical activity as a potential protective factor for preventing mild cognitive impairment [37–39]. When adults experiencing subjective memory impairment engaged in regular physical activity through a six-month program, a modest improvement in cognition was observed [37]. Moreover, meta-analysis concluded that aerobic activities are beneficial for cognition in healthy older adults [38].

A major staple food in the Korean diet is rice, which accounts for 32.7% of total calorie intake [40]. Koreans eat plain white rice, or rice mixed with multigrain (brown rice, black rice, barley, or millet *etc.*) and/or beans. White rice and brown rice have similar amounts of calories, but white rice consists mostly of starchy endosperm because a great portion of the nutrients of brown rice is eliminated during the polishing process. Several vitamins and minerals such as B vitamins (B_1, B_2, and B_6), α-tocopherol, vitamin E, iron, zinc, and selenium are lost through the polishing process. Thus, mixed-grain rice contains more B vitamins (B_1, B_2, and B_6), α-tocopherol, vitamin E, iron, zinc, and selenium than white rice. The constituents of multigrain rice, such as B vitamins, α-tocopherol, vitamin E, iron, zinc, and selenium, are thought to exert favorable effects on cognitive function [41]. However, to our knowledge, no study has directly examined the relationship between multigrain intake and cognitive function, apart from a constituent of a dietary pattern. Therefore, further studies on the relationship between whole grain intake and cognitive function are required.

The MFDF dietary pattern showed higher intakes of multigrain rice, fish, dairy products, and fruits and fruit juices. Such foods can be good dietary sources of antioxidant vitamins, B-vitamins, and *n*-3 polyunsaturated fatty acid. So far, the evidence from observational studies is insufficient to exert a definitive association between several nutrients and cognitive function [12,13,42]; however, several studies have supported the beneficial effects of higher intakes of β-carotene, B-vitamins, and n-3 fatty acids for cognitive function [11,43,44]. Fish is a good source of n-3 polyunsaturated fatty acids, which are major constituents of nerve cell membranes and have anti-inflammatory effects, possibly providing support for their protective effects against cognitive impairment [45]. B-vitamins (Vitamin B_6 and folate) can be consumed through whole grains and fruits. Many studies have reported a significant association between hyperhomocysteinemia and cognitive impairment [46]. Deficiency of folate, Vitamin B_6 or B_{12} is a major factor influencing homocysteine (Hcy) concentration [46,47]. Fruit is rich in antioxidant vitamins. In the present study, participants of the MFDF dietary pattern consumed more β-carotene compared to those demonstrating the WNC dietary pattern. β-carotene plasma levels were reported to be related to better memory performance [48]. A randomized trial reported that long-term β-carotene supplementation for 18 years may be necessary to obtain cognitive benefits [43]. Brain tissue contains easily oxidizable fatty acids which require the protection of fat-soluble antioxidant vitamins such as β-carotene. Adequate intake of β-carotene may protect brain tissue against oxidative damage by free radicals. Therefore, the sufficient intake of *n*-3 polyunsaturated fatty acids, B-vitamins, and β-carotene in the MFDF dietary pattern may explain the lower risk of cognitive impairment.

In this study, potassium and calcium intakes were significantly higher in the MFDF dietary pattern compared to the WNC dietary pattern. Fruits are rich in potassium and dairy products are a good source of calcium. Ozawa M *et al.*, reported that potassium and calcium intakes reduced the risk of vascular dementia [49]. However, Cherbuin N *et al.* observed that a higher intake of potassium was related to an increased risk of developing MCI and that there was no effect of calcium on MCI [50]. Further studies on the effects of potassium and calcium intakes on cognitive function are necessary.

MAR evaluates overall dietary quality. The MFDF dietary pattern showed a higher MAR score than the WNC dietary pattern after adjusting for sex. Several studies have reported that consumption of a healthy diet, defined by *a priori* hypotheses such as the Mediterranean diet (MeDi) score, the Healthy Eating Index (HEI), and the Recommended Food Score (RFS), was associated with better cognitive function among the elderly [51–57]. Higher quality diets may help to protect against age-related cognitive decline in the elderly.

The WNC dietary pattern, centered on staple foods such as white rice and noodles without the consumption of various foods, was identified in this study. This pattern was associated with lower cognitive function. Previous studies have reported that unbalanced dietary patterns such as "white rice, kimchi, and seaweed" [58], "white rice and kimchi" [59], and "rice-oriented" [36] dietary patterns were related to health problems in Koreans. The "White rice, kimchi, and seaweed" dietary pattern was negatively related to bone health [58], the "white rice and kimchi" dietary pattern was positively related to obesity [59], and the "rice-oriented" dietary pattern was positively related to hypertriglyceridemia and low high density lipoprotein-cholesterol [36]. Therefore, white rice-centered unbalanced dietary patterns could influence the development of health conditions. In the WNC dietary pattern, coffee intake was higher than for the MFDF dietary pattern. Some studies reported that caffeine could be helpful for preventing cognitive impairment and dementia [60]. Although the intake of caffeinated drinks such as coffee was higher in the WNC dietary pattern, it seems difficult to show beneficial effects of caffeine alone without the consumption of healthy foods.

Limitations of this study should be noted when interpreting the results. Since this was a cross-sectional study, we cannot conclude causality of dietary patterns for cognitive impairment. Although we tried to reduce the influence of participants with lower cognition by eliminating the participants who fell in the lowest 5% of MMSE-KC scores, there is still the possibility of reverse causality. Because old adults with cognitive impairment may lose their ability to prepare adequate meals, cognitive impairment can affect dietary pattern. Second, a gold standard for determination of the number of clusters has not yet been established [61], and dietary pattern analysis (cluster analysis) requires the subjective decisions of the investigator. Third, depression status was not considered as a potential confounder because a small number of subjects were included in the depression survey. In addition, although we tried to control for covariates, except for depression status, it is possible that there were residual confounders influencing cognitive function, such as unknown risks or protective factors. Despite these limitations, the dietary patterns identified in this study were similar to the previous studies on Koreans [33,34], and the result of previous studies which suggested adhering to a healthy diet could lower the risk of cognitive impairment was also confirmed [15,18].

5. Conclusions

In conclusion, this study identified two distinct dietary patterns, the MFDF dietary pattern and the WNC dietary pattern. The MFDF dietary pattern, consisting of higher intakes of multigrain rice, fish, dairy products, and fruits and fruit juices, showed lower risk of cognitive impairment among older Korean adults than the WNC dietary pattern, which was made up of higher intakes of white rice, noodles, and coffee. The present study demonstrated that dietary pattern was related to the risk of cognitive impairment among Korean older adults. However, since this was a cross-sectional study, further investigations are necessary to identify causal associations between dietary pattern and cognitive impairment among Korean older adults.

Acknowledgments: This research was supported by Basic Science Research Program through the National Research Foundation of Korea (NRF) funded by the Ministry of Science, ICT & Future Planning (2012R1A1A1041792).

Author Contributions: Y.J.Y. and J.K. designed the experiments; B.Y.C., M.K.K., J.H.N., D.H.O., and A.Y. performed the experiments; J.K. and Y.J.Y. analyzed the data; B.Y.C., M.K.K., J.H.N., and D.H.O. contributed to the cohort and gave significant comments; J.K and Y.J.Y. wrote the paper.

Conflicts of Interest: The authors declare no conflict of interest.

References

1. United Nations. World Population Ageing 2013. Available online: http://www.un.org/en/development/desa/population/publications/ageing/WorldPopulationAgeingReport2013.shtml (accessed on 20 May 2015).

2. Ferri, C.P.; Prince, M.; Brayne, C.; Brodaty, H.; Fratiglioni, L.; Ganguli, M.; Hall, K.; Hasegawa, K.; Hendrie, H.; Huang, Y.; *et al.* Alzheimer's Disease International Global prevalence of dementia: A Delphi consensus study. *Lancet* **2005**, *366*, 2112–2117.

3. Ministry of Health and Welfare. A Nationwide Survey on the states of the elderly with dementia. Available online: http://www.prism.go.kr/homepage/researchCommon/retrieveResearchDetailPopup.do; jsessionid=96BD6E6308C135F388289CD1B2C7AC32.node02?research_id=1351000-201000126 (accessed on 26 May 2015).

4. Petersen, R.C.; Smith, G.E.; Waring, S.C.; Ivnik, R.J.; Tangalos, E.G.; Kokmen, E. Mild cognitive impairment: Clinical characterization and outcome. *Arch. Neurol.* **1999**, *56*, 303–308. [CrossRef] [PubMed]

5. Ganguli, M.; Snitz, B.E.; Saxton, J.A.; Chang, C.H.; Lee, C.; Vander Bilt, J.; Hughes, T.F.; Loewenstein, D.A.; Unverzagt, F.W.; Petersen, R.C. Outcomes of mild cognitive impairment by definition: A population study. *Arch. Neurol.* **2011**, *68*, 761–767. [CrossRef] [PubMed]

6. Petersen, R.C.; Doody, R.; Kurz, A.; Mohs, R.C.; Morris, J.C.; Rabins, P.V.; Ritchie, K.; Rossor, M.; Thal, L.; Winblad, B. Current concepts in mild cognitive impairment. *Arch. Neurol.* **2001**, *58*, 1985–1992. [CrossRef] [PubMed]

7. Paleologos, M.; Cumming, R.G.; Lazarus, R. Cohort study of vitamin C intake and cognitive impairment. *Am. J. Epidemiol.* **1998**, *148*, 45–50. [CrossRef] [PubMed]

8. Goodwin, J.S.; Goodwin, J.M.; Garry, P.J. Association between nutritional status and cognitive functioning in a healthy elderly population. *JAMA* **1983**, *249*, 2917–2921. [CrossRef] [PubMed]

9. Riggs, K.M.; Spiro, A., 3rd; Tucker, K.; Rush, D. Relations of vitamin B-12, vitamin B-6, folate, and homocysteine to cognitive performance in the Normative Aging Study. *Am. J. Clin. Nutr.* **1996**, *63*, 306–314. [PubMed]

10. Eskelinen, M.H.; Ngandu, T.; Helkala, E.L.; Tuomilehto, J.; Nissinen, A.; Soininen, H.; Kivipelto, M. Fat intake at midlife and cognitive impairment later in life: A population-based CAIDE study. *Int. J. Geriatr. Psychiatry* **2008**, *23*, 741–747. [CrossRef] [PubMed]

11. Van Gelder, B.M.; Tijhuis, M.; Kalmijn, S.; Kromhout, D. Fish consumption, *n*-3 fatty acids, and subsequent 5-y cognitive decline in elderly men: The Zutphen Elderly Study. *Am. J. Clin. Nutr.* **2007**, *85*, 1142–1147. [PubMed]

12. Dangour, A.D.; Whitehouse, P.J.; Rafferty, K.; Mitchell, S.A.; Smith, L.; Hawkesworth, S.; Vellas, B. B-vitamins and fatty acids in the prevention and treatment of Alzheimer's disease and dementia: A systematic review. *J. Alzheimers Dis.* **2010**, *22*, 205–224. [PubMed]

13. Crichton, G.E.; Bryan, J.; Murphy, K.J. Dietary antioxidants, cognitive function and dementia—A systematic review. *Plant Foods Hum. Nutr.* **2013**, *68*, 279–292. [CrossRef] [PubMed]

14. Akbaraly, T.N.; Singh-Manoux, A.; Marmot, M.G.; Brunner, E.J. Education attenuates the association between dietary patterns and cognition. *Dement. Geriatr. Cogn. Disord.* **2009**, *27*, 147–154. [CrossRef] [PubMed]

15. Kesse-Guyot, E.; Andreeva, V.A.; Jeandel, C.; Ferry, M.; Hercberg, S.; Galan, P. A healthy dietary pattern at midlife is associated with subsequent cognitive performance. *J. Nutr.* **2012**, *142*, 909–915. [CrossRef] [PubMed]

16. Samieri, C.; Jutand, M.A.; Féart, C.; Capuron, L.; Letenneur, L.; Barberger-Gateau, P. Dietary patterns derived by hybrid clustering method in older people: Association with cognition, mood, and self-rated health. *J. Am. Diet. Assoc.* **2008**, *108*, 1461–1471. [CrossRef] [PubMed]

17. Corley, J.; Starr, J.M.; McNeill, G.; Deary, I.J. Do dietary patterns influence cognitive function in old age? *Int. Psychogeriatr.* **2013**, *25*, 1393–1407. [CrossRef] [PubMed]

18. Torres, S.J.; Lautenschlager, N.T.; Wattanapenpaiboon, N.; Greenop, K.R.; Beer, C.; Flicker, L.; Alfonso, H.; Nowson, C.A. Dietary Patterns are Associated with Cognition among Older People with Mild Cognitive Impairment. *Nutrients* **2012**, *4*, 1542–1551. [CrossRef] [PubMed]

19. Chan, R.; Chan, D.; Woo, J. A cross sectional study to examine the association between dietary patterns and cognitive impairment in older Chinese people in Hong Kong. *J. Nutr. Health Aging* **2013**, *17*, 757–765. [CrossRef] [PubMed]

20. Kalmijn, S.; van Boxtel, M.P.; Ocké, M.; Verschuren, W.M.; Kromhout, D.; Launer, L.J. Dietary intake of fatty acids and fish in relation to cognitive performance at middle age. *Neurology* **2004**, *62*, 275–280. [CrossRef] [PubMed]

21. Folstein, M.F.; Folstein, S.E.; McHugh, P.R. "Mini-mental state". A practical method for grading the cognitive state of patients for the clinician. *J. Psychiatr. Res.* **1975**, *12*, 189–198. [CrossRef]

22. Lee, J.H.; Lee, K.U.; Lee, D.Y.; Kim, K.W.; Jhoo, J.H.; Kim, J.H.; Lee, K.H.; Kim, S.Y.; Han, S.H.; Woo, J.I. Development of the Korean version of the Consortium to Establish a Registry for Alzheimer's Disease Assessment Packet (CERAD-K): Clinical and neuropsychological assessment batteries. *J. Gerontol. B Psychol. Sci. Soc. Sci.* **2002**, *57*, P47–P53. [CrossRef] [PubMed]

23. Lee, D.Y.; Lee, K.U.; Lee, J.H.; Kim, K.W.; Jhoo, J.H.; Kim, S.Y.; Yoon, J.C.; Woo, S.I.; Ha, J.; Woo, J.I. A normative study of the CERAD neuropsychological assessment battery in the Korean elderly. *J. Int. Neuropsychol. Soc.* **2004**, *10*, 72–81. [CrossRef] [PubMed]

24. Kim, G.; Kim, H.; Kim, K.N.; Son, J.I.; Kim, S.Y.; Tamura, T.; Chang, N. Relationship of cognitive function with B vitamin status, homocysteine, and tissue factor pathway inhibitor in cognitively impaired elderly: A cross-sectional survey. *J. Alzheimers Dis.* **2013**, *33*, 853–862. [PubMed]

25. Kim, Y.N.; Kim, D.H. Decreased serum angiogenin level in Alzheimer's disease. *Prog Neuropsychopharmacol. Biol. Psychiatry* **2012**, *38*, 116–120.

26. Kang, N.R.; Kim, M.D.; Lee, C.I.; Kwak, Y.S.; Choi, K.M.; Im, H.J.; Park, J.H. The influence of subcortical ischemic lesions on cognitive function and quality of life in late life depression. *J. Affect. Disord.* **2012**, *136*, 485–490. [CrossRef] [PubMed]

27. Ahn, Y.; Kwon, E.; Shim, J.E.; Park, M.K.; Joo, Y.; Kimm, K.; Park, C.; Kim, D.H. Validation and reproducibility of food frequency questionnaire for Korean genome epidemiologic study. *Eur. J. Clin. Nutr.* **2007**, *61*, 1435–1441. [CrossRef] [PubMed]

28. SAS Institute Inc. *SAS/STAT®9.3 User's Guide*; SAS Institute Inc: Cary, NC, USA, 2011; pp. 2241–2266.

29. The Korean Nutrition Society. *Dietary Reference Intakes for Koreans*; The Korean Nutrition Society: Seoul, Republic of Korea, 2010.

30. Botelho, P.B.; Fioratti, C.O.; Abdalla, D.S.; Bertolami, M.C.; Castro, I.A. Classification of Individuals with Dyslipidaemia Controlled by Statins According to Plasma Biomarkers of Oxidative Stress using Cluster Analysis. *Br. J. Nutr.* **2010**, *103*, 256–265. [CrossRef] [PubMed]

31. Villegas, R.; Yang, G.; Gao, Y.T.; Cai, H.; Li, H.; Zheng, W.; Shu, X.O. Dietary patterns are associated with lower incidence of type 2 diabetes in middle-aged women: The Shanghai Women's Health Study. *Int. J. Epidemiol.* **2010**, *39*, 889–899.

32. Ambrosini, G.L.; Huang, R.C.; Mori, T.A.; Hands, B.P.; O'Sullivan, T.A.; de Klerk, N.H.; Beilin, L.J.; Oddy, W.H. Dietary patterns and markers for the metabolic syndrome in Australian adolescents. *Nutr. Metab. Cardiovasc. Dis.* **2010**, *20*, 274–283. [CrossRef] [PubMed]

33. Kim, J.; Lee, Y.; Lee, S.Y.; Kim, Y.O.; Chung, Y.S.; Park, S.B. Dietary Patterns and Functional Disability in Older Korean Adults. *Maturitas* **2013**, *76*, 160–164. [CrossRef] [PubMed]

34. Lim, J.H.; Lee, Y.S.; Chang, H.C.; Moon, M.K.; Song, Y. Association between Dietary Patterns and Blood Lipid Profiles in Korean Adults with Type 2 Diabetes. *J. Korean Med. Sci.* **2011**, *26*, 1201–1208. [CrossRef] [PubMed]

35. Oh, C.; No, J.K.; Kim, H.S. Dietary pattern classifications with nutrient intake and body composition changes in Korean elderly. *Nutr. Res. Pract.* **2014**, *8*, 192–197. [CrossRef] [PubMed]

36. Song, S.J.; Lee, J.E.; Paik, H.Y.; Park, M.S.; Song, Y.J. Dietary patterns based on carbohydrate nutrition are associated with the risk for diabetes and dyslipidemia. *Nutr. Res. Pract.* **2012**, *6*, 349–356. [CrossRef] [PubMed]

37. Lautenschlager, N.T.; Cox, K.L.; Flicker, L.; Foster, J.K.; van Bockxmeer, F.M.; Xiao, J.; Greenop, K.R.; Almeida, O.P. Effect of physical activity on cognitive function in older adults at risk for Alzheimer disease: A randomized trial. *JAMA* **2008**, *300*, 1027–1037. [CrossRef] [PubMed]

38. Angevaren, M.; Aufdemkampe, G.; Verhaar, H.J.; Aleman, A.; Vanhees, L. Physical activity and enhanced fitness to improve cognitive function in older people without known cognitive impairment. *Cochrane Database Syst. Rev.* **2008**, *16*. [CrossRef]

39. Rockwood, K.; Middleton, L. Physical activity and the maintenance of cognitive function. *Alzheimers Dement.* **2007**, *3*, S38–S44. [CrossRef] [PubMed]

40. Ministry of Health and Welfare, Korea Centers for Disease Control and Prevention. Korea Health Statistics 2010: Korea National Health and Nutrition Examination Survey (KNHANES V-1). Available online: https: //knhanes.cdc.go.kr/knhanes/sub04/sub04_03.do?classType=7 (accessed on 20 May 2015).

41. Rafnsson, S.B.; Dilis, V.; Trichopoulou, A. Antioxidant nutrients and age-related cognitive decline: A systematic review of population-based cohort studies. *Eur. J. Nutr.* **2013**, *52*, 1553–1567. [CrossRef] [PubMed]

42. Sydenham, E.; Dangour, A.D.; Lim, W.S. Omega 3 fatty acid for the prevention of cognitive decline and dementia. *Cochrane Database Syst. Rev.* **2012**, *6*, CD005379. [PubMed]

43. Grodstein, F.; Kang, J.H.; Glynn, R.J.; Cook, N.R.; Gaziano, J.M. A Randomized Trial of Beta Carotene Supplementation and Cognitive Function in Men: The Physicians' Health Study II. *Arch. Intern. Med.* **2007**, *167*, 2184–2190. [CrossRef] [PubMed]

44. Walker, J.G.; Batterham, P.J.; Mackinnon, A.J.; Jorm, A.F.; Hickie, I.; Fenech, M.; Kljakovic, M.; Crisp, D.; Christensen, H. Oral folic acid and vitamin B-12 supplementation to prevent cognitive decline in community-dwelling older adults with depressive symptoms—The Beyond Ageing Project: A randomized controlled trial. *Am. J. Clin. Nutr.* **2012**, *95*, 194–203. [CrossRef] [PubMed]

45. Luchtman, D.W.; Song, C. Cognitive enhancement by omega-3 fatty acids from child-hood to old age: Findings from animal and clinical studies. *Neuropharmacology* **2013**, *64*, 550–565. [CrossRef] [PubMed]

46. Vogel, T.; Dali-Youcef, N.; Kaltenbach, G.; Andrès, E. Homocysteine, vitamin B12, folate and cognitive functions: A systematic and critical review of the literature. *Int. J. Clin. Pract.* **2009**, *63*, 1061–1067. [CrossRef] [PubMed]

47. Herrmann, W.; Obeid, R. Homocysteine: A biomarker in neurodegenerative diseases. *Clin. Chem. Lab. Med.* **2011**, *49*, 435–441. [CrossRef] [PubMed]

48. Perrig, W.J.; Perrig, P.; Stähelin, H.B. The relation between antioxidants and memory performance in the old and very old. *J. Am. Geriatr. Soc.* **1997**, *45*, 718–724. [CrossRef] [PubMed]

49. Ozawa, M.; Ninomiya, T.; Ohara, T.; Hirakawa, Y.; Doi, Y.; Hata, J.; Uchida, K.; Shirota, T.; Kitazono, T.; Kiyohara, Y. Self-reported dietary intake of potassium, calcium, and magnesium and risk of dementia in the Japanese: The Hisayama Study. *J. Am. Geriatr. Soc.* **2012**, *60*, 1515–1520. [CrossRef] [PubMed]

50. Cherbuin, N.; Kumar, R.; Sachdev, P.S.; Anstey, K.J. Dietary mineral intake and risk of mild cognitive impairment: The PATH through life project. *Front. Aging Neurosci.* **2014**, *6*. [CrossRef] [PubMed]

51. Wengreen, H.J.; Neilson, C.; Munger, R.; Corcoran, C. Diet quality is associated with better cognitive test performance among aging men and women. *J. Nutr.* **2009**, *139*, 1944–1949. [CrossRef] [PubMed]

52. Tangney, C.C.; Kwasny, M.J.; Li, H.; Wilson, R.S.; Evans, D.A.; Morris, M.C. Adherence to a Mediterranean-type dietary pattern and cognitive decline in a community population. *Am. J. Clin. Nutr.* **2011**, *93*, 601–607. [CrossRef] [PubMed]

53. Ye, X.; Scott, T.; Gao, X.; Maras, J.E.; Bakun, P.J.; Tucker, K.L. Mediterranean diet, healthy eating index 2005, and cognitive function in middle-aged and older Puerto Rican adults. *J. Acad. Nutr. Diet.* **2013**, *113*, 276–281.e3. [CrossRef] [PubMed]

54. Martinez-Lapiscina, E.H.; Clavero, P.; Toledo, E.; Estruch, R.; Salas-Salvadó, J.; San Julian, B.; Sanchez-Tainta, A.; Ros, E.; Valls-Pedret, C.; Martinez-Gonzalez, M.Á. Mediterranean diet improves cognition: The PREDIMED-NAVARRA randomized trial. *J. Neurol. Neurosurg. Psychiatry* **2013**, *84*, 1318–1325.

55. Olsson, E.; Karlström, B.; Kilander, L.; Byberg, L.; Cederholm, T.; Sjögren, P. Dietary patterns and cognitive dysfunction in a 12-year follow-up study of 70 year old men. *J. Alzheimers Dis.* **2015**, *43*, 109–119. [PubMed]

56. Scarmeas, N.; Stern, Y.; Mayeux, R.; Manly, J.J.; Schupf, N.; Luchsinger, J.A. Mediterranean diet and mild cognitive impairment. *Arch. Neurol.* **2009**, *66*, 216–225. [CrossRef] [PubMed]

57. Corrêa Leite, M.L.; Nicolosi, A.; Cristina, S.; Hauser, W.A.; Nappi, G. Nutrition and cognitive deficit in the elderly: A population study. *Eur. J. Clin. Nutr.* **2001**, *55*, 1053–1058. [CrossRef] [PubMed]
58. Shin, S.; Joung, H. A dairy and fruit dietary pattern is associated with a reduced likelihood of osteoporosis in Korean postmenopausal women. *Br. J. Nutr.* **2013**, *110*, 1926–1933. [CrossRef] [PubMed]
59. Kim, J.; Jo, I.; Joung, H. A rice-based traditional dietary pattern is associated with obesity in Korean adults. *J. Acad. Nutr. Diet.* **2012**, *112*, 246–253. [CrossRef] [PubMed]
60. Chiu, G.S.; Chatterjee, D.; Darmody, P.T.; Walsh, J.P.; Meling, D.D.; Johnson, R.W.; Freund, G.G. Hypoxia/reoxygenation impairs memory formation via adenosine-dependent activation of caspase 1. *J. Neurosci.* **2012**, *32*, 13945–13955. [CrossRef] [PubMed]
61. Togo, P.; Osler, M.; Sorensen, T.I.; Heitmann, B.L. Food intake patterns and body mass index in observational studies. *Int. J. Obes. Relat. Metab. Disord.* **2001**, *25*, 1741–1751. [CrossRef] [PubMed]

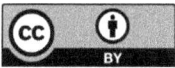

nutrients

MDPI

Article

Association between Dietary Patterns and Atopic Dermatitis in Relation to *GSTM1* and *GSTT1* Polymorphisms in Young Children

Jayong Chung [1], Sung-Ok Kwon [1], Hyogin Ahn [1], Hyojung Hwang [1], Soo-Jong Hong [2] and Se-Young Oh [1,*]

[1] Department of Food & Nutrition, Research Center for Human Ecology, College of Human Ecology, Kyung Hee University, 26, Kyungheedae-ro, Hoegi-dong, Dongdaemun-gu, Seoul 02447, Korea; jchung@khu.ac.kr (J.C.); kamelon@hanmail.net (S.-O.K.); ddottori@naver.com (H.A.); fullmoon0118@naver.com (H.H.)

[2] Department of Pediatrics, Childhood Asthma Atopy Center, Research Center for Standardization of Allergic Diseases, University of Ulsan College of Medicine 13, Gangdong-daero, Pungnap-dong, Songpa-gu, Seoul 05535, Korea; sjhong@amc.seoul.kr

* Correspondence: seyoung@khu.ac.kr; Tel.: +82-2961-0649; Fax: +82-2959-0649

Received: 11 August 2015 ; Accepted: 2 November 2015 ; Published: 13 November 2015

Abstract: Previous research suggests the association of glutathione S-transferase (*GST*) gene polymorphisms or diet, but no interactions between these factors in atopic dermatitis (AD). We conducted a community-based case-control study including 194 AD and 244 matched non-AD preschoolers. Glutathione S-transferase *M1* (*GSTM1*) and *T1* (*GSTT1*) *present/null* genotypes were evaluated uisng a multiplex PCR method. We measured dietary intakes by a validated food frequency questionnaire and constructed three dietary patterns such as "traditional healthy", "animal foods", and "sweets" diets. In stratified analyses by *GST* genotypes, the "traditional healthy" diet and reduced AD showed association only in the *GSTM1-present* group (odd ratio (OR) 0.31, 95% confidence interval (CI) 0.13–0.75). A similar pattern of the association existed in the combined *GSTM1/T1* genotype that indicated the inverse association between the "traditional healthy" diet and AD in the double *GSTM1/T1-present* genotype group (OR 0.24, 95% CI 0.06–0.93). Results from the multiplicative test analyses showed that the "traditional healthy" diet on reduced AD was significant or borderline significant in the *GSTM1-present* group (OR 0.71, 95% CI 0.54–0.92 *vs.* *GSTM1-null* group) or the *GSTM1/T1* double *present* group (OR 0.63, 95% CI 0.39–1.03 *vs.* *GSTM1/T1* double *null* group). These findings demonstrate that the *present* type of *GSTM1* may increase susceptibility to the potential effect of the "traditional healthy" diet on AD.

Keywords: dietary patterns; *GST* gene; polymorphisms; atopic dermatitis; young children

1. Introduction

Atopic dermatitis (AD) is a chronic and relapsing inflammatory skin disease. It is one of the most common allergic diseases in children, affecting up to 25% worldwide [1]. Comparable or even greater prevalence of AD (25%–34%) has been reported in a large scale study of Korean children [2]. The majority of AD starts in early childhood, and 70% of children with AD show clinical symptoms before the age of five years [3,4]. As AD is a major health concern that severely compromises quality of life in children, understanding the factors associated with the development of AD and its prevention are critical.

Multiple genetic and environmental factors are thought to contribute to the risk and development of AD. AD is usually associated with a family history of atopic disorders, such as asthma, rhinitis, and AD itself, and twin studies have shown that the genetic contribution is substantial [5]. However, a steady increase in the prevalence of AD over recent decades indicates that environmental factors also play important roles in AD pathogenesis. Although the molecular mechanisms underlying AD are not fully understood, impaired homeostasis of oxygen/nitrogen radicals as well as increased oxidative stress have been suggested to be involved in the pathophysiology of childhood AD [6,7]. In skin inflammation associated with AD, reactive oxygen species are released during the activation and infiltration of lymphocytes, monocytes, and eosinophils [8,9].

Diet has been suggested as a predictor of health such as allergic diseases and mental health in childhood [10–16], although the actual association is not clear. Previously, we have demonstrated that a higher intake of dietary antioxidant vitamins, including β-carotene and vitamin E, is associated with a reduced risk of AD among preschool-age children in Korea and suggested a possible role of oxidative stress in this association [10]. Dietary pattern providing an overall view of intake draws attention because it could minimize chance inter-correlations among many nutrients in the diet. "Processed" or "Western" diets , high in fat and sugar content, or "healthy" or "prudent" diets, containing micronutrient-rich foods, have been reported regarding child mental health, although the associations are not clear [13–16].

Genetic variations in glutathione S-transferase (*GST*) that alter enzymatic activity can have a significant impact on susceptibility to diseases whose pathogenesis involves oxidative stress, as is the case in many inflammatory diseases such as atopic dematitis (AD) [17–20]. Several genetic polymorphisms have been identified in *GST* isoforms. A limited number of studies [21,22], including one of our own [23], have examined the association of *GST* gene polymorphisms with AD, yet the findings are inconsistent.

Considering that both genetic and environmental factors are important contributors to AD development, we hypothesize that interactions between genetic determinants of antioxidant capacity and diet may play a role in AD. Therefore, in the present study, we examined the association between dietary patterns and AD in relation to glutathione S-transferase M1 (*GSTM1*) and T1 (*GSTT1*)-*present/null* polymorphisms.

2. Methods

2.1. Participants and Study Design

As shown in Figure 1, at the beginning, our participants were from a population based and matched case-control study including 781 subjects who were selected by screening eligibility from 2638 preschoolers residing in middle-income areas in large cities in Korea such as Seoul and Incheon between May and July 2006 [10,23]. We assessed the child's AD by the Korean version of ISAAC (The International Study of Asthma and Allergies in Childhood) [10,23]. Case subjects were children who had experienced AD symptoms in the form of AD diagnosis or treatment ($n = 351$), and controls were matched by the same preschools ($n = 430$), considering both age and gender. Of those 781 participants, we excluded 343 children who had no dietary intake variables ($n = 179$; 82 AD, 97 non-AD), energy intake less than 500 kcal or greater than 4,500 kcal ($n = 15$; 7 AD, 8 non-AD), modified diet by AD ($n = 36$; 26 AD, 10 non-AD) or other diseases ($n = 8$; 7 AD, 1 non-AD), or no genetic information ($n = 105$; 35 AD, 70 non-AD). A total of 438 (194 AD, 244 non-AD) children were included in our data analyses (Figure 1). Due to the exclusion of a large number of children, we did comparison analysis including the child's age (5.3 *vs.* 5.2 years), BMI (15.4 *vs.* 15.5) and gender (48.3% *vs.* 50.3% for girls), as well as household monthly income (38.4% *vs.* 33.8% for greater than 4 million Korean Won, close to 4000 US $). There was no significant group difference in these variables (Supplementary Table S1).

Data on dietary intake, AD, and other related information were collected by questionnaires. Blood samples were taken for the analyses of genetic information and total IgE concentration between September 2006 and January 2007.

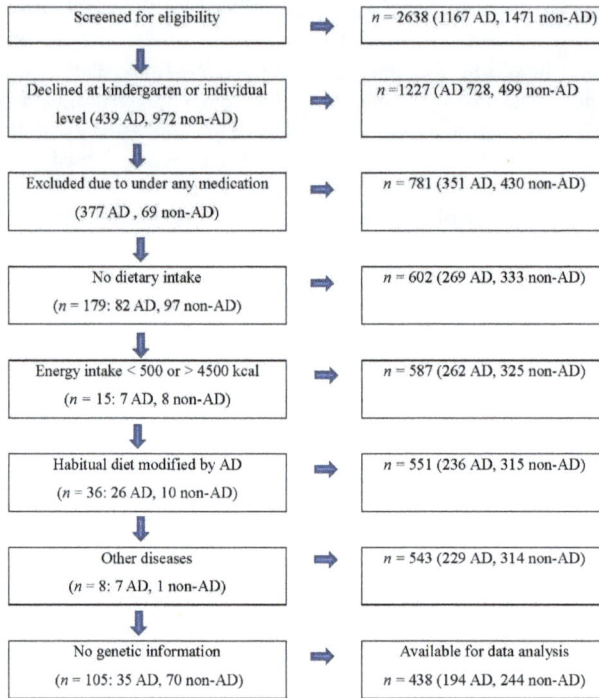

Screened for eligibility	$n = 2638$ (1167 AD, 1471 non-AD)
Declined at kindergarten or individual level (439 AD, 972 non-AD)	$n = 1227$ (AD 728, 499 non-AD
Excluded due to under any medication (377 AD , 69 non-AD)	$n = 781$ (351 AD, 430 non-AD)
No dietary intake ($n = 179$: 82 AD, 97 non-AD)	$n = 602$ (269 AD, 333 non-AD)
Energy intake < 500 or > 4500 kcal ($n = 15$: 7 AD, 8 non-AD)	$n = 587$ (262 AD, 325 non-AD)
Habitual diet modified by AD ($n = 36$: 26 AD, 10 non-AD)	$n = 551$ (236 AD, 315 non-AD)
Other diseases ($n = 8$: 7 AD, 1 non-AD)	$n = 543$ (229 AD, 314 non-AD)
No genetic information ($n = 105$: 35 AD, 70 non-AD)	Available for data analysis $n = 438$ (194 AD, 244 non-AD)

Figure 1. Sample selection process. Atopic Dermatitis (AD).

2.2. Dietary Assessment

We assessed dietary intake through a validated semi-quantitative food frequency questionnaire (FFQ) used in other studies [10,24]. Reproducibility ($r = 0.5$–0.8) and validity ($r = 0.3$–0.6) of this instrument were both acceptable [10,24]. The FFQ contains 86 food items with nine non-overlapping frequency response categories as well as three portion size options (low 0.5, medium 1, high 1.5). Using CAN PRO II (Computer-Aided Nutritional Analysis Program II), developed by the Korean Nutrition Society, the amount of each food item in the FFQ was converted into grams, after which daily intakes of nutrients were calculated.

To develop dietary patterns for this study group, we used 84 food items, excluding two rarely eaten foods (organ meat and fermented salty fish). From the 84 food items, our analysis consisted of 33 food/food groups based on nutrient profiles of each food item (Table 1).

Table 1. Thirty-three food groups used in statistical analyses with factor analysis.

Food/Food Group	Food
Beans	Soybean curd (tofu)/curd residue, soybean (boiled with soy sauce), soymilk
Beef	Sliced beef with sauces (Galbi, Bulgogi), beef (loin, tender loin), beef soup/beef broiled down in soy
Bread	White and dark breads
Cereals	Breakfast cereals
Cheese	Cheese
Chicken	Chicken (fried), chicken (boiled, braised)
Chocolate	Chocolate
Eggs	Eggs

Table 1. *Cont.*

Fast food	Hamburger, pizza, French fries
Eggs	Eggs
Fast food	Hamburger, pizza, French fries
Fats	Butter/margarine, mayonnaise
Fresh fish	White fish (pan fried, fried), white fish (grilled, broiled down in soy) blue fish (pan fried, fried), blue fish (grilled, broiled down in soy), squid/octopus, shrimps, clams/oysters
Fruit juice	Orange juice, tomato juice, other fruit juices
Fruits	Strawberries, apple, pear, mandarin/orange, tomato, banana, melon/muskmelon, watermelon, peaches/plum, grapes
Ice cream	Ice cream
Kimchi	Korean cabbage kimchi/seasoned cubed radish roots/young radish kimchi, other kinds of kimchi
Milk	Whole milk, flavored milk, low fat milk
Mulchi	Anchovy (stir-fried)
Noodles & Dumplings	Korean style noodles, spaghetti/bean sauce noodles, dumplings
Nuts	Nuts
Pork	Pork (loin, tender loin, shoulder), pork (belly)
Potatoes	Potatoes, sweet potatoes (not fried)
Processed fish	Canned tuna, fish paste
Processed meat	Ham/sausage
Ramyeon	*Ramyeon*
Rice	White rice, other grains
Rice cake	Rice cakes
Seaweeds	Dried laver, sea mustard
Snacks	Chips, crackers
Sweet bread	Sweet bread
Sweet drinks	Cocoa, soft drinks, sport drinks, traditional sweet drinks
Sweets	Candies, jam
Vegetables	Lettuce/cabbage (raw), lettuce/cabbage (cooked), radish, bean sprout/mungbean sprout, cucumber, spinach, perilla leaves, unripe hot pepper, onion, carrots, squash, mushrooms, roots of balloon flower/fernbrake
Yogurt	Yogurt, yogurt drinks

2.3. Genotyping

Genotypes for *GSTM1* and *GSTT1 present/null* polymorphisms were assessed as described by Chung *et al.* [23]. Genomic DNA was extracted from buffy coats using an AxyPrep™ Blood Genomic DNA miniprep kit (Axygen Biosciences, Union City, CA, USA), after which multiplex PCR analyses were performed. Briefly, *GSTM1*, *GSTT1*, and β-*globin* genes were simultaneously amplified by PCR along with mixed primers for each gene. PCR conditions were as follows: initial denaturation at 94 °C for 3 min, followed by 27 cycles of 94 °C for 30 s, 62 °C for 30 s, and 72 °C for 45 s, and a final extension step of 10 min at 72 °C. After amplification, PCR products were analyzed on a 2% agarose gel and stained with ethidium bromide. The presence or absence of *GSTT1* (480 bp) and *GSTM1* (215 bp) genes was determined in the presence of the control β-*globin* gene (268 bp).

2.4. Other Factors

Using a questionnaire, we measured household monthly income, parental education level, and child's age as continuous variables, and parental allergic history including AD, asthma, or rhinitis, and child's gender, nutrient supplement intake, and current exposure to smoking at home as categorical variables. Height and weight of children were measured by following recommended standard procedures [25]. Body mass index (BMI) was calculated by using height and weight measures. Serum total IgE concentrations were determined by EIA (AutoCAP system, Pharmacia, Uppsala, Sweden).

2.5. Statistical Analysis

Based on the 33 food/food groups (Table 1) with daily intake frequency values per 1000 kcal, we performed factor analysis to develop dietary patterns with varimax rotation [26]. Three dietary patterns were selected in accordance with the eigenvalue (>1.5), scree plots, and interpretability of factors. We calculated factor loadings for each food/food group across the three dietary factors, and a factor score for each subject obtained for the 33 food/food groups, in which intakes of food groups were weighted by their factor loadings and summed.

We named dietary patterns based on food/food groups with the most positive factor loadings. The "traditional healthy" pattern was identified by considering relatively higher intakes of vegetables, fruits, seaweeds, beans, anchovies, potatoes, fresh fish, *kimchi*, and cheese, as well as lower intake of *ramyeon*. The "animal foods" pattern was characterized by higher intakes of beef, pork, poultry, fish, and fast foods, in addition to noodles and rice cake. The "sweets" included higher intakes of fruit juice, sweet drinks, chocolate, snacks, and ice cream, but lower intake of rice (Table 2).

Table 2. Factor-loading matrix for defining dietary patterns by the factor analysis using 33 food or food group variables (*n* = 438).

Food/Food Groups	Traditional Healthy	Animal Foods	Sweets
Vegetables	0.62	0.13	−0.13
Fruit	0.58	−0.01	0.18
Seaweeds	0.48	0.06	−0.02
Beans	0.44	0.01	0.10
Mulchi	0.46	−0.03	−0.06
Potatoes	0.46	0.21	−0.04
Kimchi	0.38	−0.08	−0.22
Fresh fish	0.37	0.21	−0.10
Ramyeon	−0.35	0.29	−0.17
Noodles and dumplings	−0.21	0.52	0.03
Bread	0.04	0.49	0.12
Rice cake	0.15	0.48	−0.04
Chicken	−0.07	0.47	−0.02
Fast food	−0.19	0.43	0.19
Sweet bread	−0.03	0.40	0.06
Beef	0.15	0.37	0.04
Sweets	−0.01	0.36	0.35
Fats	0.11	0.33	−0.01
Pork	0.05	0.30	0.05
Processed meat	−0.21	0.28	0.09
Processed fish	0.09	0.25	0.01
Milk	0.01	−0.34	0.19
Fruit juice	0.24	0.01	0.50
Sweet drinks	−0.23	0.17	0.46
Chocolate	−0.14	0.14	0.46
Snacks	−0.28	0.14	0.41
Ice cream	0.02	0.06	0.38
Cheese	0.32	−0.13	0.33
Rice	−0.23	−0.01	−0.60
Yogurt	0.20	−0.23	0.29
Eggs	0.16	0.15	−0.27
Nuts	0.27	−0.05	0.27
Cereals	−0.04	0.02	0.16

Each dietary pattern was divided into high (Q4) and low (Q1–Q3) groups according to the quartiles of dietary pattern scores. In addition to initial crude models, multivariate logistic regression models were used to estimate the effects of dietary patterns and *GST* genotypes on AD. As potential residual confounders, parental allergic history, maternal education level, household income, and child's age, gender, BMI, total energy and nutrient supplement intakes, and secondary smoking exposure had been considered. Among these variables, household income, maternal education level, and child's secondary smoking exposure were excluded in the analytic model because these variables did not show any significant difference between AD and non-AD groups.

To investigate the association between dietary patterns and AD with respect to *GST* genotypes, stratified analyses were performed after dividing the subjects into two groups for the *GSTM1* and *GSTT1* (*null* and *present*), and three groups for the *GSTM1/T1* (double *null*, either *present*, or double *present*). The stratified analysis by *GST* genotype was conducted adjusted for the confounders in the corresponding model. Multiplicative interactions were performed using the corresponding models that included the interaction term to examine the modifying effect of *GST* genotypes on the association between dietary patterns and AD. Results were reported as odds ratios (OR) and 95% confident intervals (CI). Significance was set at $p < 0.05$. Statistical analyses were conducted with SAS version 9.3 (SAS Institute Inc., Cary, NC, USA).

2.6. Ethics Statement

This study was conducted in accordance with the guidelines detailed in the Declaration of Helsinki, and all procedures involving human subjects were approved by the Institutional Review Board of the College of Human Ecology at Kyung Hee University [10,23]. Written informed consent was obtained from all parents of participating children.

3. Results

When we compared the high (Q4) and low (Q1–Q3) groups of dietary patterns, the "traditional healthy" diet was associated with higher intakes of protein, unsaturated fat, and micronutrients (Table 3). In particular, higher intakes of β–carotene and vitamin C (2.1 and 1.5-fold difference between the high and low groups, respectively) were substantial. The "animal foods" dietary pattern showed higher intakes of macronutrients except for plant protein and saturated fatty acids (SFA), but had no associations with micronutrients excluding vitamin E. The "sweets" diet was relevant to higher intakes of energy, plant fat, SFA, retinol, and vitamin C, as well as a lower intake of plant protein.

When we compared nutrient intakes by AD, AD showed an association with lower intakes of vitamin E, folate, and possibly β-carotene (Table 4). General characteristics were similar between AD and non-AD children except for child's total IgE concentration and allergic history of parents (Table 4). In the AD group, the majority of children (80.4%) showed experience of physician's diagnosis of AD, followed by AD symptoms (45.8%–49.5%) and AD treatment (22.6%).

The proportions of children with the *null* genotype in *GSTM1* and *GSTT1* were close to 60% and 50%, respectively (Table 5). When the *GSTM1* and *GSTT1* genotypes were combined, about 30% of children carried the *null* genotype for both genes. There were no associations of AD with *GST* genotypes and dietary patterns in univariate analyses.

In stratified analyses by *GST* genotypes (Table 6), the "traditional healthy" diet and reduced AD showed association only in the *GSTM1-present* group (OR 0.31, 95% CI 0.13–0.75). A similar pattern of the association existed in the combined *GSTM1/T1* genotype, which indicated an inverse association between the "traditional healthy" diet and AD in the double *GSTM1/T1-present* genotype group (OR 0.24, 95% CI 0.06–0.93). There was a stronger association between the "traditional healthy" diet and AD (7%) in the *GSTM1/T1* double *present* group (OR 0.24) than the case of *GSTM1-present* (OR 0.31) group. Results from the multiplicative test analyses showed that the "traditional healthy" diet on reduced AD was significant or borderline significant in the *GSTM1-present* group (OR 0.71, 95% CI 0.54–0.92 *vs. GSTM1-null* group) or the *GSTM1/T1* double *present* group (OR 0.63, 95% CI 0.39–1.03 *vs. GSTM1/T1* double *null* group). These associations did not exist in the "animal foods" and "sweets" dietary patterns.

Table 3. Associations of daily nutrient intakes with dietary patterns between the low (Q1–Q3, $n = 329$) and high (Q4, $n = 109$) groups *.

Nutrient	Traditional Healthy					Animal Foods					Sweets				
	Low (Q1–Q3)		High (Q4)		p	Low (Q1–Q3)		High (Q4)		p	Low (Q1–Q3)		High (Q4)		p
	Mean	SE	Mean	SE		Mean	SE	Mean	SE		Mean	SE	Mean	SE	
Energy (kJ)	1556.3	37.1	1511.9	64.5	0.551	1583.0	37.0	1431.4	64.2	0.041	1497.5	36.8	1689.3	64.0	0.010
Animal protein (g)	32.0	0.6	39.3	1.1	<0.001	32.8	0.6	36.8	1.1	0.003	33.9	0.7	33.4	1.1	0.706
Plant protein (g)	22.6	0.3	23.8	0.5	0.048	23.1	0.3	22.5	0.5	0.363	23.7	0.3	20.5	0.5	<0.001
Animal fat (g)	28.0	0.6	32.6	1.1	<0.001	28.4	0.6	31.5	1.1	0.011	28.7	0.6	30.5	1.1	0.140
Plant fat (g)	18.5	0.4	20.8	0.7	0.004	18.0	0.4	22.4	0.7	<0.001	17.9	0.4	22.8	0.7	<0.001
Vitamin A (μg, RE)	413.6	10.3	652.4	17.8	<0.001	481.1	11.7	448.7	20.4	0.170	459.9	11.7	512.8	20.4	0.025
Retinol (μg)	229.5	5.7	258.5	9.9	0.012	240.8	5.7	224.4	10.0	0.157	216.3	5.4	298.2	9.5	<0.001
β-carotene (μg)	1247.3	55.0	2561.9	95.6	<0.001	1598.4	63.4	1502.3	110.4	0.452	1560.3	63.5	1617.3	110.7	0.656
Vitamin C (mg)	65.3	2.3	97.3	4.0	<0.001	73.8	2.4	71.6	4.2	0.659	65.6	2.3	96.4	4.0	<0.001
Folate (μg)	172.1	2.8	231.4	4.9	<0.001	188.7	3.1	181.3	5.5	0.242	186.6	3.2	187.8	5.5	0.855
Vitamin E (mg, α-TE)	8.5	0.2	12.3	0.4	<0.001	8.7	0.2	11.6	0.4	<0.001	9.5	0.2	9.2	0.4	0.513
Saturated fatty acids (g)	12.1	0.3	13.1	0.6	0.131	12.5	0.3	11.9	0.6	0.326	11.9	0.3	13.8	0.6	0.004
Monounsaturated fatty acids (g)	8.0	0.2	9.7	0.4	<0.001	8.1	0.2	9.4	0.4	0.003	8.3	0.2	8.8	0.4	0.224
Polyunsaturated fatty acids (g)	3.9	0.1	5.5	0.2	<0.001	4.0	0.1	5.2	0.2	<0.001	4.3	0.1	4.2	0.2	0.749

Abbreviations: SE = standard error, RE = retinol equivalents, TE = tochopherol equivalents; * Adjusted for energy intake except for the energy variable.

Table 4. Associations of nutrient intakes and general characteristics with atopic dermatitis (AD) in young children.

	AD (*n* = 194)		Non-AD (*n* = 244)		*p* *
	Mean	SD	Mean	SD	
Age (year)	5.4	1.2	5.3	1.3	0.270
BMI (kg/m^2)	18.3	3.5	17.9	3.4	0.260
Birth weight (kg)	3.3	0.7	3.3	0.8	0.876
Daily nutrient intake					
Energy (kJ)	6305.2	2622.3	6592.8	2957.5	0.289
Animal protein (g)	31.8	18.6	35.4	23.3	0.073
Plant protein (g)	22.4	9.4	23.3	10.2	0.324
Animal fat (g)	27.5	16.8	30.5	21.0	0.095
Plant fat (g)	18.2	10.5	19.8	11.9	0.130
Vitamin A (µg RE)	442.5	274.3	497.3	321.0	0.055
Retinol (µg)	231	158.8	241.2	161.8	0.509
β-carotene (µg)	1442.2	1244.3	1679.6	1397.8	0.065
Vitamin C (mg)	69.3	57.1	76.4	61.8	0.217
Folate (µg)	173.8	88.0	197.3	106.5	0.012
Vitamin E (mg α-TE)	8.5	5.3	10.2	7.4	0.005
Saturated fatty acids (g)	11.9	7.8	12.7	9.1	0.357
Monounsaturated fatty acids (g)	7.8	4.6	8.8	6.8	0.072
Polyunsaturated fatty acids (g)	3.9	2.4	4.6	3.5	0.009
Total IgE (U/mL) [†]	325.8	617.2	187.7	307.9	0.006
	n	(%)	*n*	(%)	
Gender (boys)	103	(53.4)	123	(50.4)	0.539
AD status [‡]					
Symptoms (*n* = 192)	88	45.8			
Itchy rash in the last year (*n* = 180)	89	49.5			
Diagnosis by physician (*n* = 194)	156	80.4			
Treatment (*n* = 190)	43	22.6			
Current exposure to smoking at home	31	(17.0)	35	(15.4)	0.645
Supplementary multivitamin use	80	(46.0)	110	(48.9)	0.564
Household income (10^4 Won/mo) [§]					
<200	28	(15.0)	30	(12.7)	0.733
200–399	90	(48.1)	113	(47.7)	
≥400	69	(36.9)	94	(39.7)	
Maternal educational level (≥16 year)	86	(44.8)	99	(40.7)	0.396
Allergic history of mother					
Asthma	9	(4.6)	13	(5.3)	0.743
Rhinitis	46	(23.7)	57	(23.4)	0.932
AD	26	(13.4)	14	(5.7)	0.006
Allergic history of father					
Asthma	9	(4.6)	6	(2.5)	0.213
Rhinitis	47	(24.2)	35	(14.3)	0.008
AD	22	(11.3)	17	(7.0)	0.110

Abbreviations: RE = retinol equivalents, TE = tochopherol equivalents; * Unadjusted; [†] *n* = 182 for AD, *n* = 232 for Non-AD; [‡] Only for AD group; [§] Approximately 10^4 Won =10 US dollars.

Table 5. Associations of the glutathione S-transferase *M1* (*GSTM1*) and *T1* (*GSTT1*) genotypes and dietary patterns with atopic dermatitis (AD).

	AD		Non-AD		*p* *
	n	%	*n*	%	
Genotypes					
GSTM1					0.466
Null	118	60.8	140	57.4	
Present	76	39.2	104	42.6	
GSTT1					0.686
Null	98	50.5	128	52.5	
Present	96	49.5	116	47.5	
GSTM1/GSTT1					0.638
Double *null*	57	29.4	75	30.7	
Either *null*	102	52.6	118	48.4	
Double *present*	35	18.0	51	20.9	
Dietary patterns					
Traditional healthy					0.466
Low (Q1-Q3)	149	45.3	180	54.7	
High (Q4)	45	41.3	64	58.7	
Animal foods					0.873
Low (Q1-Q3)	145	44.1	184	55.9	
High (Q4)	49	45.0	60	55.0	
Sweets					0.776
Low (Q1-Q3)	147	44.7	182	55.3	
High (Q4)	47	43.1	62	56.9	

* Unadjusted.

Table 6. Association between dietary pattern and atopic dermatitis (AD) by of the glutathione S-transferase *M1* (*GSTM1*) and /or *T1* (*GSTT1*) genotypes (*n* = 438) *.

			AD *vs.* Non AD			
	aOR	95% CI	*p* for Chi-Square [†]	aOR	95% CI	*p* for Interaction [‡]
Tradition healthy						
GSTM1						
Null	1.24	(0.68, 2.26)	0.495	1		
Present	0.31	(0.13, 0.75)	0.009	0.71	(0.54, 0.92)	0.011
GSTT1						
Null	0.67	(0.34, 1.30)	0.239	1		
Present	0.90	(0.45, 1.81)	0.788	1.08	(0.85, 1.37)	0.542
GSTM1/GSTT1						
Double *null*	0.93	(0.41, 2.13)	0.881	1		
Either *null*	0.97	(0.49, 1.90)	0.931	1.27	(0.90.1.37)	0.176
Double *present*	0.24	(0.06, 0.93)	0.039	0.63	(0.39, 1.03)	0.065
Animal foods						
GSTM1						
Null	1.07	(0.56, 2.08)	0.843	1		
Present	1.25	(0.62, 2.52)	0.550	1.04	(0.82, 1.32)	0.760
GSTT1						
Null	1.07	(0.55, 2.07)	0.861	1		
Present	1.18	(0.60, 2.32)	0.649	1.03	(0.81, 1.30)	0.836
GSTM1/GSTT1						
Double *null*	1.18	(0.47, 2.98)	0.741	1		
Either *null*	0.95	(0.49, 1.84)	0.891	0.88	(0.64, 1.21)	0.423
Double *present*	1.68	(0.60, 4.68)	0.329	1.17	(0.79. 1.72)	0.441
Sweets						
GSTM1						
Null	0.68	(0.36, 1.26)	0.220	1		
Present	1.53	(0.73, 3.20)	0.266	1.23	(0.96, 1.56)	0.098
GSTT1						
Null	0.85	(0.42, 1.73)	0.665			
Present	1.02	(0.54, 1.93)	0.963	1.05	(0.82,1.33)	0.712
GSTM1/GSTT1						
Double *null*	0.59	(0.24, 1.44)	0.247	1		
Either *null*	1.04	(0.52, 2.10)	0.920	1.02	(0.74, 1.41)	0.897
Double *present*	1.62	(0.61, 4.33)	0.343	1.27	(0.87, 1.86)	0.212

* Model included the main and interaction effects of the *GSTM1* and/or *GSTT1* genotype (*present vs. null*) and dietary pattern (high *vs.* low) with adjustment for child's age, sex, total energy intake, multivitamin use and BMI, and parental history of allergic diseases; [†] *P* for the stratified association between dietary patterns and AD by *GST-null* and *present* groups in the corresponding models; [‡] *P* for the multplicative association between AD and dietary pattern (high *vs.* low) in the *GST present* group compared to this association in the *GST null* group as reference (OR 1) in the corresponding models. N *null*; p *present*.

4. Discussion

Our findings suggest the association between the "traditional healthy" diet and reduced AD in children with the *GSTM1-present* genotype, and that children with *GSTT1-present* genotype may be more susceptible to this association. Such associations may not be relevant to an inactive *GST* allele such as the *GST-null* genotype.

Despite a lack of clear explanation, the absence of an association of the *GSTM1-* or *GSTT1-null* genotype with dietary components may suggest that certain polyphenols and carotenoids induce the expression of *GST* genes and increase the activities of *GST* enzymes [27–29]. Thus, the lack of an active *GST* allele would inhibit the response to dietary components that affect the expression of *GST* genes. Similar to our findings, a recent human intervention study [30] reported that a high-fruit juice and vegetable diet significantly increased erythrocyte *GST* activities and antioxidant capacity-related biomarker levels in blood from *GSTM1-* and *GSTT1-present* participants, whereas blood from *GSTM1-* and *GSTT1-null* participants was unaffected. Even though the interactions of *GST* genotypes and diet in relation to AD have not been studied yet, previous reports [31,32] that examined these interactions in other diseases support our findings. Specifically, a significant inverse association between intake of carotenoid-rich or cruciferous vegetables and cancer risk was detected in carriers of the *GSTM1-* or *GSTT1-present* genotype but not in those participants with the *GSTM1-* or *GSTT1-null* genotype.

These results, as well as our findings, suggest that carriers of the *GSTM1-* or *GSTT1-present* genotype may be more responsive to dietary changes and could benefit more from healthy dietary patterns.

There have been conflicting reports on the association of *GST present/null* genotypes with AD [21,22,33]. Consistent with our results, the *GSTM1-present* genotype has been reported to be relevant to AD only in the presence of specific environmental stimuli (prenatal smoke exposure) [34]. Detection of these gene-diet interactions suggests that it is important to determine the effects of gene polymorphisms as well as appropriate dietary information in order to account for the heterogeneity of previous findings. Further, unlike genetic determinants, diet can be modified by lifestyle intervention. Therefore, understanding the interactions between genetic and dietary factors is valuable in establishing dietary guidelines to reduce disease risk.

Several studies [10,35–38] have shown the association between nutrient/food intakes and AD, but little is known regarding specific dietary patterns relevant to AD in relation to *GST* genes. Dietary pattern analysis considers the effects of the whole diet, including interactions and synergistic effects among nutrients and foods [39]. As nutrients and foods are not consumed in isolation, dietary patterns more accurately reflect eating habits than nutrient intake levels. The "traditional healthy" pattern that showed a positive impact on reduced AD in this study is somewhat similar to the "Mediterranean diet", which mainly involves higher intakes of micronutrients [40]. Adherence to a "Mediterranean diet" during pregnancy has been demonstrated as a protective factor against atopy until an age of 6.5 years (OR 0.55, 95% CI 0.31–0.97) [41]. On the other hand, no association between the "Mediterranean diet" and AD has been reported in 6 to 7-year-old school children in Spain [42]. This discrepancy may be explained in part by a function of effect modifiers, like *GST* genes that we found in this study.

The limitations of this study are as follows. We assessed AD based on subjective measures without considering objective indices, although the ISAAC questionnaire used in this study is an internationally standardized protocol and has been widely used to determine the prevalence of allergic diseases in Korea [2,10,43]. Another limitation would be small sample size to identify a diet-gene interaction against AD. We determined sample size at the beginning of this study based on antioxidant nutrients and AD, but with little consideration of genetic characteristics. Possibly meaningful, but unmeasured or unexamined variables such as heavy metals [44] and other genes may also limit our findings [45,46].

Regardless of these limitations, this study of gene-diet interaction in AD is meaningful because it is the first study to suggest the importance of genetic susceptibility that could play a crucial role in the "traditional healthy" diet on a child's AD. A large scale prospective study is needed to confirm these findings.

5. Conclusions

We conclude that healhty diet may reduce AD only in children with the *GSTM1-present* genotype. These findings suggest genetic susceptibility to the association between diet on AD.

Supplementary Materials: Supplementary materials can be accessed at: http://www.mdpi.com/2072-6643/7/11/5473/s1.

Acknowledgments: This study was supported in part by a grant from the Basic Research Program of the Korea Science and Engineering Foundation (R01-2006-00010887-0).

Author Contributions: S.-Y.O., J.C. designed research; S.-O.K. and H.A., conducted research; S.-Y.O, J.C., S.-O.K., and H.H. analyzed data, and S.-Y.O. and J.C. wrote the paper; S.H. reviewed the paper; S.-Y.O. had primary responsibility for final content.

Conflicts of Interest: The authors declare no conflict of interest.

References

1. Eichenfield, L.F.; Tom, W.L.; Berger, T.G.; Krol, A.; Paller, A.S.; Schwarzenberger, K.; Bergman, J.N.; Chamlin, S.L.; Cohen, D.E.; Cooper, K.D. Guidelines of care for the management of atopic dermatitis: Section 2. management and treatment of atopic dermatitis with topical therapies. *J. Am. Acad. Dermatol.* **2014**, *71*, 116–132. [PubMed]
2. Lee, J.Y.; Seo, J.H.; Kwon, J.W.; Yu, J.; Kim, B.J.; Lee, S.Y.; Kim, H.B.; Kim, W.K.; Kim, K.W.; Shin, Y.J.; *et al.* Exposure to gene-environment interactions before 1 year of age may favor the development of atopic dermatitis. *Int. Arch. Allergy Immunol.* **2012**, *157*, 363–371. [CrossRef] [PubMed]
3. Williams, H.C. Atopic dermatitis. *N. Engl. J. Med.* **2005**, *352*, 2314–2324. [CrossRef] [PubMed]
4. Bieber, T. Atopic dermatitis 2.0: From the clinical phenotype to the molecular taxonomy and stratified medicine. *Allergy* **2012**, *67*, 1475–1482. [CrossRef] [PubMed]
5. Larsen, F.S. Atopic dermatitis: A genetic-epidemiologic study in a population-based twin sample. *J. Am. Acad. Dermatol.* **1993**, *28*, 719–723. [CrossRef]
6. Omata, N.; Tsukahara, H.; Ito, S.; Ohshima, Y.; Yasutomi, M.; Yamada, A.; Jiang, M.; Hiraoka, M.; Nambu, M.; Deguchi, Y. Increased oxidative stress in childhood atopic dermatitis. *Life Sci.* **2001**, *69*, 223–228. [CrossRef]
7. Tsukahara, H.; Shibata, R.; Ohshima, Y.; Todoroki, Y.; Sato, S.; Ohta, N.; Hiraoka, M.; Yoshida, A.; Nishima, S.; Mayumi, M. Oxidative stress and altered antioxidant defenses in children with acute exacerbation of atopic dermatitis. *Life Sci.* **2003**, *72*, 2509–2516. [CrossRef]
8. Kapp, A.; Zeck-Kapp, G.; Czech, W.; Schöpf, E. The chemokine rantes is more than a chemoattractant: characterization of its effect on human eosinophil oxidative metabolism and morphology in comparison with IL-5 and GM-CSF. *J. Investig. Dermatol.* **1994**, *102*, 906–914. [CrossRef] [PubMed]
9. Portugal, M.; Barak, V.; Ginsburg, I.; Kohen, R. Interplay among oxidants, antioxidants, and cytokines in skin disorders: Present status and future considerations. *Biomed. Pharmacother.* **2007**, *61*, 412–422. [CrossRef] [PubMed]
10. Oh, S.; Chung, J.; Kim, M.; Kwon, S.; Cho, B. Antioxidant nutrient intakes and corresponding biomarkers associated with the risk of atopic dermatitis in young children. *Eur. J. Clin. Nutr.* **2010**, *64*, 245–252. [CrossRef] [PubMed]
11. Saadeh, D.; Salameh, P.; Baldi, I.; Raherison, C. Diet and allergic diseases among population aged 0 to 18 years: myth or reality? *Nutrients* **2013**, *5*, 3399–3423. [CrossRef] [PubMed]
12. Nurmatov, U.; Devereux, G.; Sheikh, A. Nutrients and foods for the primary prevention of asthma and allergy: Systematic review and meta-analysis. *J. Allergy Clin. Immunol.* **2011**, *127*, 724–733. [CrossRef] [PubMed]
13. Howard, A.L.; Robinson, M.; Smith, G.J.; Ambrosini, G.L.; Piek, J.P.; Oddy, W.H. ADHD is associated with a "western" dietary pattern in adolescents. *J. Atten. Disord.* **2011**, *15*, 403–411. [CrossRef] [PubMed]
14. Millichap, J.G.; Yee, M.M. The diet factor in attention-deficit/hyperactivity disorder. *Pediatrics* **2012**, *129*, 330–337. [CrossRef] [PubMed]
15. Northstone, K.; Joinson, C.; Emmett, P.; Ness, A.; Paus, T. Are dietary patterns in childhood associated with IQ at 8 years of age? A population-based cohort study. *J. Epidemiol. Community Health* **2012**, *66*, 624–628. [CrossRef] [PubMed]
16. Smithers, L.G.; Golley, R.K.; Mittinty, M.N.; Brazionis, L.; Northstone, K.; Emmett, P.; Lynch, J.W. Dietary patterns at 6, 15 and 24 months of age are associated with IQ at 8 years of age. *Eur. J. Epidemiol.* **2012**, *27*, 525–535. [CrossRef] [PubMed]
17. Castaldi, P.J.; Cho, M.H.; Cohn, M.; Langerman, F.; Moran, S.; Tarragona, N.; Moukhachen, H.; Venugopal, R.; Hasimja, D.; Kao, E.; *et al.* The COPD genetic association compendium: A comprehensive online database of COPD genetic associations. *Hum. Mol. Genet.* **2010**, *19*, 526–534. [CrossRef] [PubMed]
18. Karban, A.; Krivoy, N.; Elkin, H.; Adler, L.; Chowers, Y.; Eliakim, R.; Efrati, E. Non-Jewish Israeli IBD patients have significantly higher glutathione S-transferase GSTT1-Null frequency. *Dig. Dis. Sci.* **2011**, *56*, 2081–2087. [CrossRef] [PubMed]
19. Thakur, H.; Gupta, L.; Sobti, R.C.; Janmeja, A.K.; Seth, A.; Singh, S.K. Association of GSTM1T1 GENES with COPD and prostate cancer in North Indian Population. *Mol. Biol. Rep.* **2011**, *38*, 1733–1739. [CrossRef] [PubMed]

20. Oniki, K.; Hori, M.; Saruwatari, J.; Morita, K.; Kajiwara, A.; Sakata, M.; Mihara, S.; Ogata, Y.; Nakagawa, K. Interactive effects of smoking and glutathione S-transferase polymorphisms on the development of non-alcoholic fatty liver Disease. *Toxicol. Lett.* **2013**, *220*, 143–149. [CrossRef] [PubMed]

21. Vavilin, V.; Safronova, O.; Lyapunova, A.; Lyakhovich, V.; Kaznacheeva, L.; Manankin, N.; Molokova, A. Interaction of GSTM1, GSTT1, and GSTP1 genotypes in determination of predisposition to atopic dermatitis. *Bull. Exp. Biol. Med.* **2003**, *136*, 388–391. [CrossRef] [PubMed]

22. Cho, H.; Uhm, Y.; Kim, H.; Ban, J.; Chung, J.; Yim, S.; Choi, B.; Lee, M. Glutathione S-transferase M1 (GSTM1) polymorphism is associated with atopic dermatitis susceptibility in a Korean population. *Int. J. Immunogenet.* **2011**, *38*, 145–150. [CrossRef] [PubMed]

23. Chung, J.; Oh, S.; Shin, Y. Association of glutathione-S-transferase polymorphisms with atopic dermatitis risk in preschool age children. *Clin. Chem. Lab. Med.* **2009**, *47*, 1475–1481. [CrossRef] [PubMed]

24. Shin, K.O.; Oh, S.; Park, H.S. Empirically derived major dietary patterns and their associations with overweight in Korean Preschool Children. *Br. J. Nutr.* **2007**, *98*, 416–421. [CrossRef] [PubMed]

25. World Health Organization. *Physical Status: The Use of and Interpretation of Anthropometry*; Report of a WHO Expert Committee; World Health Organization: Geneva, Switzerland, 1995.

26. Cody, R.; Smith, J. *Applied Statistics and the SAS Programming Language*, 5th ed.; Prentice-Hall: Upper Saddle River, NJ, USA, 2005.

27. Bhuvaneswari, V.; Velmurugan, B.; Nagini, S. Induction of glutathione-dependent hepatic biotransformation enzymes by lycopene in the hamster cheek pouch carcinogenesis model. *J. Biochem. Mol. Biol. Biophys.* **2002**, *6*, 257–260. [PubMed]

28. Munday, R.; Munday, J.S.; Munday, C.M. Comparative effects of mono-, di-, tri-, and tetrasulfides derived from plants of the Allium Family: Redox cycling *in vitro* and hemolytic activity and phase 2 enzyme induction *in vivo*. *Free Radic. Biol. Med.* **2003**, *34*, 1200–1211. [CrossRef]

29. Kuo, W.; Chou, F.; Young, S.; Chang, Y.; Wang, C. Geniposide activates GSH S-transferase by the induction of GST M1 and GST M2 Subunits involving the transcription and phosphorylation of MEK-1 Signaling in rat hepatocytes. *Toxicol. Appl. Pharmacol.* **2005**, *208*, 155–162. [CrossRef] [PubMed]

30. Yuan, L.; Zhang, L.; Ma, W.; Zhou, X.; Ji, J.; Li, N.; Xiao, R. Glutathione S-transferase M1 and T1 gene polymorphisms with consumption of high fruit-juice and vegetable diet affect antioxidant capacity in healthy adults. *Nutrition* **2013**, *29*, 965–971. [CrossRef] [PubMed]

31. Joseph, M.A.; Moysich, K.B.; Freudenheim, J.L.; Shields, P.G.; Bowman, E.D.; Zhang, Y.; Marshall, J.R.; Ambrosone, C.B. Cruciferous vegetables, genetic polymorphisms in glutathione S-transferases M1 and T1, and prostate cancer risk. *Nutr. Cancer* **2004**, *50*, 206–213. [CrossRef] [PubMed]

32. Wang, L.I.; Giovannucci, E.L.; Hunter, D.; Neuberg, D.; Su, L.; Christiani, D.C. Dietary intake of cruciferous vegetables, glutathione S-transferase (GST) polymorphisms and lung cancer risk in a Caucasian population. *Cancer Causes Control* **2004**, *15*, 977–985. [CrossRef] [PubMed]

33. Safronova, O.; Vavilin, V.; Lyapunova, A.; Makarova, S.; Lyakhovich, V.; Kaznacheeva, L.; Manankin, N.; Batychko, O.; Gavalov, S. Relationship between glutathione S-transferase P1 polymorphism and bronchial asthma and atopic dermatitis. *Bull. Exp. Biol. Med.* **2003**, *136*, 73–75. [CrossRef] [PubMed]

34. Wang, I.; Guo, Y.L.; Lin, T.; Chen, P.; Wu, Y. GSTM1, GSTP1, prenatal smoke exposure, and atopic dermatitis. *Ann. Allergy Asthma Immunol.* **2010**, *105*, 124–129. [CrossRef] [PubMed]

35. Miyake, Y.; Sasaki, S.; Tanaka, K.; Hirota, Y. Consumption of vegetables, fruit, and antioxidants during pregnancy and wheeze and eczema in infants. *Allergy* **2010**, *65*, 758–765. [CrossRef] [PubMed]

36. Okuda, M.; Bando, N.; Terao, J.; Sasaki, S.; Sugiyama, S.; Kunitsugu, I.; Hobara, T. Association of serum carotenoids and tocopherols with atopic diseases in japanese children and adolescents. *Pediatr. Allergy Immunol.* **2010**, *21*, e705–e710. [CrossRef] [PubMed]

37. Nwaru, B.I.; Erkkola, M.; Lumia, M.; Kronberg-Kippilä, C.; Ahonen, S.; Kaila, M.; Ilonen, J.; Simell, O.; Knip, M.; Veijola, R. Maternal intake of fatty acids during pregnancy and allergies in the offspring. *Br. J. Nutr.* **2012**, *108*, 720–732. [CrossRef] [PubMed]

38. Rosenlund, H.; Magnusson, J.; Kull, I.; Håkansson, N.; Wolk, A.; Pershagen, G.; Wickman, M.; Bergström, A. Antioxidant intake and allergic disease in children. *Clin. Exp. Allergy* **2012**, *42*, 1491–1500. [CrossRef] [PubMed]

39. Fung, T.T.; Hu, F.B.; Holmes, M.D.; Rosner, B.A.; Hunter, D.J.; Colditz, G.A.; Willett, W.C. Dietary patterns and the risk of postmenopausal breast cancer. *Int. J. Cancer* **2005**, *116*, 116–121. [CrossRef] [PubMed]

40. Chatzi, L.; Kogevinas, M. Prenatal and childhood mediterranean diet and the development of asthma and allergies in children. *Public Health Nutr.* **2009**, *12*, 1629–1634. [CrossRef] [PubMed]

41. Chatzi, L.; Torrent, M.; Romieu, I.; Garcia-Esteban, R.; Ferrer, C.; Vioque, J.; Kogevinas, M.; Sunyer, J. Mediterranean diet in pregnancy is protective for wheeze and atopy in childhood. *Thorax* **2008**, *63*, 507–513. [CrossRef] [PubMed]

42. Suarez-Varela, M.M.; Alvarez, L.G.; Kogan, M.D.; Ferreira, J.C.; Martinez Gimeno, A.; Aguinaga Ontoso, I.; Gonzalez Diaz, C.; Arnedo Pena, A.; Dominguez Aurrecoechea, B.; Busquets Monge, R.M.; *et al.* Diet and prevalence of atopic eczema in 6 to 7-year-old schoolchildren in Spain: ISAAC Phase III. *J. Investig. Allergol. Clin. Immunol.* **2010**, *20*, 469–475. [PubMed]

43. Lee, S. Prevalence of childhood asthma in Korea: International study of asthma and allergies in childhood. *Allergy Asthma Immunol. Res.* **2010**, *2*, 61–64. [CrossRef] [PubMed]

44. Kim, J.H.; Jeong, K.S.; Ha, E.; Park, H.; Ha, M.; Hong, Y.; Lee, S.; Lee, K.Y.; Jeong, J.; Kim, Y. Association between prenatal exposure to cadmium and atopic dermatitis in infancy. *J. Korean Med. Sci.* **2013**, *28*, 516–521. [CrossRef] [PubMed]

45. Alvarez, A.E.; de Lima Marson, F.A.; Bertuzzo, C.S.; Arns, C.W.; Ribeiro, J.D. Epidemiological and genetic characteristics associated with the severity of acute viral bronchiolitis by respiratory syncytial virus. *J. Pediatr.* **2013**, *89*, 531–543. [CrossRef] [PubMed]

46. Jung, Y.; Seo, J.; Kim, H.Y.; Kwon, J.; Kim, B.; Kim, H.; Lee, S.; Jang, G.C.; Song, D.J.; Kim, W.K. The relationship between asthma and bronchiolitis is modified by TLR4, CD14, and IL-13 polymorphisms. *Pediatr. Pulmonol.* **2015**, *50*, 8–16. [CrossRef] [PubMed]

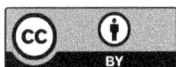

nutrients

MDPI

Article

Cross-Sectional Associations between Empirically-Derived Dietary Patterns and Indicators of Disease Risk among University Students

Stacy A. Blondin [1,*], Megan P. Mueller [1], Peter J. Bakun [1], Silvina F. Choumenkovitch [1], Katherine L. Tucker [2] and Christina D. Economos [1]

[1]   Tufts University Friedman School of Nutrition Science and Policy, 150 Harrison Avenue, Boston, MA 02111, USA; m.mueller@tufts.edu (M.P.M.); peter.bakun@tufts.edu (P.J.B.); silvina.choumenkovitch@tufts.edu (S.F.C.); christina.economos@tufts.edu (C.D.E.)

[2]   Clinical Laboratory & Nutritional Sciences, Center for Population Health & Health Disparities, University of Massachusetts at Lowell, 3 Solomont Way, Suite 4, Lowell, MA 01854, USA; katherine_tucker@uml.edu

*   Correspondence: stacy.blondin@tufts.edu; Tel.: +1-760-458-2426

Received: 22 November 2015; Accepted: 10 December 2015; Published: 24 December 2015

Abstract: The transition from adolescence to adulthood is a unique period during which lifelong dietary habits are shaped. Dietary patterns (DPs) among young adults attending college have not been adequately described, and associations between DPs and indicators of disease risk are not well understood in this age group. Dietary data were collected from undergraduates participating in the Tufts Longitudinal Health Study (TLHS; 1998–2007) by Food Frequency Questionnaire (FFQ; n = 1323). DPs were derived using principal components analysis with varimax rotation. Scree plots; eigenvalues; factor loadings; and previous studies were used to determine and label the DPs retained. Cross-sectional relationships between DP scores and anthropometric measures (percent body fat (PBF) and (BMI) and lipid biomarkers (total; HDL and LDL cholesterol; and triglycerides) were assessed with multivariable regression models; adjusted for demographics; physical activity; smoking; intention to gain/lose weight; and total energy intake. Effect modification by sex was tested. Three DPs were identified: Prudent; Western; and Alcohol. Greater adherence to the Prudent DP was associated with favorable anthropometric outcomes. The Alcohol DP was associated with a favorable lipid profile. Associations between the Western DP and blood lipids differed by sex; with unfavorable impact observed only among males. Our findings add to the literature linking DPs in young adults with measurable adiposity and cardiometabolic outcomes; suggesting that improving nutrition among college students could reduce chronic disease risk.

Keywords: dietary patterns; principle component analysis; college students; BMI; percent body fat; blood lipids; Tufts Longitudinal Health Study

1. Introduction

Dietary composition represents the largest risk factor for mortality and disease burden in the United States, responsible for 26% of deaths and 14% of disability-adjusted life years (Murray *et al.*, 2013). The most important dietary risks in the United States include low intakes of fruit, vegetables, nuts and seeds and high intakes of sodium, added sugars, processed meats, and *trans* fats. Because dietary intake is a modifiable lifestyle behavior, interventions to help individuals make positive dietary choices throughout the lifespan have the potential to substantially improve the quality and duration of life.

The transition between adolescence and adulthood, characterized by increasing independence, autonomy, and responsibility, is often the first time period in which individuals make autonomous decisions about "how, what, where, and when to eat" [1] and is, therefore, a crucial life-stage for establishing life-long health behaviors and habits, including healthy eating patterns [2]. For many, the transition into adulthood results in a shift in composition and quality of the diet. In fact, most studies have found that diet quality may worsen during this transition [1]. Data from the 2005–2006 and 2003–2004 NHANES suggest that the 13–18 and 19–39 year age groups consume the most caloric beverages [3] and are most likely to fall short of meeting fruit and vegetable serving recommendations [4]. Longitudinal studies support these findings, showing that consumption of fruit, vegetables, and milk generally decreases, while intake of sweetened beverages and snack foods tends to increase [5–7]. The transition to young adulthood has also been associated with increased frequency of fast food consumption and reduced frequency of breakfast consumption [8,9].

An increasing proportion of young adults are attending colleges and universities in the US, such that 20.2 million are expected to enroll in a degree-granting program in 2015, up by 4.9 million since 2000 (15% increase 1992–2002, 24% increase 2002–2012). With more than half of the college-going population attending four-year universities (13.2 million) and most enrolling full time (12.6 million) [10], the college population is of particular interest as a target group for health promotion- and disease-prevention interventions. To date, the majority of studies on diet-related health outcomes among college students have focused on weight status and/or trajectory, especially weight gain during the transition period from home to college during the freshman year [11–14].

A recent meta-analysis of studies from 1960 to 2013 (*n* = 49) on weight gain during the college years reported adjusted mean effect sizes of 1.55 kg increase in body weight and 1.17% increase in percent body fat (PBF) [12]. Others have explored potential factors that predict weight gain during college, such as place of residency, physical activity, psycho-social and sociodemographic factors, and body image/self-perception [15–24]. Though dietary behavior and intake among college students have been topics of longstanding interest [25–34], the extent to which variability in dietary patterns contribute to weight status among first-year college students has received limited attention. Most studies have investigated whether college students meet dietary guideline recommendations and/or whether specific foods or food groups influence weight status. However, considering individual dietary components in isolation provides a limited picture of how synergies among foods and nutrients in combination (*i.e.*, the diet as a whole) influence health outcomes [95].

Given the relative dearth of literature examining associations between dietary patterns and health outcomes among college students, the aim of this analysis was to investigate cross-sectional associations between empirically-derived dietary patterns and anthropometric and biomarker disease indicators among four-year university students. Identifying lifestyle factors that influence college students' health, including dietary patterns, could inform policies, programs, and interventions designed to reduce lifelong chronic disease risk of current and future generations. Although this life stage has been recognized as a critical time period for establishing nutrition behaviors carried into adulthood [2], and dietary patterns have been recognized as an important determinant of health [35,36], additional research is needed to elucidate relationships between the two.

2. Materials and Methods

2.1. Sample and Study Design

The Tufts Longitudinal Health Study (TLHS) is a prospective cohort study on the health and health-related behaviors of undergraduate students at Tufts University, a private research university in Medford, MA. All undergraduate students enrolling from 1998 to 2007 were eligible and recruited to participate. Members of each incoming freshmen class received a soft and hard version of the study's informed consent form, with information about the objectives, potential risks and benefits, and procedures in late July/early August, prior to the start of the academic year. Students who read, signed, and returned the form were enrolled in the study. Participants completed a 40-item Health Behavior Survey (HBS) before arriving at school and were invited to participate in a follow-up health assessment each spring. During the spring health assessment, students completed the HBS, a Food Frequency Questionnaire (FFQ), anthropometric and physical fitness measurements, and an optional blood draw. These assessments took place in April (approximately eight months after baseline HBS administration) and were repeated freshman through senior year. All procedures were performed in accordance with human subject research standards and approved by the Tufts University Institutional Review Board.

For this analysis, we restricted the sample to students who completed the health assessment during freshman year between 1998 and 2007, which included the largest number of participants (*n* = 1096). Approximately 99.3% of these students lived on campus and all were required to purchase a campus dining hall meal plan (97.2% reported eating in the dining hall frequently). As only a subset of participants completed blood assessments, we only excluded those with missing anthropometric data and/or missing data on diet, demographics, or physical activity (*n* = 313). We excluded data from students entering college in 2003 (*n* = 84) due to inconsistencies in the data. Individuals with negative, outlying, and/or implausible values for exposure or outcome variables based on age/sex appropriate population distributions were excluded (*n* = 16). In total, 683 participants had complete information on measures of body fatness, dietary data, and covariates of interest and 191 had complete blood lipid data, dietary data, and covariates of interest (Figure 1).

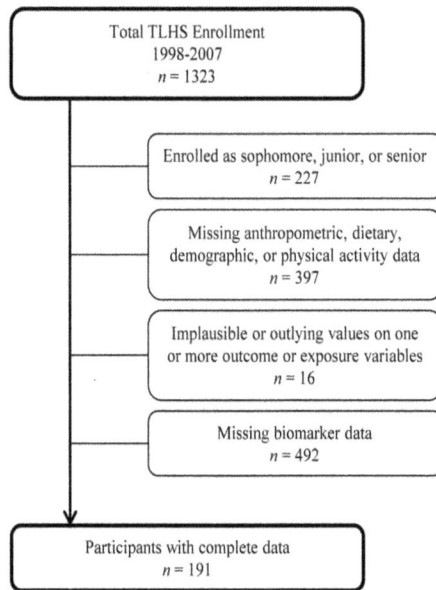

Figure 1. Flow chart depicting analytic sample deduction (boxes to the right indicate the number of participants excluded for each reason).

2.2. Assessments

2.2.1. Outcome Variables: Health Indices

Anthropometric Measurements

Anthropometric variables of interest included weight, height, body mass index (BMI), and body composition. BMI was calculated as weight (kg)/height (m^2) from measured height and weight (collected from the spring assessment). Participants removed their shoes and wore light clothing for measurement procedures. Weight was measured using a portable balance beam scale

(Healthometer, Boca Raton, FL, USA) and recorded to the nearest 1/4 pound. Height was measured using a portable stadiometer (Model 214, Seca Weighing and Measuring Systems, Hanover, MD, Germany) and recorded to the nearest 1/8 inch. Agreement between measured and self-reported weight and height was strong ($r = 0.997$, $p < 0.001$ for weight and $r = 0.957$, $p < 0.001$ for height) [37].

Body composition was determined via Bioelectrical Impedance Analysis (BIA). Total body resistance (ohms) and reactance (ohms) were measured on participants lying supine, with four surface self-adhesive spot electrodes and a standard conduction current of 800 1A and 50 kHz (BIA Model 101, RJL Systems, Detroit, MI, USA) following standard procedures. The laboratory-reported intra-operator ($n = 4$ operators; $n = 4$ subjects; triplicate measures) CV was 2.15% for resistance and 3.70% for reactance, and the inter-operator ($n = 6$ participants; 2–3 measures each) CV was 2.70% for resistance and 3.25% for reactance.

Fat Free Mass (FFM) was calculated using the race-combined equations developed by Sun *et al.*, (2003) Equation (1) for men and women, and a two compartment model was used to calculate total body fat (BF) and PBF by subtracting FFM from total mass [38].

$$FFM_{Males} = \_9.88 + 0.65 stature^2/resistance + 0.26^* \ weight + 0.02^* \ resistance$$
$$FFM_{Females} = \_11.03 + 0.70 \ stature^2/resistance + 0.17^* \ weight + 0.02^* \ resistance$$

(1)

Lipid Biomarkers

Blood samples were collected in 2000–2002, 2004, 2006, and 2007. Blood was drawn after a 12-h overnight fast. Serum lipid profiles (total cholesterol, HDL cholesterol, and triglycerides) and glucose were measured by ACEi Clinical Chemistry Systems (Schiapparelli Biosystems, Fairfield, NJ, USA) using standard reagent kits. LDL cholesterol was calculated via the Friedewald equation [39].

2.2.2. Exposure/Predictor Variables: Dietary Intake and Dietary Patterns

Dietary data were collected using an adapted version of the Fred Hutchinson Cancer Research Center Food Frequency Questionnaire (Version 06.10.88, Cancer Prevention Research Program, Fred Hutchinson Cancer Research Center, Seattle, WA, USA). Participants were asked to report how frequently they consumed each food item listed (ranging from 2 or more per day to never/less than once per month) in each of 8 main food categories (fruit/juices, breakfast, vegetables, meat/fish/poultry, breads/snacks/spreads, dairy, sweets, and beverages). They were also asked to indicate the amount of each food they usually consumed (small, medium, or large) relative to a specified medium serving size (e.g., ½ cup). FFQs were scanned using a Scantron OpScan6 optical mark reader and linked to the Minnesota Nutrition Data System (NDS) [40] for food grouping, serving size, and nutrient intake using a SAS program maintained by the Epidemiology and Dietary Assessment Research Program, USDA Human Nutrition Research Center on Aging at Tufts University, Boston, MA, USA.

The FFQ food items (~100) were condensed into 43 food groups, adapted from Hu *et al.* (1999) [41] (Table S1). For each observation, the number of medium serving sizes of foods within each group were summed across all relevant food items. Dietary patterns were derived using principal components analysis (PCA). The resulting scree plot was used to visually assess the variability captured by each factor (Figure S1). Eigenvalues, factor loading values, and previous studies were used to determine and label the dietary patterns. Three factors with eigenvalues >2 were identified and then orthogonally rotated (varimax rotation was applied to obtain uncorrelated factors). Food groups in each factor with loadings ⩾0.3 in absolute value were used to interpret the factors. Each participant received a score for each dietary pattern.

2.2.3. Confounding and Effect Modifying Variables

Physical Activity

Self-reported physical activity and exercise habits were measured using the Cooper Institute for Aerobics Research Aerobics Center Longitudinal Study (ACLS) questionnaire [42–44]. For each activity included on the questionnaire (e.g., walking, stair climbing, jogging/running, bicycling, swimming, weight training, *etc.*), participants were asked to self-report the number of sessions they engaged in, the average duration of each session, and the distance and/or speed traveled in each session (as relevant), over the past three months for activities engaged in at least once a week.

Total Metabolic Equivalent of Task (MET) minutes were calculated for each student from physical activity information collected via the ACLS. The number of sessions per week was multiplied by the average session duration to calculate the total number of minutes engaged in each activity per week, and distance was divided by the duration of each session to calculate average speed for endurance activities (e.g., running, swimming, biking, walking, *etc.*). The total number of minutes engaged in each activity at each intensity value (as available/applicable) was then multiplied by the corresponding MET value [45]. When there was not an exact match in the MET compendium for an ACLS activity, we used the MET value for the most closely related activity or took an average of the MET values for the most closely related category of activities. Because a wide variety of activities were listed for the "other" category (e.g., singing *versus* rowing), we used the average MET value for all of the activities included in the compendium.

Total Energy

Total energy intake per day was calculated from the FFQ data by summing the total kJ per person per day across all food groups.

Demographic Variables

The HBS was developed from existing population-based surveys and pilot tested with more than 100 college-age students in 1998 and 1999. Questions were adapted and compiled from validated instruments and questionnaires previously used in large studies of college age students, including the National College Health Risk Behavior Survey (NCHRBS), American College Health Association (ACHA) National College Health Assessment, Youth Risk Behavior Surveillance System (YRBSS), and Colorado State University Wellness Lifestyle Profile [46–48]. Students self-reported their height/weight and answered questions about age, sex, and race/ethnicity.

Age was coded as a continuous variable, sex dichotomized into male and female, and self-reported race/ethnicity responses collapsed from Asian/Pacific American, Black/African American, Hispanic/Latin American, White/Caucasian, Bi-racial/Multiracial, Native American, Other into five categories: Caucasian, African American, Hispanic, Asian, and Other. Smoking status was dichotomized into smokers and non-smokers, based on self-report of current smoking behavior. Participants' intention to gain or lose weight were dichotomous variables based on yes/no survey question responses.

2.3. Statistical Analysis

All analyses were performed with SAS statistical software (Version 9.3, Cary, NC, USA). p values < 0.05 were considered statistically significant. Distributions identified as non-normal based on the Shapiro-Wilk test for normality [49] were log-transformed (BMI, LDL, triglycerides, and total cholesterol). When log transforming non-normally-distributed outcome variables did not affect coefficient directionality or model significance, non-logged estimates were reported to enhance interpretability of results.

Regression Models

Multivariable regression models were used to examine cross-sectional relationships between empirically derived dietary pattern scores and BMI and lipid biomarkers. Models were adjusted for age, sex, race, physical activity (MET minutes), and total energy intake (kJ/day). KJ values <2510.4 and >20,920 were excluded, based on approximations from previous literature [50,51]. Tukey's test was used to identify outliers for all predictor and outcome variables [52]. Outlying values for physical activity were included because they were plausible and their inclusion did not affect the directionality or significance of the results. Sensitivity analyses were run with physical activity quantified as total minutes of activity per week and with dietary pattern score categorized into quartiles. Sex was evaluated as an effect modifier; main effects were reported when no significant interaction was present. All biomarkers (HDL, LDL, and total cholesterol, and triglycerides) were treated as continuous variables.

3. Results

3.1. Sample Demographics

The analytic sample included 683 participants with HBS and biomarker data collected during their freshman year at Tufts University. Sample demographics are presented in Table 1. Briefly, participants were predominantly non-Hispanic white (76.1%), and the majority were female (68.1%). The mean age was 18.5 ± 6.0 years and ranged from 17 to 21 years. Participants were generally healthy (mean anthropometric and biomarkers within normal ranges), non-smoking, and physically active.

Table 1. Overall sample characteristics (*n* = 683).

Characteristic	
Male (%)	31.9
Age years	18.5 ± 0.6
Race/Ethnicity	
Caucasian (%)	76.1
African American (%)	3.4
Hispanic (%)	3.7
Other (%)	16.8
Current smokers (%)	4.1
Freshman (%)	100.0
Intention to lose weight (%)	52.3
Intention to gain weight (%)	11.2
MET minutes PA per week	2324.4 ± 2276.6
Total Daily Energy Intake (kJ)	7824.5 ± 3172.3
Percent Body Fat (%)	24.3 ± 6.9
BMI (kg/m^2)	22.8 ± 3.0
Lipid Profile (*n* = 191)	
LDL (mg/dL)	93.8 ± 27.9
HDL (mg/dL)	54.0 ± 12.0
Total cholesterol (mg/dL)	167.0 ± 32.6
Triglycerides (mg/dL)	96.3 ± 42.1

All values are mean ± sd unless otherwise noted.

3.2. Dietary Pattern Characterization

Three dietary patterns were identified and labeled: Western, Prudent, and Alcohol. These patterns explained 10.3%, 9.3% and 4.8% of total variance, respectively. Food groups with PCA factor loading values ⩾0.3 are listed for each dietary pattern in Table 2. Negative values reflect inverse correlations (e.g., legumes and other vegetables for the Alcohol dietary pattern). The highest values (absolute values >0.5) were observed for red meat, French fries, refined grains, processed meats, and snacks for the Western dietary pattern; fruit, vegetables (including subtypes), and whole grains for the Prudent pattern; and liquor and beer, for the Alcohol dietary pattern. In general the Western pattern was characterized by refined and energy-dense foods high in fat and sugar; the Prudent pattern by whole, plant-based foods and healthy fats and oils; and the Alcohol pattern by caloric beverages, especially those containing alcohol and, to a lesser extent, coffee (mean intake 4.68 fl oz per day among those in the highest quartile). The average medium serving sizes consumed by participants in the lowest and highest quartile of dietary pattern scores for the top five foods in each of the three patterns are listed in Table 3.

3.3. Dietary Patterns and Indicators of Disease Risk

Adherence to the Prudent dietary pattern was inversely associated with percent body fat and BMI after adjustment for biological and behavioral variables (Table 4). The crude, positive association between the Prudent dietary pattern and HDL was no longer significant after further adjustment. Significant dietary pattern score by sex interaction terms were observed for the Western dietary pattern and selected health indices (Table 4 and stratified models in Table 5). In crude models, the Western dietary pattern was positively associated with PBF among males and with HDL among females, although significance was reduced in adjusted models.

In general, associations between the Western dietary pattern and disease indicators were stronger and more adverse among males. The Western dietary pattern was positively associated with triglycerides among males in all three models. Although significant positive associations with LDL cholesterol and triglycerides among males were attenuated with the inclusion of lifestyle variables in Model 3, positive borderline significant associations ($p < 0.1$) were observed between Western dietary pattern and LDL cholesterol, total cholesterol, and triglycerides (Table 5). When looking at differences in food group consumption among males and females with scores in the upper quartile of Western dietary pattern, the most statistically significant differences ($p < 0.001$) were observed for beer, high energy drinks, processed meats, red meat, pizza, and sweets/desserts (Table S2). The greatest absolute differences (≥ 0.25 servings/day) were observed for fruit juice, sweets/desserts, beer, processed meats, and red meat. Of the differences with the greatest statistical significance and absolute value, the processed meat and red meat food groups had the highest factor loadings for the Western dietary pattern (>0.5), followed by sweets/desserts (0.31). Differences in pizza consumption were also notable, with an absolute difference of 0.16 servings per day. Though the difference in beer servings consumed was considerable (0.25 per day), the factor loading was relatively low (0.14).

Alcohol dietary pattern adherence was positively associated with HDL cholesterol and inversely associated with LDL cholesterol. These relationships were strengthened with adjustment for additional variables. Borderline positive associations were observed for the Alcohol dietary pattern and PBF in Model 1 and BMI in Model 2.

Table 2. Factor loading matrix for the three major dietary patterns identified from the Food Frequency Questionnaire (FFQ).

		Dietary Pattern			
Western		Prudent		Alcohol	
Foods or Food Groups	Factor Loading	Foods or Food Groups	Factor Loading	Foods or Food Groups	Factor Loading
Red meat	0.66	Fruit	0.74	Liquor	0.55
French fries	0.59	Dark yellow-orange vegetables	0.60	Beer	0.48
Refined grains	0.58	Other vegetables	0.57	Wine	0.46
Processed meats	0.56	Whole grains	0.55	Coffee	0.38
Snacks	0.51	Cruciferous vegetables	0.52	Low-energy drinks	0.30
Potatoes	0.49	Green leafy vegetables	0.51	Legumes	−0.38
Pizza	0.48	Legumes	0.51	Other vegetables	−0.40
Butter	0.45	Non-cream soups	0.47		
High energy drinks	0.45	Tomatoes	0.44		
Pasta	0.45	Yogurt	0.43		
Creamy dressings	0.42	Nuts	0.38		
High fat dairy products	0.42	Breakfast cereal	0.35		
Ice cream	0.42	Fish and seafood	0.34		
Poultry	0.42				
Margarine	0.38				
Other fats and oils	0.38				
Fruit juice	0.37				
Sweets and desserts	0.31				

Table 3. Mean daily intake of participants with scores in the top and bottom quartile (Q4 and Q1, respectively) of the three dietary patterns for the foods/food groups with the highest factor loadings.

	Dietary Pattern								
Western			**Prudent**			**Alcohol**			
Foods/Food Groups	Daily Intake		Foods/Food Groups	Daily Intake (Cups)		Food/Food Groups	Daily Intake (fl oz)		
	Q1	Q4		Q1	Q4		Q1	Q4	
Red meat (ounces)	0.25	2.64	Fruit [3]	0.25	1.31	Liquor	0.06	0.63	
French fries (cups)	0.07	0.68	Dark yellow-orange vegetables [4]	0.04	0.27	Beer	0.00	5.4	
Refined grains (pieces) [1]	0.56	1.89	Other vegetables	0.04	0.29	Wine	0.05	0.40	
Processed meats (pieces) [2]	0.12	1.02	whole grains [5]	0.11	0.52	Coffee	0.36	4.68	
Snacks (cups)	0.07	0.33	Cruciferous vegetables	0.03	0.25	Low-energy drinks	0.72	7.44	

Mean daily intake was calculated by multiplying the mean servings consumed per day from each food group by the mean serving size (the most common serving size unit); [1] Serving sizes of food items in the refined grains group included 1 piece, 1 medium, 2 each, 6 small or 3 large, 1-4 ¼" diameter pastry, 1 large. The most common serving size listed was 1 piece; [2] Processed meats servings sizes were determined based on the serving sizes for bacon and pork sausage links: 2 links or pieces; [3] Serving sizes of food items in the fruit group included 1 medium, ½ cup, 1 each, ¼ cup, 3 each, ¼ of 5" diameter, ½ of 10" diameter, ½ of 4" diameter. The most common serving size listed was ½ cup; [4] Serving sizes of food items in the dark yellow-orange group included ½ cup and 1 medium. The most common serving size listed was ½ cup; [5] Serving sizes of food items in the whole grains group included 2 slices, 6 small, ½ cup, ¾ cup, 1 cup. The most common serving sizes listed were in cups, so the items with servings listed in cups were averaged.

Table 4. Associations between dietary pattern scores and anthropometric and biomarker outcomes.

Outcomes	Model 1 β	se	p	Model 2 β	se	p	Model 3 β	se	p
Western									
Body fat (%)		(p-interaction = 0.0426)		−0.08	0.37	0.818	0.31	0.36	0.381
BMI (kg/m²)		(p-interaction = 0.0247)		−0.10	0.21	0.640	0.21	0.20	0.305
HDL (mg/dL)		(p-interaction = 0.0128)		−1.89	1.58	0.234	−1.55	1.60	0.336
LDL(mg/dL)		(p-interaction = 0.0460)			(p-interaction = 0.0134)			(p-interaction = 0.0148)	
Triglycerides(mg/dL)		(p-interaction = 0.0210)			(p-interaction = 0.0190)			(p-interaction = 0.0139)	
Total Cholesterol(mg/dL)	1.40	2.46	0.569		(p-interaction = 0.0271)			(p-interaction = 0.0303)	
Prudent									
Body fat (%)	0.36	0.26	0.176	−0.26	0.22	0.236	−0.42	0.21	0.046 *
BMI (kg/m²)	−0.18	0.11	0.114	−0.15	0.12	0.217	−0.29	0.12	0.017 *
HDL (mg/dL)	2.17	0.88	0.014 *	1.29	0.92	0.165	1.19	0.96	0.216
LDL(mg/dL)	1.48	2.07	0.476	1.03	2.34	0.660	0.79	2.47	0.748
Triglycerides(mg/dL)	0.18	3.13	0.954	−1.88	3.48	0.590	−1.96	3.55	0.581
Total Cholesterol(mg/dL)	3.70	2.41	0.126	1.95	2.68	0.467	1.60	2.82	0.572
Alcohol									
Body fat (%)	0.46	0.27	0.083 +	0.33	0.22	0.130	0.15	0.21	0.482
BMI (kg/m²)	0.19	0.12	0.105	0.24	0.12	0.052 +	0.13	0.12	0.280
HDL (mg/dL)	2.49	0.92	0.007 *	1.94	0.92	0.036 *	2.16	0.93	0.021 *
LDL(mg/dL)	−4.07	2.16	0.061 +	−5.43	2.31	0.020 *	−5.46	2.38	0.023 *
Triglycerides (mg/dL)	1.39	3.29	0.673	−0.33	3.49	0.924	−0.59	3.48	0.866
Total Cholesterol (mg/dL)	−1.29	2.55	0.612	−3.55	2.67	0.186	−3.40	2.75	0.218

Model 1: unadjusted; Model 2: adjusted for age, race, sex, energy; Model 3: adjusted for age, race, sex, energy, smoking status, physical activity, and weight gain/loss intentions; * $p < 0.05$, + $p < 0.1$; Interaction term *p* values are reported for models with significant modification by gender.

Table 5. Western dietary pattern regression models stratified by sex (β (standard error), *p*-value).

	% Body Fat	BMI	HDL	LDL	Triglycerides	Total Cholesterol
			Model 1			
Males	0.58 (0.35), *p* = 0.1	0.21 (0.21), *p* = 0.30	−0.72 (1.31), *p* = 0.58	8.34 (3.4), *p* = 0.02 *	14.1 (4.54), *p* = 0.003 *	NA
Females	−0.21 (0.30), *p* = 0.5	−0.21 (0.17), *p* = 0.21	2.48 (1.37), *p* = 0.07 +	−2.58 (3.28), *p* = 0.43	−2.43 (5.22), *p* = 0.64	NA
			Model 2			
Males	NA	NA	NA	13.0 (6.55), *p* = 0.05 +	24.7 (8.59), *p* = 0.01 *	14.5 (6.99), *p* = 0.04 *
Females	NA	NA	NA	−0.84 (5.26), *p* = 0.87	−1.83 (8.14), *p* = 0.82	−1.08 (6.24), *p* = 0.86
			Model 3			
Males	NA	NA	NA	12.2 (6.75), *p* = 0.08 +	23.7 (8.19), *p* = 0.005 *	13.98 (7.22), *p* = 0.06 +
Females	NA	NA	NA	−1.38 (5.53), *p* = 0.80	−4.98 (8.28), *p* = 0.55	−1.88(6.54), *p* = 0.77

Model 1: unadjusted; Model 2: adjusted for age, race, sex, energy; Model 3: adjusted for age, race, sex, energy, smoking status, physical activity, and weight gain/loss intentions; * *p* < 0.05, + *p* < 0.1.

4. Discussion

Findings from this analysis suggest that variability in dietary pattern adherence among freshmen attending a four-year university is associated with observable differences in select anthropometric and lipid biomarkers. Specifically, greater adherence to a Prudent dietary pattern, characterized by high consumption of plant-based foods, was favorably associated with body composition, while greater adherence to a dietary pattern characterized by higher, but modest, levels of alcohol consumption was favorably associated with blood lipid concentrations (mean intake less than one standard alcoholic beverage equivalents per day (0.95 standard drinks equaling 14 g pure alcohol)). Conversely, adherence to a Western dietary pattern had no impact on anthropometric outcomes but adverse impacts on lipid biomarkers among males.

Previous research supports Prudent dietary pattern adherence as protective and Western dietary pattern adherence as predisposing toward a variety of chronic disease outcomes, including type 2 diabetes, obesity, cancer, heart disease, anxiety/depression, and mortality among adults [41,53–62] and mental and metabolic health among adolescents [63–66]. Our findings extend the inverse associations between the Prudent pattern and anthropometric/biomarker indices to a younger population. Although previous empirically derived dietary pattern analyses in this population are lacking, our results are consistent with studies linking consumption of specific foods and food groups with health outcomes (e.g., Rose 2007 [67]).

A recent analysis of the Coronary Artery Risk Development in Young Adults (CARDIA) study data in young adults (18–30 years) reported a protective role of Mediterranean dietary pattern adherence against metabolic syndrome risk (abdominal obesity, elevated triglycerides, and low HDL cholesterol) in longitudinal models [68]. Although the CARDIA study was not restricted to young adults and employed researcher-defined dietary pattern parameters, similarities between the Mediterranean dietary pattern—rich in fruit, vegetables, whole grains, nuts, and fish and low in red and processed meat—in the aforementioned study and the Prudent pattern in ours are evident. Another study, investigating the relationship between nutrient intakes and adiposity in the National Heart, Lung, and Blood Institute Growth and Health Study cohort of 2371 black and white girls, (9–10 years of age at baseline) reported that the "healthy pattern", characterized by high intake of fruit, vegetables, dairy, grains without added fats, mixed dishes and soups, and low intake of sweetened drinks, other sweets, fried foods, burgers, and pizza, was related to more favorable nutrient intakes and a smaller increase in waist circumference at age 19–20 years [69]. Although this population differed in age range and demographic profile, the findings were consistent with ours, since both studies supported a positive association between Prudent pattern adherence and adiposity outcomes among youth.

The deleterious association between the Western dietary patterndietary pattern score and cardiovascular disease biomarkers among males also agrees with previous research in adult populations [41,70]. Despite these adverse results, no associations were seen with adiposity outcomes among males in our study. Given the young age and generally healthy profile of our population, the lack of findings could suggest that adherence to the Western dietary pattern may affect lipid biomarkers of disease independently and/or prior to measurable changes in anthropometric outcomes in some cases, which may be important in early detection of cardiometabolic disease risk.

Interestingly, associations between the Western dietary pattern adherence and disease indicators in females were non-significant in adjusted models. Differences in the mean number of medium servings consumed from each food group by males and females scoring in the highest quartile of the Western dietary pattern (Table S2) may have accounted in part for the effect modification. It is also possible that biological differences in females (e.g., hormonal or neuro-endocrine differences) may mitigate or delay the adverse impacts seen in males. These hypotheses and other potential explanations merit further research.

Finally, the protective relationships observed between adherence to the Alcohol dietary pattern and lipid biomarkers are consistent with literature supporting a link between moderate consumption of alcohol and reduced risk for cardiovascular disease [71,72]. While previous studies have identified "alcohol" or "drinker" patterns using empirically-derived dietary pattern methodology [73–76], the emergence of this pattern has generally been reported less consistently than variations of Prudent (healthy) and Western (unhealthy) patterns. However, increases in alcohol consumption during college has been observed, though its intake is likely to vary considerably within this population [77], which could help explain the emergence of a dietary pattern defined by alcohol consumption [78,79]. Nonetheless, even among students in the top quartile of dietary pattern adherence, average daily intake was relatively low (0.95 standard drinks). We did not observe significant associations between Alcohol dietary pattern adherence and anthropometric outcomes in our study, and few previous studies have looked specifically at alcohol consumption and overweight/obesity risk. However, several have considered relationships between alcohol consumption, especially binge drinking behavior, and eating patterns, body satisfaction, and weight loss intentions [80–82]. Findings from these studies suggest that alcohol abuse may be associated with disordered eating and/or lower diet quality. In one study, binge drinking was associated with poor diets, unhealthy weight control, body dissatisfaction, and sedentary behavior; although no independent associations between alcohol consumption and adiposity were reported, differences in alcohol-related eating behavior were associated with increased risk of overweight/obesity and, therefore, may moderate the association [83]. Students who "usually" or "always" ate before and/or during drinking were more likely to be overweight (RR: 1.24 (1.03–1.50)), with differences by year in school and weight status observed. In the general adult population a systematic review of previous studies did not support a positive association between alcohol consumption and adiposity [84]. Although positive findings between alcohol intake and weight gain have been reported, they have been primarily detected among high consumers; in contrast, some studies have suggested that light-to-moderate alcohol intake may protect against weight gain [84], which could also explain the lack of association seen here. In other studies, consumption of distilled alcoholic beverages has been positively associated with weight gain, whereas wine intake has shown a possible inverse association [84].

Future analyses should consider the frequency, amount, and type of alcohol consumed in relation to adiposity outcomes specifically among college students, as drinking patterns in this population differ from that of the general population [77,85,86]. It is also possible that alcohol consumption coincides with compensatory eating and/or exercise behaviors among college students [87]. Finally, though coffee was less strongly associated with the Alcohol pattern and mean intakes were relatively low (<6 fl oz per day), coffee consumption was found to be associated with increased total cholesterol, LDL cholesterol, and triglycerides in a systematic review of randomized trials [88], despite moderate consumption being consistently associated with reduced chronic disease risk in observational studies [89]. Further research linking beverage consumption and diet-related behavior could further clarify these relationships.

While findings from this study contribute to the scientific discussion on dietary patterns and health outcomes in an understudied age group, several limitations are apparent. First, the cross-sectional nature of the analysis limits our capacity to draw causal and temporal inferences from our findings. While models controlled for important variables hypothesized to confound or modify the relationship between dietary patterns and disease indicators, including total energy intake and physical activity, several relied upon self-report data, which are vulnerable to inherent biases. Moreover, it is possible that residual confounding could have affected the magnitude and/or significance of associations. For example, because dietary data were not collected for the time period prior to degree program matriculation, we could not account for the potential influence of childhood/adolescent dietary patterns on current dietary pattern and/or health status. Likewise, despite the relative sociodemographic homogeneity of our sample, we were not able to control for socioeconomic status in our models. Previous research suggests that income and education may influence diet quality among young adults [90] and, therefore, should be considered. We restricted our sample to freshman, nearly all of whom lived on campus and were required to purchase a University meal plan, regardless. Though previous literature on linking place of residence and dining habits with diet quality and health outcomes is mixed [23,91–93], results may or may not generalize to students living and/or dining off campus, which was more common among upperclassmen. The race/ethnicity of our sample was also predominantly non-Hispanic white, which may limit generalizability to more diverse populations.

Furthermore, it is possible that the variables that were measured and controlled in our analysis contain measurement error. Dietary intake was self-reported by FFQ and, consequently, subject to biases, such as recall error and observer/social desirability effects. Similarly, physical activity was assessed by self-report. However, the ACLS has been used in previous studies [42–44,94], and MET minutes were calculated to capture physical activity intensity and duration. We used the updated 2011 compendium, which included 800 unique activity-intensity levels [45], allowing for comprehensive and precise estimates of energy expenditure. Finally, although we relied on well-established methodology and conducted sensitivity analyses, PCA involves subjective decision-making (e.g., the total number of food groups included, number of patterns retained, pattern labeling, *etc.*), which could affect our results and their interpretation. For example, the percentage of the total variance explained by the derived factors is strongly influenced by the number of food groups included in the analysis and may also affect the precision of regression estimates [96–98]. Accordingly, we weighed eigenvalues and factor interpretability more heavily in deciding how many and which factors to retain for this analysis [98,99].

Despite these potential limitations, this study has notable strengths. In particular, the sample size was large (*n* = 683), even when limiting the analytic sample to students with complete data, including blood samples (*n* = 191). The comprehensiveness and measurement validity of our outcome variables, including measured height and weight, BIA-assessed body composition, and biomarkers collected via blood sample add merit to our findings. Finally, this study is one of few to evaluate associations between total diet and health status of first-year college students.

5. Conclusions

These results provide insight into potential associations between dietary patterns among college students and disease indices. The evidence could be strengthened by future studies using longitudinal methods to identify whether changes in dietary pattern adherence over multiple college years are associated with changes in anthropometric and biomarker measurements. It would also be of interest to identify predictors of dietary pattern choice. Understanding the relationship between diet and health among young adults attending colleges and universities is important for developing programs, policies, and behavior change strategies to improve quality of life and reduce diet-related disease burden at the population level.

Acknowledgments: The authors would like to thank Gail Rogers for her guidance on dietary patterns analysis methods and Rebecca Boulos for her assistance with data management. Funding for this research was provided primarily by Tufts University. This material is based upon work supported by the National Institute of Food and Agriculture, U.S. Department of Agriculture, under Agreement No. 2012-38420-30200.

Author Contributions: Stacy Blondin and Megan Mueller conceptualized, designed, and conducted all analyses. Stacy Blondin led the drafting and revising of the manuscript. Peter Bakun assisted with data management. Silvina Choumenkovitch contributed to analysis design. Christina Economos designed, led, and collected data for the original study and provided guidance on data analysis and interpretation of results. Katherine Tucker oversaw the dietary data management and analysis in the original study and provided guidance on data analysis and interpretation of results. All authors were involved in revising the manuscript for important intellectual content and have given approval of the final version.

Conflicts of Interest: The authors declare no conflict of interest.

References

1. VanKim, N.A.; Larson, N.; Laska, M.N. Emerging adulthood: A critical age for preventing excess weight gain? *Adolesc. Med. State Art Rev.* **2012**, *23*, 571–588. [PubMed]
2. Nelson, M.C.; Story, M.; Larson, N.I.; Neumark-Sztainer, D.; Lytle, L.A. Emerging adulthood and college-aged youth: An overlooked age for weight-related behavior change. *Obesity* **2008**, *16*, 2205–2211. [CrossRef] [PubMed]
3. Popkin, B.M. Patterns of beverage use across the lifecycle. *Physiol. Behav.* **2010**, *100*, 4–9. [CrossRef] [PubMed]
4. Kimmons, J.; Gillespie, C.; Seymour, J.; Serdula, M.; Blanck, H.M. Fruit and vegetable intake among adolescents and adults in the United States: Percentage meeting individualized recommendations. *Medscape J. Med.* **2009**, *11*, 26. [PubMed]
5. Lytle, L.A.; Seifert, S.; Greenstein, J.; McGovern, P. How do children's eating patterns and food choices change over time? Results from a cohort study. *Am. J. Health Promot.* **2000**, *14*, 222–228. [CrossRef] [PubMed]
6. Demory-Luce, D.; Morales, M.; Nicklas, T.; Baranowski, T.; Zakeri, I.; Berenson, G. Changes in food group consumption patterns from childhood to young adulthood: The Bogalusa Heart Study. *J. Am. Diet. Assoc.* **2004**, *104*, 1684–1691. [CrossRef] [PubMed]
7. Larson, N.I.; Neumark-Sztainer, D.; Hannan, P.J.; Story, M. Trends in adolescent fruit and vegetable consumption, 1999–2004: Project EAT. *Am. J. Prev. Med.* **2007**, *32*, 147–150. [CrossRef] [PubMed]
8. Niemeier, H.M.; Raynor, H.A.; Lloyd-Richardson, E.E.; Rogers, M.L.; Wing, R.R. Fast food consumption and breakfast skipping: Predictors of weight gain from adolescence to adulthood in a nationally representative sample. *J. Adolesc. Health* **2006**, *39*, 842–849. [CrossRef] [PubMed]
9. Vikraman, S.; Fryar, C.D.; Ogden, C.L. Caloric Intake from Fast Food among Children and Adolescents in the United States, 2011–2012. *NCHS Data Brief* **2015**, *213*, 1–8. [PubMed]
10. U.S. Department of Education Institute of Education Sciences National Center for Education Statistics. Fast Facts: Back to School Statistics. Available online: http://nces.ed.gov/fastfacts/display.asp?id=372 (accessed on 12 December 2015).
11. Vella-Zarb, R.A.; Elgar, F.J. The "freshman 5": A meta-analysis of weight gain in the freshman year of college. *J. Am. Coll. Health* **2009**, *58*, 161–166. [CrossRef] [PubMed]
12. Fedewa, M.V.; Das, B.M.; Evans, E.M.; Dishman, R.K. Change in weight and adiposity in college students: A systematic review and meta-analysis. *Am. J. Prev. Med.* **2014**, *47*, 641–652. [CrossRef] [PubMed]
13. Vadeboncoeur, C.; Townsend, N.; Foster, C. A meta-analysis of weight gain in first year university students: Is freshman 15 a myth? *BMC Obes.* **2015**, *2*. [CrossRef] [PubMed]
14. Bodenlos, J.S.; Gengarelly, K.; Smith, R. Gender differences in freshmen weight gain. *Eating Behav.* **2015**, *19*, 1–4. [CrossRef] [PubMed]
15. Kapinos, K.A.; Yakusheva, O.; Eisenberg, D. Obesogenic environmental influences on young adults: Evidence from college dormitory assignments. *Econ. Hum. Biol.* **2014**, *12*, 98–109. [CrossRef] [PubMed]
16. Yakusheva, O.; Kapinos, K.; Weiss, M. Peer effects and the freshman 15: Evidence from a natural experiment. *Econ. Hum. Biol.* **2011**, *9*, 119–132. [CrossRef] [PubMed]
17. Gillen, M.M.; Lefkowitz, E.S. The "freshman 15": Trends and predictors in a sample of multiethnic men and women. *Eating Behav.* **2011**, *12*, 261–266. [CrossRef] [PubMed]
18. Finlayson, G.; Cecil, J.; Higgs, S.; Hill, A.; Hetherington, M. Susceptibility to weight gain. Eating behaviour traits and physical activity as predictors of weight gain during the first year of university. *Appetite* **2012**, *58*, 1091–1098. [CrossRef] [PubMed]
19. Lowe, M.R.; Annunziato, R.A.; Markowitz, J.T.; Didie, E.; Bellace, D.L.; Riddell, L.; Maille, C.; McKinney, S.; Stice, E. Multiple types of dieting prospectively predict weight gain during the freshman year of college. *Appetite* **2006**, *47*, 83–90. [CrossRef] [PubMed]
20. Pliner, P.; Saunders, T. Vulnerability to freshman weight gain as a function of dietary restraint and residence. *Physiol. Behav.* **2008**, *93*, 76–82. [CrossRef] [PubMed]
21. Provencher, V.; Polivy, J.; Wintre, M.G.; Pratt, M.W.; Pancer, S.M.; Birnie-Lefcovitch, S.; Adams, G.R. Who gains or who loses weight? Psychosocial factors among first-year university students. *Physiol. Behav.* **2009**, *96*, 135–141. [CrossRef] [PubMed]
22. Freedman, M.R. Gender, residence and ethnicity affect freshman BMI and dietary habits. *Am. J. Health Behav.* **2010**, *34*, 513–524. [CrossRef] [PubMed]

23. Pelletier, J.E.; Laska, M.N. Campus food and beverage purchases are associated with indicators of diet quality in college students living off campus. *Am. J. Health Promot.* **2013**, *28*, 80–87. [CrossRef] [PubMed]

24. Chin, J.; Chang, K. College students' attitude toward body weight control, health-related lifestyle and dietary behavior by self-perception on body image and obesity index. *J. Korean Soc. Food Sci. Nutr.* **2005**, *34*, 1559–1565.

25. Querido, J.; Morrell, J. How does inaccurate perception of weight compared to actual BMI status affect the diet score of college students? *FASEB J.* **2015**, *29*, LB315.

26. Brevard, P.B.; Ricketts, C.D. Residence of college students affects dietary intake, physical activity, and serum lipid levels. *J. Am. Diet. Assoc.* **1996**, *96*, 35–38. [CrossRef]

27. Anding, J.D.; Suminski, R.R.; Boss, L. Dietary intake, body mass index, exercise, and alcohol: Are college women following the dietary guidelines for Americans? *J. Am. Coll. Health* **2001**, *49*, 167–171. [CrossRef] [PubMed]

28. Huang, Y.; Song, W.O.; Schemmel, R.A.; Hoerr, S.M. What do college students eat? Food selection and meal pattern. *Nutr. Res.* **1994**, *14*, 1143–1153. [CrossRef]

29. Dinger, M.K.; Waigandt, A. Dietary intake and physical activity behaviors of male and female college students. *Am. J. Health Promot.* **1997**, *11*, 360–362. [CrossRef] [PubMed]

30. Haberman, S.; Luffey, D. Weighing in college students' diet and exercise behaviors. *J. Am. Coll. Health* **1998**, *46*, 189–191. [CrossRef] [PubMed]

31. Graham, D.J.; Laska, M.N. Nutrition label use partially mediates the relationship between attitude toward healthy eating and overall dietary quality among college students. *J. Acad. Nutr. Dietet.* **2012**, *112*, 414–418. [CrossRef]

32. Block, J.P.; Gillman, M.W.; Linakis, S.K.; Goldman, R.E. "If It Tastes Good, I'm Drinking It": Qualitative Study of Beverage Consumption Among College Students. *J. Adolesc. Health* **2013**, *52*, 702–706. [CrossRef] [PubMed]

33. Tully, L.R.; Morrell, J.S.; Mastriano, C.M. Multivitamin/mineral usage, MyPlate adherence, and diet quality among college students. *FASEB J.* **2013**, *27*, lb255.

34. Kelly, N.R.; Mazzeo, S.E.; Bean, M.K. Systematic review of dietary interventions with college students: Directions for future research and practice. *J. Nutr. Educ. Behav.* **2013**, *45*, 304–313. [CrossRef] [PubMed]

35. Newby, P.; Tucker, K.L. Empirically derived eating patterns using factor or cluster analysis: A review. *Nutr. Rev.* **2004**, *62*, 177–203. [CrossRef] [PubMed]

36. Newby, P.K.; Muller, D.; Tucker, K.L. Associations of empirically derived eating patterns with plasma lipid biomarkers: A comparison of factor and cluster analysis methods. *Am. J. Clin. Nutr.* **2004**, *80*, 759–767. [PubMed]

37. Economos, C.D.; Hildebrandt, M.L.; Hyatt, R.R. College freshman stress and weight change: Differences by gender. *Am. J. Health Behav.* **2008**, *32*, 16–25. [CrossRef] [PubMed]

38. Sun, S.S.; Chumlea, W.C.; Heymsfield, S.B.; Lukaski, H.C.; Schoeller, D.; Friedl, K.; Kuczmarski, R.J.; Flegal, K.M.; Johnson, C.L.; Hubbard, V.S. Development of bioelectrical impedance analysis prediction equations for body composition with the use of a multicomponent model for use in epidemiologic surveys. *Am. J. Clin. Nutr.* **2003**, *77*, 331–340. [PubMed]

39. Fukuyama, N.; Homma, K.; Wakana, N.; Kudo, K.; Suyama, A.; Ohazama, H.; Tsuji, C.; Ishiwata, K.; Eguchi, Y.; Nakazawa, H.; Tanaka, E. Validation of the friedewald equation for evaluation of plasma LDL-cholesterol. *J. Clin. Biochem. Nutr.* **2008**, *43*, 1–5. [CrossRef] [PubMed]

40. Center, N.C. *Minnesota Nutrition Data System (NDS) Software*; University of Minnesota: Minneapolis, MN, USA, 1992.

41. Hu, F.B.; Rimm, E.B.; Stampfer, M.J.; Ascherio, A.; Spiegelman, D.; Willett, W.C. Prospective study of major dietary patterns and risk of coronary heart disease in men. *Am. J. Clin. Nutr.* **2000**, *72*, 912–921. [PubMed]

42. Finley, C.E.; LaMonte, M.J.; Waslien, C.I.; Barlow, C.E.; Blair, S.N.; Nichaman, M.Z. Cardiorespiratory fitness, macronutrient intake, and the metabolic syndrome: The Aerobics Center Longitudinal Study. *J. Am. Diet. Assoc.* **2006**, *106*, 673–679. [CrossRef] [PubMed]

43. Eisenmann, J.C.; Wickel, E.E.; Welk, G.J.; Blair, S.N. Relationship between adolescent fitness and fatness and cardiovascular disease risk factors in adulthood: The Aerobics Center Longitudinal Study (ACLS). *Am. Heart J.* **2005**, *149*, 46–53. [CrossRef] [PubMed]

44. Stofan, J.R.; DiPietro, L.; Davis, D.; Kohl, H.W., III; Blair, S.N. Physical activity patterns associated with cardiorespiratory fitness and reduced mortality: The Aerobics Center Longitudinal Study. *Am. J. Public Health* **1998**, *88*, 1807–1813. [CrossRef] [PubMed]
45. Ainsworth, B.E.; Haskell, W.L.; Herrmann, S.D.; Meckes, N.; Bassett, D.R., Jr.; Tudor-Locke, C.; Greer, J.L.; Vezina, J.; Whitt-Glover, M.C.; Leon, A.S. 2011 Compendium of Physical Activities: A second update of codes and MET values. *Med. Sci. Sports Exerc.* **2011**, *43*, 1575–1581. [CrossRef] [PubMed]
46. Douglas, K.A.; Collins, J.L.; Warren, C.; Kann, L.; Gold, R.; Clayton, S.; Ross, J.G.; Kolbe, L.J. Results from the 1995 national college health risk behavior survey. *J. Am. Coll. Health* **1997**, *46*, 55–67. [CrossRef] [PubMed]
47. Kolbe, L.J.; Kann, L.; Collins, J.L. Overview of the youth risk behavior surveillance system. *Public Health Rep.* **1993**, *108* (Suppl. S1), 2–10. [PubMed]
48. Brener, N.D.; Kann, L.; McManus, T.; Kinchen, S.A.; Sundberg, E.C.; Ross, J.G. Reliability of the 1999 youth risk behavior survey questionnaire. *J. Adolesc. Health* **2002**, *31*, 336–342. [CrossRef]
49. Shapiro, S.S.; Wilk, M.B. An analysis of variance test for normality (complete samples). *Biometrika* **1965**, 591–611. [CrossRef]
50. Ning, H.; van Horn, L.; Shay, C.M.; Lloyd-Jones, D.M. Associations of dietary fiber intake with long-term predicted cardiovascular disease risk and C-reactive protein levels (from the National Health and Nutrition Examination Survey Data (2005–2010)). *Am. J. Cardiol.* **2014**, *113*, 287–291. [CrossRef] [PubMed]
51. Fallaize, R.; Forster, H.; Macready, A.L.; Walsh, M.C.; Mathers, J.C.; Brennan, L.; Gibney, E.R.; Gibney, M.J.; Lovegrove, J.A. Online dietary intake estimation: Reproducibility and validity of the Food4Me food frequency questionnaire against a 4-day weighed food record. *J. Med. Internet Res.* **2014**, *16*. [CrossRef] [PubMed]
52. Tukey, J.W. Exploratory data analysis. Addison-Wesley: Boston, MA, USA, 1977.
53. Fung, T.T.; Willett, W.C.; Stampfer, M.J.; Manson, J.E.; Hu, F.B. Dietary patterns and the risk of coronary heart disease in women. *Arch. Intern. Med.* **2001**, *161*, 1857–1862. [CrossRef] [PubMed]
54. Fung, T.; Hu, F.B.; Fuchs, C.; Giovannucci, E.; Hunter, D.J.; Stampfer, M.J.; Colditz, G.A.; Willett, W.C. Major dietary patterns and the risk of colorectal cancer in women. *Arch. Intern. Med.* **2003**, *163*, 309–314. [CrossRef] [PubMed]
55. Van Dam, R.M.; Rimm, E.B.; Willett, W.C.; Stampfer, M.J.; Hu, F.B. Dietary patterns and risk for type 2 diabetes mellitus in US men. *Ann. Intern. Med.* **2002**, *136*, 201–209. [CrossRef] [PubMed]
56. Jacka, F.N.; Pasco, J.A.; Mykletun, A.; Williams, L.J.; Hodge, A.M.; O'Reilly, S.L.; Nicholson, G.C.; Kotowicz, M.A.; Berk, M. Association of Western and traditional diets with depression and anxiety in women. *Am. J. Psychiatry* **2010**, *167*, 305–311. [CrossRef] [PubMed]
57. Kerver, J.M.; Yang, E.J.; Bianchi, L.; Song, W.O. Dietary patterns associated with risk factors for cardiovascular disease in healthy US adults. *Am. J. Clin. Nutr.* **2003**, *78*, 1103–1110. [PubMed]
58. Heidemann, C.; Schulze, M.B.; Franco, O.H.; van Dam, R.M.; Mantzoros, C.S.; Hu, F.B. Dietary patterns and risk of mortality from cardiovascular disease, cancer, and all causes in a prospective cohort of women. *Circulation* **2008**, *118*, 230–237. [CrossRef] [PubMed]
59. Esmaillzadeh, A.; Kimiagar, M.; Mehrabi, Y.; Azadbakht, L.; Hu, F.B.; Willett, W.C. Dietary patterns, insulin resistance, and prevalence of the metabolic syndrome in women. *Am. J. Clin. Nutr.* **2007**, *85*, 910–918. [PubMed]
60. Schulze, M.B.; Fung, T.T.; Manson, J.E.; Willett, W.C.; Hu, F.B. Dietary patterns and changes in body weight in women. *Obesity* **2006**, *14*, 1444–1453. [CrossRef] [PubMed]
61. Schulze, M.B.; Hoffmann, K.; Manson, J.E.; Willett, W.C.; Meigs, J.B.; Weikert, C.; Heidemann, C.; Colditz, G.A.; Hu, F.B. Dietary pattern, inflammation, and incidence of type 2 diabetes in women. *Am. J. Clin. Nutr.* **2005**, *82*, 675–684. [PubMed]
62. Brennan, S.F.; Cantwell, M.M.; Cardwell, C.R.; Velentzis, L.S.; Woodside, J.V. Dietary patterns and breast cancer risk: A systematic review and meta-analysis. *Am. J. Clin. Nutr.* **2010**, *91*, 1294–1302. [CrossRef] [PubMed]
63. Howard, A.L.; Robinson, M.; Smith, G.J.; Ambrosini, G.L.; Piek, J.P.; Oddy, W.H. ADHD is associated with a "Western" dietary pattern in adolescents. *J. Atte. Disord.* **2011**, *15*, 403–411. [CrossRef] [PubMed]
64. Oddy, W.H.; Robinson, M.; Ambrosini, G.L.; Therese, A.; de Klerk, N.H.; Beilin, L.J.; Silburn, S.R.; Zubrick, S.R.; Stanley, F.J. The association between dietary patterns and mental health in early adolescence. *Prev. Med.* **2009**, *49*, 39–44. [CrossRef] [PubMed]

65. Oddy, W.H.; Herbison, C.E.; Jacoby, P.; Ambrosini, G.L.; O'Sullivan, T.A.; Ayonrinde, O.T.; Olynyk, J.K.; Black, L.J.; Beilin, L.J.; Mori, T.A. The Western dietary pattern is prospectively associated with nonalcoholic fatty liver disease in adolescence. *Am. J. Gastroenterol.* **2013**, *108*, 778–785. [CrossRef] [PubMed]

66. Ambrosini, G.L.; Huang, R.; Mori, T.A.; Hands, B.P.; O'Sullivan, T.A.; de Klerk, N.H.; Beilin, L.J.; Oddy, W.H. Dietary patterns and markers for the metabolic syndrome in Australian adolescents. *Nutr. Metab. Cardiovasc. Dis.* **2010**, *20*, 274–283. [CrossRef] [PubMed]

67. Rose, N.; Hosig, K.; Davy, B.; Serrano, E.; Davis, L. Whole-grain intake is associated with body mass index in college students. *J. Nutr. Educ. Behav.* **2007**, *39*, 90–94. [CrossRef] [PubMed]

68. Zamora, D.; Gordon-Larsen, P.; Jacobs, D.R., Jr.; Popkin, B.M. Diet quality and weight gain among black and white young adults: The Coronary Artery Risk Development in Young Adults (CARDIA) Study (1985–2005). *Am. J. Clin. Nutr.* **2010**, *92*, 784–793. [CrossRef] [PubMed]

69. Ritchie, L.D.; Spector, P.; Stevens, M.J.; Schmidt, M.M.; Schreiber, G.B.; Striegel-Moore, R.H.; Wang, M.C.; Crawford, P.B. Dietary patterns in adolescence are related to adiposity in young adulthood in black and white females. *J. Nutr.* **2007**, *137*, 399–406. [PubMed]

70. Fung, T.T.; Rimm, E.B.; Spiegelman, D.; Rifai, N.; Tofler, G.H.; Willett, W.C.; Hu, F.B. Association between dietary patterns and plasma biomarkers of obesity and cardiovascular disease risk. *Am. J. Clin. Nutr.* **2001**, *73*, 61–67. [PubMed]

71. Brien, S.E.; Ronksley, P.E.; Turner, B.J.; Mukamal, K.J.; Ghali, W.A. Effect of alcohol consumption on biological markers associated with risk of coronary heart disease: Systematic review and meta-analysis of interventional studies. *BMJ* **2011**, *342*. [CrossRef] [PubMed]

72. Chiva-Blanch, G.; Arranz, S.; Lamuela-Raventos, R.M.; Estruch, R. Effects of wine, alcohol and polyphenols on cardiovascular disease risk factors: Evidences from human studies. *Alcohol Alcohol.* **2013**, *48*, 270–277. [CrossRef] [PubMed]

73. Schulze, M.B.; Hoffmann, K.; Kroke, A.; Boeing, H. Dietary patterns and their association with food and nutrient intake in the European Prospective Investigation into Cancer and Nutrition (EPIC)—Potsdam study. *Br. J. Nutr.* **2001**, *85*, 363–373. [CrossRef] [PubMed]

74. Engeset, D.; Alsaker, E.; Ciampi, A.; Lund, E. Dietary patterns and lifestyle factors in the Norwegian EPIC cohort: The Norwegian Women and Cancer (NOWAC) study. *Eur. J. Clin. Nutr.* **2005**, *59*, 675–684. [CrossRef] [PubMed]

75. Varraso, R.; Garcia-Aymerich, J.; Monier, F.; le Moual, N.; de Batlle, J.; Miranda, G.; Pison, C.; Romieu, I.; Kauffmann, F.; Maccario, J. Assessment of dietary patterns in nutritional epidemiology: Principal component analysis compared with confirmatory factor analysis. *Am. J. Clin. Nutr.* **2012**, *96*, 1079–1092. [CrossRef] [PubMed]

76. Magalhaes, B.; Peleteiro, B.; Lunet, N. Dietary patterns and colorectal cancer: Systematic review and meta-analysis. *Eur. J. Cancer Prev.* **2012**, *21*, 15–23. [CrossRef] [PubMed]

77. White, A.; Hingson, R. The burden of alcohol use: Excessive alcohol consumption and related consequences among college students. *Alcohol Res. Curr. Rev.* **2014**, *35*, 201–218.

78. Malinauskas, B.M.; Aeby, V.G.; Overton, R.F.; Carpenter-Aeby, T.; Barber-Heidal, K. A survey of energy drink consumption patterns among college students. *Nutr. J.* **2007**, *6*, 35–41. [CrossRef] [PubMed]

79. Lenk, K.M.; Erickson, D.J.; Nelson, T.F.; Winters, K.C.; Toomey, T.L. Alcohol policies and practices among four-year colleges in the United States: Prevalence and patterns. *J. Stud. Alcohol. Drugs* **2012**, *73*, 361–367. [CrossRef] [PubMed]

80. Barry, A.E.; Whiteman, S.; Piazza-Gardner, A.K.; Jensen, A.C. Gender differences in the associations among body mass index, weight loss, exercise, and drinking among college students. *J. Am. Coll. Health* **2013**, *61*, 407–413. [CrossRef] [PubMed]

81. Antin, T.M.; Paschall, M.J. Weight perception, weight change intentions, and alcohol use among young adults. *Body Image* **2011**, *8*, 149–156. [CrossRef] [PubMed]

82. Kelly-Weeder, S. Binge drinking and disordered eating in college students. *J. Am. Acad. Nurse Pract.* **2011**, *23*, 33–41. [CrossRef] [PubMed]

83. Nelson, M.C.; Lust, K.; Story, M.; Ehlinger, E. Alcohol use, eating patterns, and weight behaviors in a university population. *Am. J. Health Behav.* **2009**, *33*, 227–237. [CrossRef] [PubMed]

84. Sayon-Orea, C.; Martinez-Gonzalez, M.A.; Bes-Rastrollo, M. Alcohol consumption and body weight: A systematic review. *Nutr. Rev.* **2011**, *69*, 419–431. [CrossRef] [PubMed]

85. Dawson, D.A.; Goldstein, R.B.; Saha, T.D.; Grant, B.F. Changes in alcohol consumption: United States, 2001–2002 to 2012–2013. *Drug Alcohol Depend.* **2015**, *148*, 56–61. [CrossRef] [PubMed]

86. Chen, C.M.; Yi, H.; Faden, V.B. *Surveillance Report# 101: Trends in Underage Drinking in the United States, 1991–2013*; Division of Epidemiology and Prevention Research, Alcohol Epidemiologic Data System; NIAAA: Rockville, MD, USA, 2015.

87. Bryant, J.B.; Darkes, J.; Rahal, C. College students' compensatory eating and behaviors in response to alcohol consumption. *J. Am. Coll. Health* **2012**, *60*, 350–356. [CrossRef] [PubMed]

88. Cai, L.; Ma, D.; Zhang, Y.; Liu, Z.; Wang, P. The effect of coffee consumption on serum lipids: A meta-analysis of randomized controlled trials. *Eur. J. Clin. Nutr.* **2012**, *66*, 872–877. [CrossRef] [PubMed]

89. *Scientific Report of the 2015 Dietary Guidelines for Americans Advisory Committee*; US Department of Agriculture; US Department of Health and Human Services: Washington DC, WA, USA, 2015.

90. Deshmukh-Taskar, P.; Nicklas, T.; Morales, M.; Yang, S.; Zakeri, I.; Berenson, G. Tracking of overweight status from childhood to young adulthood: The Bogalusa Heart Study. *Eur. J. Clin. Nutr.* **2006**, *60*, 48–57. [CrossRef] [PubMed]

91. Levitsky, D.A.; Halbmaier, C.A.; Mrdjenovic, G. The freshman weight gain: A model for the study of the epidemic of obesity. *Int. J. Obes.* **2004**, *28*, 1435–1442. [CrossRef] [PubMed]

92. Brunt, A.R.; Rhee, Y.S. Obesity and lifestyle in US college students related to living arrangemeents. *Appetite* **2008**, *51*, 615–621. [CrossRef] [PubMed]

93. Small, M.; Bailey-Davis, L.; Morgan, N.; Maggs, J. Changes in eating and physical activity behaviors across seven semesters of college: Living on or off campus matters. *Health Educ. Behav.* **2013**, *40*, 435–441. [CrossRef] [PubMed]

94. Eisenmann, J.C.; Welk, G.J.; Wickel, E.E.; Blair, S.N. Stability of variables associated with the metabolic syndrome from adolescence to adulthood: The Aerobics Center Longitudinal Study. *Am. J. Hum. Biol.* **2004**, *16*, 690–696. [CrossRef] [PubMed]

95. Jacobs, D.R.; Tapsell, L.C. Food synergy:The key to a healthy diet. *Proc. Nutr. Soc.* **2013**, *72*, 200–206.

96. McCann, S.E.; Marshall, J.R.; Brasure, J.R.; Graham, S.; Freudenheim, J.L. Analysis of patterns of food intake in nutritional epidemiology: Food classification in principal components analysis and the subsequent impact on estimates for endometrial cancer. *Public Health Nutr.* **2001**, *4*, 989–997.

97. Hamer, M.; McNaughton, S.; Bates, C.; Mishra, G. Dietary patterns, assessed from a weighed food record, and survival among elderly participants from the United Kingdom. *Eur. J. Clin. Nutr.* **2010**, *64*, 853–861.

98. Hu, F.B.; Rimm, E.B.; Stampfer, M.J.; Ascherio, A.; Spiegelman, D.; Willett, W.C. Prospective study of major dietary patterns and risk of coronary heart disease in men. *Am. J. Clin. Nutr.* **2000**, *72*, 912–921.

99. Michels, K.B.; Schulze, M.B. Can dietary patterns help us detect diet-disease associations? *Nutr. Res. Rev.* **2005**, *18*, 241–248.

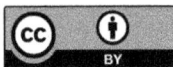

nutrients

MDPI

Article

Nutrient Patterns and Their Food Sources in Older Persons from France and Quebec: Dietary and Lifestyle Characteristics

Benjamin Allès [1,2,3,4,*], Cécilia Samieri [1,2], Simon Lorrain [1,2], Marthe-Aline Jutand [1,2], Pierre-Hugues Carmichael [3], Bryna Shatenstein [5,6], Pierrette Gaudreau [7,8], Hélène Payette [9,10], Danielle Laurin [3,4,†] and Pascale Barberger-Gateau [1,2,†]

[1] Centre INSERM U897-Epidemiologie-Biostatistique, University of Bordeaux, ISPED, Bordeaux, F-33000, France; cecilia.samieri@isped.u-bordeaux2.fr (C.S.); Simon.Lorrain@isped.u-bordeaux2.fr (S.L.); marthe-aline.jutand@isped.u-bordeaux2.fr (M.-A.J.); Pascale.Barberger-Gateau@isped.u-bordeaux2.fr (P.B.-G.)

[2] Centre INSERM U897-Epidemiologie-Biostatistique, INSERM, ISPED, Bordeaux, F-33000, France

[3] Québec Center of Excellence on Aging, CHU de Québec Research Center, Quebec City, QC G1S 4L8, Canada; pierre-hugues.carmichael.cha@ssss.gouv.qc.ca (P.-H.C.); danielle.laurin@pha.ulaval.ca (D.L.)

[4] Faculty of Pharmacy, Laval University, Quebec City, QC G1V 0A6, Canada

[5] Département de Nutrition, Université de Montréal, Montréal, QC H3T 1A8, Canada; bryna.shatenstein@umontreal.ca

[6] Centre de Recherche, Institut Universitaire de Gériatrie de Montréal, CIUSSS du Centre-est-de-l'Île-de-Montréal, Montréal, QC H3W 1W5, Canada

[7] Department of Medicine, University of Montreal, Montreal, QC H3C 3J7, Canada; pierrette.gaudreau@umontreal.ca

[8] Centre Hospitalier de l'Université de Montréal Research Center (CRCHUM), Montréal, QC H2X 0A9, Canada

[9] Research Center on Aging—Centre Intégré Universitaire de Santé et des Services Sociaux de l'Estrie—Centre Hospitalier Universitaire de Sherbrooke (CIUSS de l'Estrie-CHUS), Sherbrooke, QC J1H 4C4, Canada; Helene.Payette@usherbrooke.ca

[10] Faculty of Medicine and Health Sciences, University of Sherbrooke, Sherbrooke, QC J1K 2R1, Canada

* Correspondence: b.alles@eren.smbh.univ-paris13.fr; Tel.: +33-1-48-38-73-64

† These authors contributed equally to this work.

Received: 5 October 2015; Accepted: 31 March 2016; Published: 19 April 2016

Abstract: *Background*: Dietary and nutrient patterns have been linked to health outcomes related to aging. Food intake is influenced by environmental and genetic factors. The aim of the present study was to compare nutrient patterns across two elderly populations sharing a common ancestral cultural background, but living in different environments. *Methods*: The diet quality, lifestyle and socioeconomic characteristics of participants from the Three-City Study (3C, France, *n* = 1712) and the Québec Longitudinal Study on Nutrition and Successful Aging (NuAge, Quebec, Canada, *n* = 1596) were analyzed. Nutrient patterns and their food sources were identified in the two samples using principal component analysis. Diet quality was compared across sample-specific patterns by describing weekly food intake and associations with the Canadian Healthy Eating Index (C-HEI). *Results*: Three nutrient patterns were retained in each study: a healthy, a Western and a more traditional pattern. These patterns accounted for 50.1% and 53.5% of the total variance in 3C and NuAge, respectively. Higher education and non-physical occupations over lifetime were associated with healthy patterns in both studies. Other characteristics such as living alone, having a body mass index lower than 25 and being an ex-smoker were associated with the healthy pattern in NuAge. No association between these characteristics and the nutrient patterns was noted in 3C. The healthy and Western patterns from each sample also showed an inverse association with C-HEI. *Conclusion*: The two healthy patterns showed important similarities: adequate food variety, consumption of healthy foods and associations with common sociodemographic factors. This work highlights that nutrient patterns derived using *a posteriori* methods may be useful to compare the nutritional quality of the diet of distinct populations.

Keywords: diet; nutritional quality; aged; nutrition; socioeconomic factors

---

1. Introduction

Nutrition is known to play a role in healthy aging. Numerous epidemiological and clinical studies have reported the benefits of specific nutrients, taken individually, in reducing the risk of chronic diseases in older persons [1,2]. However, this approach does not take into account the concept of food synergy, implying that a nutrient is never consumed alone and is interacting with many other nutrients or molecules [3]. The identification of dietary and nutrient patterns, which better reflect the complexity of dietary intake, to investigate the relationship between health and nutrition could overcome this limitation. Dietary patterns or the combinations of foods and beverages in diets, and nutrient patterns or the combinations of nutrients derived from data collected through dietary surveys, take into account the antagonist, additive and synergistic effects within the "food matrix" [3,4]. Only a few studies investigated nutrients taken as a whole, using dietary and nutrient patterns [5]. As reported in a study from the European Prospective Investigation into Cancer and Nutrition (EPIC), nutrients may characterize specific nutritional profiles enhancing comparisons between populations [6]. The EPIC has derived from food frequency questionnaire (FFQ) nutrient patterns within general European populations, highlighting that it was a better way to compare dietary intake from international populations than dietary patterns [6].

In recent reviews [7–9], healthy dietary or nutrient patterns characterized by higher consumptions of fruits and vegetables have been related to lower risks of cancer, diabetes, cardiovascular disease and Alzheimer's disease, whereas Western or unhealthy patterns have been associated with increased risks. These reviews reported only a few studies investigating the relationships between the dietary or nutrient patterns and sociodemographic characteristics or the nutritional quality of the diet. Indeed, dietary and nutrient patterns are influenced by sociodemographic factors such as age, sex, socioeconomic status, and lifestyle [10]. In fact, among those factors, the Academy of Nutrition and Dietetics notes that food habits are especially determined by factors as living arrangements, finances, transportation, and disability [11]. Concerning the role of socioeconomic position in diet quality, the main hypothesis is that a higher socioeconomic status allows access to a more balanced diet than a lower status, but discordant results have been reported in some studies [12–15], and in other European countries and the US [10,16,17]. In Canada, individuals in the highest socioeconomic classes have the highest consumption of fruits and vegetables, following an income-education socioeconomic gradient [13]. Similar results have been observed in France [15]. Eating habits, diet quality and even nutritional risk in older people are influenced by living arrangement, especially loneliness or being widowed, but inconsistently [2,12,18].

To our knowledge, no comparison of dietary or nutrient patterns derived from two distinct populations of older people has been published yet. Additionally, no comparison studies have been conducted in two populations sharing a common ancestral cultural background. The aim of this study was to derive and validate nutrient patterns in two samples of older persons living in France and in Quebec, Canada. The nutritional quality of the diets of both study samples was described using nutrient intakes and their food sources. Finally, the link between nutrition and sociodemographic factors was explored and some comparisons between France and Quebec were enabled by this data harmonization.

2. Experimental Section

2.1. Study Populations

The 3C study: The French 3C study is a 12-year longitudinal cohort study of vascular risk factors for dementia which included 9294 community dwellers in Bordeaux ($n = 2104$), Dijon ($n = 4931$) and Montpellier ($n = 2259$), France. Individuals aged 65 years and over living in the community were randomly selected from electoral rolls. Methodological details of the study have been described elsewhere [19]. Baseline examination was carried out in 1999–2000; subjects were re-evaluated in 2001–2002 (wave 1) [19]. At baseline, standard data collection included sociodemographic and lifestyle characteristics, medical history, comprehensive neuropsychological testing, physical examination and blood sampling. In wave 1, there were 1712 participants (participation rate of 81.4%) from the Bordeaux sample asked to answer an extensive dietary survey conducted by trained dieticians, which included a 24-h dietary recall (excluding weekend days) and a food frequency questionnaire (FFQ). The present study is based on data from 3C wave 1 in Bordeaux.

NuAge study: The NuAge study is a four-year longitudinal study designed to evaluate the role of nutrition on physical and cognitive status, functional autonomy and social participation [20]. The study included 1793 individuals aged 67–84 years at baseline in 2003–2005. Participants in good general physical health and cognitively normal (Modified Mini-Mental State Examination score above 80 out of 100) were selected from a random sample obtained from the Quebec Medicare database using stratified sampling by age and sex [21]. After baseline examination, participants were re-examined annually over a three-year period. Trained dietitians and nurses assessed participants in face-to-face interviews or by direct measurement, at the research centers. Dietary data were collected through a FFQ at baseline and three annual 24-h dietary recalls. Further methodological details have been published elsewhere [20].

2.2. Dietary Assessments, Harmonization of Nutrient and Food Intake

In 3C, individual nutrient intakes were computed from the 24-h recall using the BILNUT® software (Cerelles, France), which converts food intake data into nutrient intake data using French food composition tables [22]. These tables were augmented for fatty acids from the Food Composition and Nutrition tables [23]. As the 24-h recall was open-ended, additional data were also obtained by consulting a French table developed by the National Institute of Health and Medical Research (Inserm) and the University of Montreal [24], the USDA National Nutrient Database, food packaging, and directly contacting food manufacturers. Extended information about the dietary habits of the Bordeaux sample have been described in detail elsewhere [25,26]. Moreover, a qualitative FFQ, including 148 food and non-alcoholic beverage items, was administered during the same dietary survey [26]. Based on the FFQ, weekly frequency of consumption of 40 categories of foods and beverages for each of the three main meals and three between-meal snacks was recorded in 11 classes. The FFQ data were used to compare the frequency of food group consumptions between different nutrient patterns, and could not be used to estimate nutrient intake because portion size was not assessed.

In NuAge, daily nutrient intake levels were computed from the first of the three 24-h recalls at baseline using the CANDAT-Nutrient Calculation System (version 10, London, ON, Canada) based on the 2005 version of the Canadian Nutrient File, augmented by a database of 1200 additional foods that was developed on-site [27]. A 78-item validated semi-quantitative FFQ [28] was also administrated at recruitment to assess usual food intake. As in 3C, FFQ data enabled description of average food intake within each nutrient pattern.

Eleven food groups based on common food items to the two studies were defined. Nutrient-dense beverages such as sugary drinks were included in the sweet products group. As water and other hot beverages are not nutrient-dense beverages, they were not considered as contributors to nutrient intake. In addition, 21 nutrients whose consumption was available in 3C and NuAge were selected to derive nutrient patterns in both studies.

2.3. Nutritional Quality of the Diet

The Canadian Healthy Eating Index (C-HEI), based on the Healthy Eating Index (HEI) [29], a nine-item index, was used to assess diet quality using adherence to dietary guidelines in both samples. The C-HEI is based on intake of four food groups: grain products, fruits and vegetables, milk products, meat and alternatives, and five other items: % of energy as total fat intake and saturated fat intake, cholesterol, salt and diet variety [30]. The score ranges from 0 to 100, with higher scores indicating whether the nutritional quality of the diet is closer to the Canadian guidelines for healthy eating [30].

2.4. Data Harmonization for Sociodemographic and Lifestyle Variables

In both studies, living arrangement was categorized according to two modalities: living alone *vs.* in a couple or cohabitation. Smoking status was classified as current, ex-smoker, or never smoker. Education was categorized as 0–6 years, 7–9 years, 10–13 years and ≥14 years.

In 3C, monthly income was reported in four pre-determined categories according to the French economic situation in 1999–2000 [25]. Yearly income was further computed (converting French francs, the past French currency, to Euros), and created a three-category variable: low income (<18,000 euros (€)/year), moderate income (18,000–27,000 €/year) and high income (≥27,000 €/year). In NuAge, income was reported as a continuous variable. Because of differences in cost of living in 1999–2000 in France (baseline 3C) *versus* in 2003–2005 in Quebec (baseline NuAge), income values were not directly comparable. To allow comparability, the validated Big Mac Index was used [31] to convert income categories from 3C to corresponding categories in NuAge (<17,040 Canadian dollar (CAD), 17,040–25,560 CAD and ≥25,560 CAD). This conversion tool uses values of a McDonald's Big Mac hamburger [31,32] at a given time in a given country, a food item consumed in many countries worldwide. Participants' main occupation during their active years was collected according to the French occupation classification (International Standard Classification of Occupations 1988 (ISCO88)) [33] in 3C and the national Canadian occupation classification in NuAge [34]. In both studies, a variable was created indicating whether the occupation was physical (manufacturing, mining, and construction workers, *etc.*), non-physical (administration, trade managers, *etc.*) or mixed (arts, culture, sales, *etc.*). Body mass index (BMI) was computed as the weight (kg)/height squared (m^2).

In 3C, missing data in food intake from the FFQ (66 participants, 3.7% of the sample) were imputed using Multivariate Imputation as described by Samieri *et al.* [35]. With respect to NuAge, 92 implausible FFQs among 1688 subjects (5%) with both 24-h recall and FFQs identified using a set of criteria developed by Shatenstein *et al.* [36] were excluded, leaving 1596 subjects for the final analysis. In both studies, missing values for covariates representing less than 5% of the sample were excluded, and dummy variables were created for variables with a frequency of missing values between 5% and 10%.

2.5. Statistical Analyses

Nutrient patterns are obtained using principal component factor analysis (FA-PCA). This procedure is performed on the correlation matrix of the 21 standardized nutrients common to both studies. In each sample, three principal components representing three independent nutrient patterns were identified according to their eigenvalues using scree plot to assess Cattel's criterion (all eigenvalues for chosen factors above 1), interpretability and percentage of variance explained. Varimax rotation was performed to improve the interpretability of the factor loadings [37]. Component scores are obtained from the computed nutrient patterns and adjusted for energy using the residual method of Willett and Stampfer [38]. As a consequence, these component scores have an average of 0 and subjects who consumed less than the average on the defining nutrients would have a negative component score.

Tucker's congruence coefficient was computed to compare statistical similarities between the two sets of nutrient patterns [39]. A coefficient close to 1 signals a very high degree of similarity between two nutrient patterns; an accepted cut-off for good congruence is greater than 0.85.

Mean nutrient intake and food groups across quartiles of the obtained nutrient patterns were described for the two study samples. The relationship between the C-HEI, the dependent variable, and the component scores was assessed using separate linear regression adjusted for sex, following bivariate analyses of variance (ANOVA). Multivariate linear regression models were adjusted to assess the relationships between nutrient pattern scores and lifestyle characteristics in each sample controlling for age. Furthermore, the relationships between socioeconomic characteristics and nutrient pattern scores were compared between the two samples using interaction terms in a single model.

3. Results

Compared with 3C participants, those from NuAge were significantly younger, more likely to be men and showed a lower proportion of subjects with six or less years of education (Table 1). NuAge participants were significantly less likely to be in the lower income category and more likely to report a non-physical occupation over lifetime and to be living as a couple or in cohabitation, suggesting they had a better socioeconomic position than those in 3C. Significantly higher BMI values and energy intake for both men and women were found in the NuAge study, as well as a higher proportion of ex-smokers.

Table 1. Characteristics of the 3C study sample (*n* = 1712) and the NuAge study sample (*n* = 1596).

	3C		NuAge		*p* *
Age, years (mean SD)	76.5	5.1	74.3	4.2	<0.001
Sex (*n* %)					
Men	644	37.6	763	49.1	<0.001
Women	1068	63.4	833	51.9	
Education, years (*n* %) [†]					
0–6	227	13.3	156	9.8	
7–9	376	22.0	402	25.1	<0.001
10–13	458	26.8	547	34.3	
14+	650	38.0	491	30.8	
Yearly income (*n* %)					
Missing or refused to answer	138	8.1	155	9.7	
Lower income (<17,040 CAN$)	645	37.7	315	19.7	
Moderate income (17,040 to 25,560 CAN$)	426	24.9	914	57.3	<0.001
Higher income (>25,560 CAN$)	503	29.4	212	13.3	
Main occupation over lifetime (*n* %) [‡]					
Physical occupation	466	27.3	392	24.7	
Non-physical occupation	495	28.9	699	44.0	<0.001
Mixed occupation	749	43.8	497	31.3	
Living arrangement (*n* %) [§]					
Alone	917	53.7	505	31.7	
Couple or cohabitation	791	46.3	1090	69.3	<0.001
BMI (*n* %)					
BMI < 25	744	43.5	431	27.0	
25 ⩽ BMI < 30	700	40.9	759	47.6	<0.001
BMI ⩾ 30	268	15.7	406	25.4	
Energy intake (mean SD)					
Men	1706	539	2131	672	<0.001
Women	1517	457	1726	540	
Smoking (*n* %) [‖]					
Non-smoker	1051	61.6	835	52.3	
Ex-smoker	552	32.3	654	41.0	<0.001
Smoker	104	6.1	107	6.7	

BMI: Body mass index, SD: standard deviation; * *p* for χ^2 for categorical variables and *t* test for linear variables; BMI: Body mass index, SD: standard deviation; [†] 1 missing value for 3C; [‡] 2 missing values for 3C, 8 for NuAge; [§] 4 missing values for 3C, 1 for NuAge; [‖] 5 missing values for 3C.

In 3C, the FA-PCA yielded a three-component solution that accounted for 50.1% of the total variance (Table 2). The first component explained 21.6% of the variance, and was characterized by, in decreasing order, higher intake of potassium, dietary fiber, magnesium, folates, vitamin B_6, carbohydrates, vitamin C, iron, vitamin E and carotene (all factor loadings >0.20). The second component explained 18.6% of the variance, and reflected high intake of monounsaturated fatty acids (MUFA), saturated fatty acids (SFA), phosphorus, proteins, *n*-3 polyunsaturated fatty acids (PUFA), calcium, *n*-6 PUFA, vitamin D and vitamin E (equally loaded between components 1 and 2). The third component with 9.9% of the explained variance was related to vitamin B_{12} and vitamin A intake. The mean nutrient intakes across quartiles of each factor score are described in Table S1. As expected, increasing intakes across quartiles of factor score were observed for nutrients with positive factor loadings from FA-PCA. Additionally, the third nutrient pattern had the highest consumption of alcohol.

Table 2. Nutrient patterns obtained by factor analysis using principal component analysis of nutrient intakes.

	3C			NuAge			
Nutrient	Factor 1 Healthy	Factor 2 Western	Factor 3 Traditional South-West of France	Nutrient	Factor 1 Healthy	Factor 2 Western	Factor 3 Traditional
Potassium	0.83	0.30	−0.01	Potassium	0.86	0.28	0.22
Fiber	0.78	0.10	−0.03	Fiber	0.81	0.17	0.02
Magnesium	0.75	0.46	−0.03	Magnesium	0.81	0.35	0.16
Folates	0.70	0.07	0.44	Vitamin B_6	0.73	0.25	0.29
Vitamin B_6	0.67	0.37	0.19	Vitamin C	0.66	−0.09	−0.04
Carbohydrates	0.61	0.34	−0.09	Carbohydrates	0.57	0.49	0.02
Vitamin C	0.58	−0.17	0.09	Phosphorus	0.57	0.52	0.39
Iron	0.49	0.34	0.35	Iron	0.57	0.48	0.28
Carotene	0.42	−0.17	0.00	Carotene	0.48	−0.10	−0.01
Zinc	0.14	0.08	0.08	Vitamin E	0.48	0.32	0.01
Vitamin E	0.31	0.31	0.07	MUFA	0.13	0.86	0.09
Proteins	0.47	0.67	0.05	SFA	0.00	0.82	0.16
MUFA	0.10	0.77	0.06	PUFA-*n*3	0.11	0.68	−0.09
SFA	0.10	0.76	0.03	Proteins	0.41	0.57	0.39
Phosphorus	0.51	0.72	0.04	Calcium	0.41	0.46	0.25
PUFA-n3	−0.06	0.58	0.06	Folates	0.00	0.45	−0.01
Calcium	0.32	0.55	−0.09	PUFA-*n*6	0.21	0.40	−0.11
PUFA-n6	0.19	0.49	0.09	Vitamin D	0.24	0.27	0.26
Vitamin D	−0.17	0.42	0.11	Vitamin B_{12}	0.01	−0.04	0.92
Vitamin A	0.05	0.01	0.91	Vitamin A	0.02	−0.10	0.83
Vitamin B_{12}	0.08	0.14	0.91	Zinc	0.25	0.42	0.49
Variance explained (%)	21.6	18.6	9.9		22.8	19.2	11.5

SFA: saturated fatty acids, MUFA: monounsaturated fatty acids, PUFA: polyunsaturated fatty acids.

In NuAge, the FA-PCA yielded also a three-component solution that accounted for 53.5% of the total variance (Table 2). The first component explained 22.8% of the variance, and was related, in decreasing order, by high intake of potassium, magnesium and dietary fiber (equally loaded), vitamin B_6, vitamin C, phosphorus, iron and carbohydrates (equally loaded), vitamin E and carotene (equally loaded). The second component accounted for 19.2% of the variance and was related to high intake of MUFA, SFA, *n*-3 PUFA, proteins, folates, calcium, *n*-6 PUFA and vitamin D. The third component with 11.5% of the explained variance was related to high intake of vitamin B_{12}, vitamin A and zinc. Similarly to the 3C study, increasing intake across quartiles of factor score were observed for nutrients with positive factor loadings from FA-PCA (Table S2).

The congruence coefficient between the first nutrient patterns of both 3C and NuAge was 0.83, indicating a borderline similarity. A moderate similarity (congruence coefficient of 0.76) was found between the second nutrient patterns of both samples, and a low similarity (congruence coefficient of 0.60) was found between the third nutrient patterns.

Mean intakes of food groups were described according to quartiles of energy-adjusted factor scores for each factor in each sample. In 3C (Table 3), the first pattern was significantly associated with greater consumption of vegetables, legumes, fruits, cereals, potatoes, fish and seafood, and with lower intake of charcuterie and alcohol. This pattern showed a relatively balanced diet and was therefore labelled healthy. Conversely, higher score on the second pattern was associated with higher intake of charcuterie and dairy products, and lower intake of vegetables, legumes, fruits, cereals, potatoes, biscuits and other sweet foods and alcohol. This pattern was labelled Western. The third pattern characterized by high intake of meat, charcuterie, fish/seafood and alcohol was typical of Bordeaux regional food behavior. Accordingly, this third pattern was labelled "traditional—South-West of France". This pattern is also characterized by lower intake of dairy products and biscuits/sweet foods.

Similar results were observed in NuAge (Table 4). The first pattern, significantly associated with higher intake of vegetables, legumes, fruits, cereals, fish/seafood, and dairy products, and with lower intake of potatoes, charcuterie, and biscuits and other sweet foods, was labelled healthy. Conversely, the second pattern associated with lower consumption of vegetables, legumes, fruits, fish/seafood, and alcohol, and higher intake of biscuits and other sweet food, was labelled Western. A third pattern was associated with higher intake of fish/seafood and dairy product intakes, and lower intake of biscuits and sweet food consumption. Considering the customary consumption of fish/seafood products on Fridays by older people in Quebec, it was labelled traditional.

Sex-specific associations between factor scores and the C-HEI for both 3C and NuAge models are shown in Figure 1 ($r^2 = 0.35$ in 3C and 0.15 in NuAge in models adjusted for sex (both F test p-values < 0.05)). In both studies, higher healthy pattern scores were associated with higher adherence to the C-HEI. No interaction was detected between sex and nutrient pattern scores on C-HEI scores. The mean increase in C-HEI score for each increase of 1 unit of the healthy pattern score was 3.88 in 3C (95% confidence interval (CI) = (1.68, 5.58)), and 2.70 in NuAge (95% CI = (1.85, 3.54)). Conversely, there was a significant inverse relationship between C-HEI scores and factor scores for Western patterns in both studies. The mean decrease in C-HEI score for each increase of 1 unit of the Western pattern score was -2.51 in 3C (95% CI = (-5.29, -1.34)), and -1.07 in NuAge (95% CI = (-1.92, -0.23)). The traditional South-West of France pattern in 3C was inversely associated with C-HEI: the mean decrease in C-HEI for each increase of 1 unit of the traditional pattern score was -1.36 (95% CI = (-5.38, -1.56)). The traditional pattern in NuAge was not associated with the C-HEI score. Compared to men, women showed higher C-HEI scores for every nutrient pattern ($\beta_{women-3C} = 6.13$, 95% CI = (5.21, 7.04) and $\beta_{women-NuAge} = 2.98$, 95% CI = (2.09, 3.87)).

Associations between socioeconomic, health and lifestyle characteristics and the nutrient patterns were examined in both studies. In 3C, results from bivariate analyses were confirmed in multivariate models for each of the nutrient pattern scores (Table 5). Indeed, the same statistically significant associations were observed except for main occupation in the Western pattern. The healthy pattern was significantly associated with higher education (only statistically significant for the 10–13 years of education category), whereas the Western pattern was significantly associated with female sex. No association was found for yearly income, living arrangement, BMI and smoking status. In NuAge (Table 6), results from bivariate analysis were confirmed in multivariate linear models for each nutrient pattern score, with the exception of occupation, which was not associated with the Western pattern in multivariate model. The healthy pattern was significantly positively associated with higher education (only statistically significant for the 14+ years of education category), lower BMI, and non-physical occupation, and negatively associated with living in a couple or cohabitation and smoking. The Western pattern was significantly associated with smoking, lower education and higher BMI.

When comparing the relationships between the two studies, significant interactions were found for education ($p < 0.01$ for Healthy pattern), main occupation during lifetime ($p < 0.01$ for Healthy pattern and $p = 0.02$ for Western pattern), sex ($p < 0.01$ for Western pattern) and BMI ($p < 0.01$ for Healthy pattern and $p = 0.03$ for Western pattern).

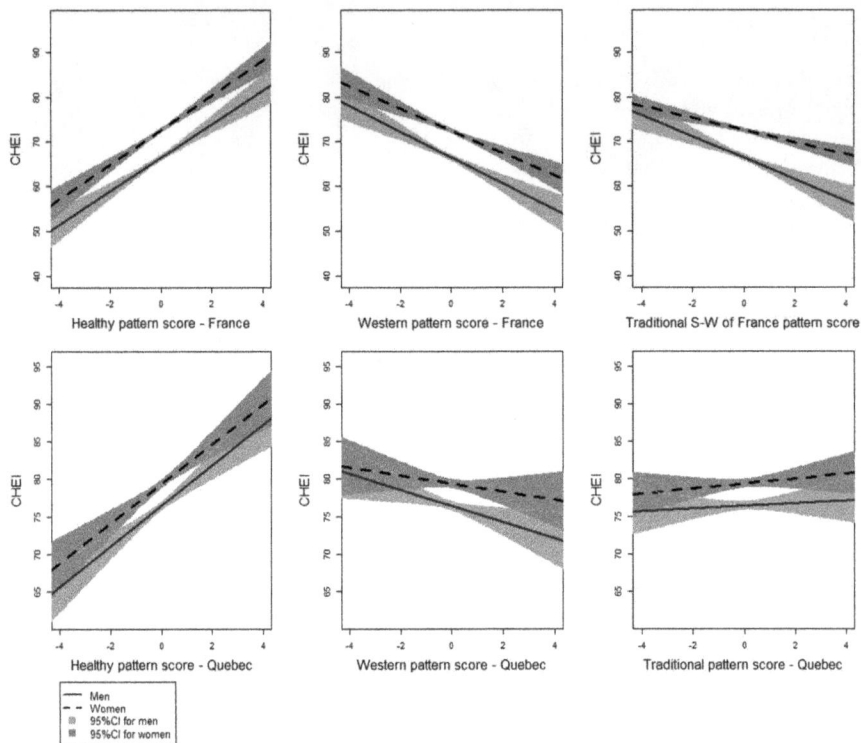

Figure 1. Linear relationships between energy-adjusted nutrient pattern scores and C-HEI scores by sex (n_{3C} = 1712. n_{NuAge} = 1596)*. * For reasons of clarity, 21 subjects in 3C and 12 subjects in NuAge are not presented in their respective traditional pattern score plots.

Table 3. Mean food group intakes according to quartiles of component scores obtained by factor analysis—principal component analysis of nutrient intake data in 3C (n = 1712), from food frequency questionnaires.

Food Groups (Servings Per Week)	Healthy Pattern Score					Western Pattern Score					Traditional—South-West of France Pattern Score				
	Q1 (Lowest) n = 428	Q2 n = 428	Q3 n = 428	Q4 (Highest) n = 428	p*	Q1 n = 428	Q2 n = 428	Q3 n = 428	Q4 n = 428	p*	Q1 n = 428	Q2 n = 428	Q3 n = 428	Q4 n = 428	p*
Vegetables	16.5	18.5	20.1	21.7	<0.001	20.3	19.3	19.0	18.2	<0.001	18.7	19.4	19.5	19.1	0.38
Legumes	0.6	0.6	0.6	0.7	0.04	0.7	0.6	0.6	0.6	0.009	0.6	0.6	0.6	0.6	0.93
Fruits	11.1	12.6	14.3	16.1	<0.001	15.5	13.8	13.1	11.7	<0.001	13.9	14	12.5	13.6	0.006
Cereals	18.8	19.6	20.5	20.4	<0.001	20.7	20.5	19.5	18.6	<0.001	20.3	20	19.4	19.7	0.14
Potatoes	2.6	2.5	2.7	2.8	0.03	2.8	2.6	2.5	2.5	0.04	2.8	2.7	2.5	2.5	0.01
Meat	4.8	4.8	4.8	4.8	0.98	4.7	4.9	4.9	4.7	0.66	4.6	4.5	5	5	0.002
Fish/seafood	2.7	2.8	2.8	3.1	0.004	2.9	2.8	2.8	2.9	0.55	2.6	2.8	3.1	3	<0.001
Charcuterie	2.1	1.7	1.4	1.4	<0.001	1.5	1.7	1.5	1.9	0.04	1.5	1.5	1.7	2	<0.001
Dairy products	18.1	18.1	18	18.7	0.48	17.2	17.8	18.5	19.5	<0.001	20.3	18.5	17.5	16.5	<0.001
Biscuits and other sweet food	11.5	11.5	11.1	10.2	0.06	12.2	11.2	11.1	9.7	<0.001	11.7	11.6	10.9	10	0.001
Alcohol	14.4	11.7	11.2	12.6	0.02	15.8	13.4	9.9	10.8	<0.001	11	10.9	13.1	14.9	<0.001

* p for ANOVA test.

Table 4. Mean food group intakes according to quartiles of component scores obtained by factor analysis—principal component analysis of nutrient intake data in NuAge (n = 1596), from food frequency questionnaires.

Food Groups (Serving per Week)	Healthy Pattern Score					Western Pattern Score					Traditional Pattern Score				
	Q1 (Lowest) n = 399	Q2 n = 399	Q3 n = 399	Q4 (Highest) n = 399	p*	Q1 n = 399	Q2 n = 399	Q3 n = 399	Q4 n = 399	p*	Q1 n = 399	Q2 n = 399	Q3 n = 399	Q4 n = 399	p*
Vegetables	25.2	29.5	31.7	36.2	<0.001	35.2	31.5	28.8	27.1	<0.001	31	30.6	30.2	30.9	0.86
Legumes	0.7	1	1.1	1.4	<0.001	1.2	1	1.1	0.9	0.02	1.2	1	1	1	0.11
Fruits	11.2	13.1	15.8	18	<0.001	17.4	14.6	13.9	12.2	<0.001	15.2	14.3	14.3	14.3	0.18
Cereals	13.8	14.8	14.2	15.7	<0.001	15.2	14.4	14.5	14.4	0.11	14.2	15	14.7	14.7	0.35
Potatoes	4.2	3.8	3.9	3.3	<0.001	3.6	3.7	3.8	3.9	0.33	3.9	3.6	3.7	3.9	0.42
Meat	3	3.1	3	2.8	0.36	2.8	3	2.9	3	0.4	2.8	3	2.9	3.1	0.38
Fish/seafood	1.5	1.8	1.8	2.3	<0.001	2.2	1.8	1.7	1.6	<0.001	1.7	1.8	1.9	2	0.04
Charcuterie	1.8	1.5	1.5	1.2	<0.001	1.4	1.4	1.7	1.7	0.13	1.4	1.5	1.5	1.6	0.15
Dairy products	21.4	21.5	20.9	23.6	<0.001	21.7	22.4	21	22.4	0.44	19.4	20.8	22.5	24.8	<0.001
Biscuits and other sweet food	20.7	17.2	14.9	13.8	<0.001	16.2	16.1	16.1	18.1	0.03	17.3	17.6	16.5	15.1	0.02
Alcohol	3.8	3.8	3.5	3.9	0.97	4.9	4	2.8	3.2	<0.001	4	3.4	3.6	3.9	0.17

Table 5. Associations between social, health and lifestyle characteristics of the subjects and nutrient patterns in 3C (n = 1712).

	Healthy Pattern				Western Pattern				Traditional—South-West of France Pattern			
	Unadjusted		Adjusted		Unadjusted		Adjusted		Unadjusted		Adjusted	
	Mean Residual Score	p*	β	95% CI	Mean Residual Score	p*	β	95% CI	Mean Residual Score	p*	β	95% CI
Sex												
Men	0.018		Reference		−0.093		Reference		−0.014		Reference	
Women	0.013	0.58	−0.03	−0.14; 0.08	0.046	<0.001	0.12	0.03; 0.20	0.028	0.39	0.06	−0.06; 0.16
Education												
0–6 years	−0.134		Reference		0.059		Reference		−0.055		Reference	
7–9 years	−0.052	0.01	0.05	−0.09; 0.15	0.027	0.24	−0.02	−0.13; 0.09	−0.007	0.86	0.01	−0.16; 0.17
10–13 years	0.122		0.20	0.05; 0.35	−0.011		−0.02	−0.13; 0.09	0.016		0.04	−0.13; 0.20
14+ years	0.021		0.12	−0.03; 0.27	−0.046		−0.04	−0.16; 0.07	0.037		0.03	−0.15; 0.20
Yearly income †												
Lower income	−0.154		Reference		0.094		Reference		0.111		Reference	
Moderate income	0.006	0.23	0.03	−0.09; 0.15	0.025	0.15	−0.02	−0.11; 0.07	−0.062	0.36	0.05	−0.08; 0.19
Higher income	0.058		−0.04	−0.18; 0.19	−0.025		−0.01	−0.11; 0.09	0.000		0.13	−0.03; 0.28
Missing or refused to answer	0.010		−0.11	−0.28; 0.05	−0.041		0.04	−0.09; 0.16	0.060		−0.04	−0.23; 0.15
Main occupation over lifetime												
Physical occupation	−0.045		Reference		0.023		Reference		0.004		Reference	
Non-physical occupation	−0.025	0.15	0.01	−0.09; 0.12	0.050	0.03	0.01	−0.07; 0.09	−0.020	0.86	−0.03	−0.16; 0.09
Mixed occupation	0.047		0.08	−0.03; 0.19	−0.046		−0.02	−0.11; 0.06	0.011		−0.02	−0.15; 0.11
Living arrangement												
Alone	0.017		Reference		−0.026		Reference		−0.005		Reference	
Couple or cohabitation	−0.017	0.43	−0.02	−0.12; 0.07	0.030	0.08	−0.01	−0.07; 0.07	0.008	0.77	0.05	−0.06; 0.16
BMI												
BMI ≥ 30	0.039		Reference		−0.018		Reference		−0.010		Reference	
25 ≤ BMI < 30	−0.010	0.76	−0.04	−0.14; 0.04	−0.007	0.94	0.02	−0.04; 0.09	0.028	0.77	0.05	−0.05; 0.15
BMI < 25	0.028		0.01	−0.10; 0.14	0.009		0.01	−0.07; 0.11	0.013		0.04	−0.10; 0.19
Smoking												
Non-smoker	0.036		Reference		0.016		Reference		0.030		Reference	
Ex-smoker	−0.007	0.76	0.07	−0.11; 0.25	−0.055	0.14	0.01	−0.12; 0.14	−0.021	0.89	−0.01	−0.21; 0.20
Smoker	−0.072		0.01	−0.18; 0.18	0.001		0.02	−0.11; 0.16	0.004		−0.01	−0.22; 0.20

* p for t test for sex and ANOVA for other variables; † Lower income: <18,294 €, Moderate income: 18,294 to 27,440 €, Higher income: >27,440 €; Bivariate analyses were performed using mean residual score separately for each social, health or lifestyle variables.; Multivariate linear models were adjusted for social, health and lifestyle (all variables presented in this table) variables altogether in a same model.

Table 6. Associations between social, health and lifestyle characteristics of the subjects and nutrient patterns in NuAge (n = 1596).

	Healthy pattern				Western pattern				Traditional pattern			
	Unadjusted		Adjusted		Unadjusted		Adjusted		Unadjusted		Adjusted	
	Mean Residual Score	p*	β	95% CI	Mean Residual Score	p*	β	95% CI	Mean Residual Score	p*	β	95% CI
Sex												
Women	0.033	0.13	Reference		0.017	0.23	Reference		0.001	0.98	Reference	
Men	−0.036		0.03	[−0.08; 0.14]	−0.020		0.05	[−0.01; 0.13]	−0.001		0.06	[−0.06; 0.18]
Education												
0–6 years	−0.175	<0.001	Reference		0.034	<0.001	Reference		−0.014	0.22	Reference	
7–9 years	−0.169		−0.02	[−0.19; 0.14]	0.083		0.04	[−0.06; 0.15]	−0.082		−0.08	[−0.26; 0.11]
10–13 years	−0.028		0.05	[−0.12; 0.22]	0.019		−0.01	[−0.11; 0.10]	0.052		0.07	[−0.11; 0.26]
14+ years	0.226		0.27	[0.09; 0.46]	−0.100		−0.12	[−0.23; −0.01]	0.014		0.05	[−0.15; 0.25]
Yearly income †												
Lower income	−0.092	0.05	Reference		0.003	0.91	Reference		−0.045	0.36	Reference	
Moderate income	−0.068		0.08	[−0.08; 0.26]	0.013		−0.02	[−0.12; 0.09]	0.014		0.05	[−0.14; 0.24]
Higher income	0.055		0.11	[−0.05; 0.27]	−0.010		0.03	[−0.07; 0.14]	0.026		0.06	[−0.12; 0.23]
Missing or refused to answer	−0.068		0.01	[−0.18; 0.19]	0.015		0.01	[−0.09; 0.15]	−0.100		−0.06	[−0.27; 0.15]
Main occupation over lifetime												
Physical occupation	−0.219	<0.001	Reference		0.076	0.006	Reference		0.003	0.91	Reference	
Non-physical occupation	0.107		0.16	[0.03; 0.29]	−0.040		0.07	[−0.01; 0.16]	−0.009		−0.07	[−0.22; 0.07]
Mixed occupation	0.018		0.13	[−0.01; 0.27]	−0.010		0.02	[−0.05; 0.08]	0.015		−0.02	[−0.18; 0.13]
Living arrangement												
Alone	0.081	0.02	Reference		−0.020	0.50	Reference		0.009	0.80	Reference	
Couple	−0.037		−0.11	[−0.21; −0.01]	0.006		0.01	[−0.05; 0.08]	−0.005		−0.01	[−0.12; 0.11]
BMI												
BMI ≥ 30	0.137	<0.001	Reference		−0.070	<0.001	Reference		−0.017	0.4	Reference	
25 ≤ BMI < 30	−0.002		0.23	[0.11; 0.36]	−0.010		−0.16	[−0.24; −0.08]	0.034		0.04	[−0.07; 0.17]
BMI < 25	−0.142		0.12	[0.01; 0.23]	0.102		−0.10	[−0.17; −0.03]	−0.044		−0.03	[−0.17; 0.10]
Smoking												
Non smoker	0.008	0.001	Reference		0.010	0.03	Reference		−0.041	0.21	Reference	
Ex-smoker	0.030		−0.04	[−0.15; 0.04]	−0.030		0.04	[−0.18; 0.11]	0.051		0.05	[−0.15; 0.25]
Smoker	−0.247		−0.30	[−0.49; −0.12]	0.115		0.17	[0.05; 0.28]	0.007		0.09	[−0.01; 0.01]

* p for t test for sex and ANOVA for other variables; † Lower income: <17,040 CAD (Canadian dollars), moderate income: 17,040–25,560 CAD, Higher income: >25,560 CAD; Bivariate analyses were performed using mean residual score separately for each social, health or lifestyle variables; Multivariate linear models were adjusted for social, health and lifestyle (all variables presented in this table), variables altogether in a same model.

4. Discussion

This study identified distinct nutrient patterns in older persons living in France and in Quebec, Canada: a healthy pattern and a Western pattern, both relatively similar in the two populations in terms of nutrient/food characteristics, especially for the healthy pattern. In both studies, the healthy pattern was reflecting good food variety and balance. Conversely, in both studies, there was a poorer variety of nutrients in the Western pattern. Very few nutrients were highly loaded in each traditional pattern, but further examination of food consumption and nutritional quality of the diet led to description of specific underlying food habits. In this study, nutrient patterns rather than dietary patterns allowed us to characterize and compare more efficiently nutritional quality of the diet of both study samples as nutrient intakes were assessed in each study using French and Canadian food composition tables, respectively.

In the 3C study sample, we labelled the second dietary pattern "Western" although this pattern may be less characteristic of a Western diet, compared to the Western dietary pattern described by Popkin [40] and identified, for example, by Hu *et al.* in an epidemiological study [4]. However, similar to the findings of Hu *et al.*, nutrients in fruits and vegetables such as fibers, carotene and vitamin C have low loadings on this Western pattern, which is in opposition to a prudent or healthy pattern. *A posteriori* dietary patterns are dependent on the sample of analysis, limiting external validity [9]. Although the Western pattern identified in 3C has a different quality of the diet compared to Western patterns from previous studies, it could still be characteristic of a Western diet within our two samples.

Surprisingly, nutrient patterns found in the current study sample from NuAge using data from a 24-h recall (*n* = 1596) differ in some ways from dietary patterns identified in another sample from NuAge using data from the FFQ [41]. In their analysis, Parrott *et al.* [41] reported dietary patterns that were labelled "prudent" and "Western". The two dietary patterns accounted for 10.4% of the total variance of the diet, contrasting with our three nutrient patterns accounting for 53.5% of the variance. These discrepancies may be related to several methodological issues. In our study, we used quantitative nutrient intake variables from 24-h recall to derive nutrient patterns, whereas Parrott *et al.* [41] used qualitative food intake variables from FFQ in a smaller sample to derive dietary patterns. In contrast to the latter study, we adjusted the nutrient patterns for energy intake, a major confounding factor for dietary patterns.

Previous work by Samieri *et al.* within the 3C cohort allowed the identification of five clusters of dietary patterns [35]. In their analysis, a healthy dietary pattern was reported associated with higher education and higher income. Even if comparison is limited because the dietary patterns were derived from FFQ in their study, this result suggests a good internal validity of our results.

A study from the EPIC cohort also studied the relationship between nutrient patterns and their food sources, and their association with sociodemographic characteristics [6]. Among the four nutrient patterns obtained in this study, the nutritional quality of the diet of the second pattern seemed similar to the healthy pattern derived in our study. Indeed, the healthy dietary pattern from the EPIC study was associated with higher consumption of fruits, vegetables and fish. This nutrient pattern was associated with a higher level of education. The similarities between these results from the EPIC study and ours, in adequation with hypotheses from previous studies [13,15], highlight that level of education might play a role in nutritional quality of the diet.

Two dietary patterns with inverse quality have been previously reported in other studies of elderly people. This duality was described among a sample of 205 American older persons with a mean age of 78 years from the Geisinger Rural Aging Study (GRAS) [42], using 24-h records as dietary assessment. The authors reported a prudent pattern characterized by high intake of fruits, vegetables, white meat, dairy and whole grain products and low consumption of fried fish. In that study, the Western pattern consisted of high consumption of sweets and candy, processed meats and salty snacks. The prudent pattern was strongly positively correlated with a higher mean adequacy ratio of essential nutrients, whereas the Western pattern was inversely correlated with this ratio. Correlations with global nutritional quality of the diet indices were not reported.

In a sample of 4693 older people (mean age 60 years) from the UK Whitehall II study, using dietary data from a FFQ, Akbaraly *et al.* [43] also identified a whole food pattern and a processed food pattern, similar to the healthy and Western patterns identified in our study. As in the NuAge sample, higher adherence to the whole food pattern was associated with a higher level of education and being ex-smokers. The reverse was true for the processed food pattern.

Similar findings were also reported by Kesse-Guyot *et al.* [44] in a French population of 3054 subjects studied at midlife, aged on average 52 years old at nutritional assessment. The authors described a healthy pattern derived from dietary data from a 24-h dietary record that was also correlated with high consumption of fruits, dairy products, vegetables, and fish. This healthy pattern was inversely correlated with meat and processed meat, which is similar to the healthy patterns from both 3C and NuAge samples.

Food habits in South-West of France, leading to the phenomenon known as the French paradox [45], are typically related to consumption of charcuterie and wine as well as fish/seafood, especially in the Bordeaux area due to the proximity of the Atlantic Ocean. Thus, a traditional food pattern has been previously reported composed of both recommended and non-recommended food and associated nutrients [46].

In Quebec, the traditional food pattern was related to higher intake of dairy products and fish, which used to be part of their traditional diet. This pattern may be explained in part by an advertising campaign promoting dairy products for the prevention of osteoporosis, a wider distribution of fish to markets and publicity for the prevention of cardiovascular disease and memory deficits with advancing age. However, this dietary pattern explicated a small amount of the total variance.

To assess nutritional quality of the diet, we chose the C-HEI because items necessary to compute this score are based on food groups and nutrient intake data that were available in both NuAge and 3C samples. Thus, the healthy patterns appeared to be associated with healthy food habits in each country, in line with the Canadian dietary guidelines, whereas the Western patterns may reflect an unbalanced diet with low adherence to these guidelines. Among those following the traditional pattern in 3C, adherence to these healthy eating guidelines was moderate, whereas in Quebec, the traditional pattern was associated with a better adherence. In NuAge, participants reported a higher weekly consumption of vegetables and lower consumption of charcuterie. This resulted in lower saturated fat intakes and may explain the higher adherence to dietary guidelines observed among those characterized by the traditional pattern.

Greater adherence to Canadian dietary guidelines was found in women but no statistical interactions on C-HEI score were observed, thus sex was not a modifier of this association and may be a potential confounder. Although it has been suggested that sex differences are important in dietary pattern analyses [41,47], our results do not support this evidence.

Socioeconomic position, lifestyle and other habits such as smoking are potentially associated with nutrient patterns. In both 3C and NuAge, higher education was associated with a healthy pattern as found in some studies [13,15,41]. However, comparisons between the two samples revealed that the association between higher education and healthy pattern seemed to be stronger in the NuAge sample (data not shown). We also compared the results of the associations between healthy pattern and additional socio-economic characteristics in the two samples. They were associated with healthy pattern only in NuAge, suggesting that socioeconomic position may have a significant influence on dietary choices in this population, similar to the results from Parrott *et al.* [41]. People with a higher level of education may have better nutrition knowledge and greater earning power, even though income was not statistically associated in our study, allowing them to choose expensive healthy food [16,48]. These findings are altogether consistent with the hypothesis that nutritional quality of the diet is associated with socioeconomic position. Higher education may play a greater role among these factors as it has been found associated with nutritional quality of the diet in both samples from our study.

In NuAge, the Western pattern was associated with higher BMI values but factor scores were adjusted for energy intake suggesting that that diet probably yielded this association. Mean total energy intake was 20% to 25% higher in NuAge than in 3C sample. Mean energy intake in NuAge reach Canadian recommendations for sedentary people under 71 but are above recommendations for people 71 years and over [49]; this may explain higher BMIs in this sample but could also be due to higher proportion of men in the NuAge sample. However, the cross-sectional design of this study does not allow us to ascertain temporality of the relationship between BMI and identified patterns.

Some limitations to our findings must be recognized. One of them is that dietary data were based on a single 24-h recall. However, it has been suggested that a single recall can provide an accurate estimation of average nutrient intake in large study samples [50]. In order to improve comparability between studies, we decided to use only the first 24-h recall to derive nutrient patterns in NuAge as in 3C. Analyses showed that percentage of explained variance of diet from the three nutrient patterns in NuAge was very similar when using three 24-h recalls (data not shown). Regarding the FFQ, for a same food group, we gathered frequencies of consumption of food items that were not estimated using the same method. For example, for the vegetable food group in NuAge, there were 13 items asking for separate categories of the most frequently consumed vegetables (beans, tomatoes, carrots, salad, *etc.*), whereas in 3C there were 12 items of vegetable consumption separated into two items for raw and two items for cooked vegetables, for each of the three meals. This may have introduced an information bias that could have underestimated vegetable consumption in the 3C sample. Conversely, closed lists of food items in FFQs as in NuAge tend to overestimate consumption. Thus, numbers of servings per week are not directly comparable between the two samples. This was an additional reason for deriving nutrient-based rather than food-based patterns. The qualitative FFQ in 3C did not allow us to describe quantities in food intake.

Although the FA-PCA allowed the identification of three dietary patterns, the aim of this method is not to classify subjects into distinct groups of nutrient intake. Indeed, individuals that have very similar intakes of different major food groups and are classified as belonging to one of the latent nutrient categories would also belong at the low end of a different latent category. Thus, the result of this analysis should be interpreted with caution.

To our knowledge, this is the first analysis using nutrient intake data from two observational studies. As mentioned, France and Quebec have a common ancestral cultural background, but Quebec has further developed food habits influenced by North American culture. Indeed, according to historians, as people from Quebec were French settlers, they inherited French food habits during the 17th century and were lately influenced by English Canadian people during late 18th century and beginning of the 19th century [51]. Thus, their diet is now a mix of those cultures. This may partially explain why Quebec and South-West of France appear to share common healthy food habits as opposed to a Western pattern characterized by lower food diversity. This research addressed identification of potential confounders of nutrient patterns as well as data harmonization between these two cohorts in order to further contribute to the investigation of associations between nutrient patterns and health outcomes. Moreover, this study highlights the need to choose the best source of dietary data to derive nutritional patterns. In fact, dietary assessment method (e.g., FFQ *vs.* 24-h recall) may also change the resulting dietary patterns within a population. Thus, describing characteristics of nutrient patterns instead of food patterns to compare nutritional quality of the diet between populations may be the best method to assess reproducibility of the results, an important part of causality in studies.

5. Conclusions

Overall, our findings add to previous literature suggesting, in various Western populations, a relatively consistent opposition between healthy and Western patterns. Further investigations are needed to enhance the methodology of dietary comparisons between populations. Finally, comparisons of the nutritional quality of the diet between countries may enhance the internationalization of dietary guidelines among populations sharing a common ancestral cultural background.

Nutrients **2016**, *8*, 225

Supplementary Materials: The following are available online at http://www.mdpi.com/2072-6643/8/4/225/s1, Table S1: Mean daily nutrient intakes according to quartiles of component scores obtained by factor analysis—principal component analysis of nutrient intake data in 3C (*n* = 1712) from 24-h recall, Table S2: Mean daily nutrient intakes according to quartiles of component scores obtained by factor analysis—principal component analysis of nutrient intake data in NuAge (*n* = 1596) from first 24-h recall.

Acknowledgments: The authors thank Katherine Gray-Donald for her critical review of the draft. This research received no specific grant from any funding agency in the public, commercial or not-for-profit sectors. Benjamin Allès was supported for this joint PhD work by a funding from Region Aquitaine and Faculty of Pharmacy, Université Laval and awards from Programme Frontenac and Jean Walter-Zellidja, Académie française. D. Laurin was supported by a scientist award from the Fonds de la recherche du Québec—Santé (FRQS). The NuAge study was funded by the Canadian Institutes of Health Research (CIHR) and the Quebec Network for Research on Aging, a thematic network of the FRQS. The 3C study is conducted under a partnership agreement between the *Institut National de la Santé et de la Recherche Médicale* (INSERM), the University Bordeaux 2 Victor Segalen and Sanofi-Aventis. The *Fondation pour la Recherche Médicale* funded the preparation and initiation of the study. The 3C study is also supported by the *Caisse Nationale Maladie des Travailleurs Salariés, Direction Générale de la Santé*, MGEN, *Institut de la Longévité, Conseils Régionaux d'Aquitaine et Bourgogne, Fondation de France*, Ministry of Research-INSERM Programme "*Cohortes et collections de données biologiques*", *Agence Nationale de la Recherche* COGINUT ANR-06-PNRA-005, the *Fondation Plan Alzheimer* (FCS 2009–2012), and the *Caisse Nationale pour la Solidarité et l'Autonomie* (CNSA).

Author Contributions: B. Allès made the review of the literature and drafted the manuscript. D. Laurin and P. Barberger-Gateau contributed to the drafting of the manuscript and supervised this research project, they equally contributed to this work. These authors act as equivalent co-senior author. B. Allès conducted statistical analyses with contribution of S. Lorrain and P.-H. Carmichael and with help from C. Samieri and M.-A. Jutand. H. Payette, B. Shatenstein and P. Gaudreau were implicated in the main NuAge study concept and design. All authors made a critical review of the draft.

Conflicts of Interest: P. Barberger-Gateau reports grants and non-financial support from Danone Research, Vifor Pharma and the CNIEL (Centre National Interprofessionnel de l'Industrie Laitière), personal fees and non-financial support from Nutricia, grants and non-financial support from Groupe Lipides et Nutrition, non-financial support from ILSI Europe.

References

1. De Groot, C.P.G.M.; van Staveren, W.A. Nutritional concerns, health and survival in old age. *Biogerontology* **2010**, *11*, 597–602. [CrossRef] [PubMed]
2. De Morais, C.; Oliveira, B.; Afonso, C.; Lumbers, M.; Raats, M.; de Almeida, M.D.V. Nutritional risk of European elderly. *Eur. J. Clin. Nutr.* **2013**, *67*, 1215–1219. [CrossRef] [PubMed]
3. Jacobs, D.R.; Gross, M.D.; Tapsell, L.C. Food synergy: An operational concept for understanding nutrition. *Am. J. Clin. Nutr.* **2009**, *89*, 1543S–1548S. [CrossRef] [PubMed]
4. Hu, F.B.; Rimm, E.B.; Stampfer, M.J.; Ascherio, A.; Spiegelman, D.; Willett, W.C. Prospective study of major dietary patterns and risk of coronary heart disease in men. *Am. J. Clin. Nutr.* **2000**, *72*, 912–921. [PubMed]
5. Mozaffarian, D.; Ludwig, D.S. Dietary guidelines in the 21st century—A time for food. *JAMA* **2010**, *304*, 681–682. [CrossRef] [PubMed]
6. Moskal, A.; Pisa, P.T.; Ferrari, P.; Byrnes, G.; Freisling, H.; Boutron-Ruault, M.-C.; Cadeau, C.; Nailler, L.; Wendt, A.; Kühn, T.; *et al.* Nutrient patterns and their food sources in an International Study Setting: Report from the EPIC study. *PLoS ONE* **2014**, *9*, e98647. [CrossRef] [PubMed]
7. Allès, B.; Samieri, C.; Féart, C.; Jutand, M.-A.; Laurin, D.; Barberger-Gateau, P. Dietary patterns: A novel approach to examine the link between nutrition and cognitive function in older individuals. *Nutr. Res. Rev.* **2012**, *25*, 207–222. [CrossRef] [PubMed]
8. Slattery, M.L. Analysis of dietary patterns in epidemiological research. *Appl. Physiol. Nutr. Metab.* **2010**, *35*, 207–210. [CrossRef] [PubMed]
9. Gu, Y.; Scarmeas, N. Dietary patterns in Alzheimer's disease and cognitive aging. *Curr. Alzheimer Res.* **2011**, *8*, 510–519. [CrossRef] [PubMed]
10. Mullie, P.; Clarys, P.; Hulens, M.; Vansant, G. Dietary patterns and socioeconomic position. *Eur. J. Clin. Nutr.* **2010**, *64*, 231–238. [CrossRef] [PubMed]
11. Kuczmarski, M.F.; Weddle, D.O.; American Dietetic Association. Position paper of the American Dietetic Association: Nutrition across the spectrum of aging. *J. Am. Diet. Assoc.* **2005**, *105*, 616–633. [PubMed]
12. Payette, H.; Shatenstein, B. Determinants of healthy eating in community-dwelling elderly people. *Can. J. Public Health* **2005**, *96* (Suppl. 3), S27–S31, S30–S35. [PubMed]

13. Azagba, S.; Sharaf, M.F. Disparities in the frequency of fruit and vegetable consumption by socio-demographic and lifestyle characteristics in Canada. *Nutr. J.* **2011**, *10*, 118. [CrossRef] [PubMed]

14. Ricciuto, L.; Tarasuk, V.; Yatchew, A. Socio-demographic influences on food purchasing among Canadian households. *Eur. J. Clin. Nutr.* **2006**, *60*, 778–790. [CrossRef] [PubMed]

15. Darmon, N.; Drewnowski, A. Does social class predict diet quality? *Am. J. Clin. Nutr.* **2008**, *87*, 1107–1117. [PubMed]

16. Wardle, J.; Parmenter, K.; Waller, J. Nutrition knowledge and food intake. *Appetite* **2000**, *34*, 269–275. [CrossRef] [PubMed]

17. Aggarwal, A.; Monsivais, P.; Cook, A.J.; Drewnowski, A. Does diet cost mediate the relation between socioeconomic position and diet quality? *Eur. J. Clin. Nutr.* **2011**, *65*, 1059–1066. [CrossRef] [PubMed]

18. Wham, C.A.; Teh, R.O.; Robinson, M.; Kerse, N.M. What is associated with nutrition risk in very old age? *J. Nutr. Health Aging* **2011**, *15*, 247–251. [CrossRef] [PubMed]

19. Three-City Study Group. Vascular factors and risk of dementia: Design of the Three-City Study and baseline characteristics of the study population. *Neuroepidemiology* **2003**, *22*, 316–325.

20. Gaudreau, P.; Morais, J.A.; Shatenstein, B.; Gray-Donald, K.; Khalil, A.; Dionne, I.; Ferland, G.; Fülöp, T.; Jacques, D.; Kergoat, M.-J.; *et al.* Nutrition as a determinant of successful aging: Description of the Quebec longitudinal study Nuage and results from cross-sectional pilot studies. *Rejuvenation Res.* **2007**, *10*, 377–386. [CrossRef] [PubMed]

21. Teng, E.L.; Chui, H.C. The Modified Mini-Mental State (3MS) examination. *J. Clin. Psychiatry* **1987**, *48*, 314–318. [PubMed]

22. Favier, J.-C.; Ireland-Ripert, J.; Toque, C.; Feinberg, M. *Répertoire Général des Aliments. Table de Composition. 2e Edititon, Revue et Augmentée*INRA-AFSSA-CIQUAL-TEC & DOC., INRA Editions ed; Quae: Versailles, France, 1995.

23. Souci, F.W.; Fachmann, W.; Kraut, H. *Food Consumption and Nutrition Tables, 6th rev. edn. Medpharm*; Scientific Publishers: Stuttgart, Germany, 2000.

24. Renaud, S.; Godsey, F.; Ortchanian, E.; Baudier, F. *Table de Composition des Aliments*; Astra-Calve: Courbevoie, France, 1979.

25. Larrieu, S.; Letenneur, L.; Berr, C.; Dartigues, J.F.; Ritchie, K.; Alperovitch, A.; Tavernier, B.; Barberger-Gateau, P. Sociodemographic differences in dietary habits in a population-based sample of elderly subjects: The 3C study. *J. Nutr. Health Aging* **2004**, *8*, 497–502. [PubMed]

26. Féart, C.; Jutand, M.A.; Larrieu, S.; Letenneur, L.; Delcourt, C.; Combe, N.; Barberger-Gateau, P. Energy, macronutrient and fatty acid intake of French elderly community dwellers and association with socio-demographic characteristics: Data from the Bordeaux sample of the Three-City Study. *Br. J. Nutr.* **2007**, *98*, 1046–1057. [CrossRef] [PubMed]

27. Johnson-Down, L.; Ritter, H.; Starkey, L.J.; Gray-Donald, K. Primary food sources of nutrients in the diet of Canadian adults. *Can. J. Diet. Pract. Res.* **2006**, *67*, 7–13. [CrossRef] [PubMed]

28. Shatenstein, B.; Payette, H.; Nadon, S.; Gray-Donald, K. An approach for evaluating lifelong intakes of functional foods in elderly people. *J. Nutr.* **2003**, *133*, 2384–2391. [PubMed]

29. Kennedy, E.T.; Ohls, J.; Carlson, S.; Fleming, K. The Healthy Eating Index: Design and applications. *J. Am. Diet. Assoc.* **1995**, *95*, 1103–1108. [CrossRef]

30. Shatenstein, B.; Nadon, S.; Godin, C.; Ferland, G. Diet quality of Montreal-area adults needs improvement: Estimates from a self-administered food frequency questionnaire furnishing a dietary indicator score. *J. Am. Diet. Assoc.* **2005**, *105*, 1251–1260. [CrossRef] [PubMed]

31. Ong, L.L. Burgernomics: The economics of the Big Mac standard. *J. Int. Money Financ.* **1997**, *16*, 865–878. [CrossRef]

32. The Economist. Big Mac Index. 14 January 2012. Available online: http://www.economist.com/node/21542808 (accessed on 12 February 2011).

33. International Labor Organization (ILO). United Nations, International Standard Classification of Occupations ISCO 88. 1991. Available online: http://www.ilo.org/public/english/bureau/stat/isco/ (accessed on 12 February 2011).

34. Statistics Canada, Ottawa, ON, Canada. National Occupational Classification (NOC) 2006. Available online: http://www.statcan.gc.ca/eng/subjects/standard/noc/2011/noc-s2006-noc2011 (accessed on 23 January 2011).

Nutrients **2016**, *8*, 225

35. Samieri, C.; Jutand, M.-A.; Féart, C.; Capuron, L.; Letenneur, L.; Barberger-Gateau, P. Dietary patterns derived by hybrid clustering method in older people: Association with cognition, mood, and self-rated health. *J. Am. Diet. Assoc.* **2008**, *108*, 1461–1471. [CrossRef] [PubMed]

36. Shatenstein, B.; Huet, C.; Jabbour, M. Plausibility assessment and quality assurance of food frequency questionnaires completed in studies of diet and health. In Proceedings of the International Conference on Diet and Activity Methods (ICDAM), Washington, DC, USA, 5–7 June 2009; pp. S4–S6, S281–S282.

37. Kleinbaum, D.G.; Kupper, L.L.; Muller, K.E. *Applied Regression Analysis and Other Multivariable Methods*; 3rd Revised edition; Wadsworth Publishing Co Inc.: Belmont, CA, USA, 1997.

38. Willett, W.; Stampfer, M.J. Total energy intake: Implications for epidemiologic analyses. *Am. J. Epidemiol.* **1986**, *124*, 17–27. [PubMed]

39. Frémeaux, A.E.; Hosking, J.; Metcalf, B.S.; Jeffery, A.N.; Voss, L.D.; Wilkin, T.J. Consistency of children's dietary choices: Annual repeat measures from 5 to 13 years (EarlyBird 49). *Br. J. Nutr.* **2011**, *106*, 725–731. [CrossRef] [PubMed]

40. Popkin, B.M. Contemporary nutritional transition: Determinants of diet and its impact on body composition. *Proc. Nutr. Soc.* **2011**, *70*, 82–91. [CrossRef] [PubMed]

41. Parrott, M.D.; Shatenstein, B.; Ferland, G.; Payette, H.; Morais, J.A.; Belleville, S.; Kergoat, M.-J.; Gaudreau, P.; Greenwood, C.E. Relationship between Diet Quality and Cognition Depends on Socioeconomic Position in Healthy Older Adults. *J. Nutr.* **2013**, *143*, 1767–1773. [CrossRef] [PubMed]

42. Bailey, R.L.; Mitchell, D.C.; Miller, C.K.; Still, C.D.; Jensen, G.L.; Tucker, K.L.; Smiciklas-Wright, H. A dietary screening questionnaire identifies dietary patterns in older adults. *J. Nutr.* **2007**, *137*, 421–426. [PubMed]

43. Akbaraly, T.N.; Singh-Manoux, A.; Marmot, M.G.; Brunner, E.J. Education attenuates the association between dietary patterns and cognition. *Dement. Geriatr. Cogn. Disord.* **2009**, *27*, 147–154. [CrossRef] [PubMed]

44. Kesse-Guyot, E.; Andreeva, V.A.; Jeandel, C.; Ferry, M.; Hercberg, S.; Galan, P. A healthy dietary pattern at midlife is associated with subsequent cognitive performance. *J. Nutr.* **2012**, *142*, 909–915. [CrossRef] [PubMed]

45. Renaud, S.; de Lorgeril, M. Wine, alcohol, platelets, and the French paradox for coronary heart disease. *Lancet* **1992**, *339*, 1523–1526. [CrossRef]

46. Samieri, C.; Ginder Coupez, V.; Lorrain, S.; Letenneur, L.; Allès, B.; Féart, C.; Paineau, D.; Barberger-Gateau, P. Nutrient patterns and risk of fracture in older subjects: Results from the Three-City Study. *Osteoporos. Int.* **2013**, *24*, 1295–1305. [CrossRef] [PubMed]

47. Northstone, K. Dietary patterns: The importance of sex differences. *Br. J. Nutr.* **2012**, *108*, 393–394. [CrossRef] [PubMed]

48. Shatenstein, B.; Ferland, G.; Belleville, S.; Gray-Donald, K.; Kergoat, M.-J.; Morais, J.; Gaudreau, P.; Payette, H.; Greenwood, C. Diet quality and cognition among older adults from the NuAge study. *Exp. Gerontol.* **2012**, *47*, 353–360. [CrossRef] [PubMed]

49. Health Canada, Minister of Health Canada. Eating Well with Canada's Food Guide 2008. Available online: http://www.hc-sc.gc.ca/fn-an/alt_formats/hpfb-dgpsa/pdf/food-guide-aliment/view_eatwell_vue_bienmang-eng.pdf (accessed on 23 January 2011).

50. Willett, W. *Nutritional Epidemiology*; Oxford University Press: New York, NY, USA, 1998.

51. Desloges, Y. The Quebecois and their food "identity": From Cartier to Expo 67. *Cuizine J. Can. Food Cult.* **2011**, *3*. (In French) [CrossRef]

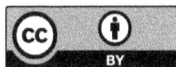

MDPI AG

St. Alban-Anlage 66

4052 Basel, Switzerland

Tel. +41 61 683 77 34

Fax +41 61 302 89 18

http://www.mdpi.com

Nutrients Editorial Office

E-mail: nutrients@mdpi.com

http://www.mdpi.com/journal/nutrients

www.ingramcontent.com/pod-product-compliance
Lightning Source LLC
Chambersburg PA
CBHW051720210326
41597CB00032B/5550